Fluids, Electrolytes, and Acid–Base Balance

Reviews & Rationales

Mary Ann Hogan, RN, CS, MSN

Clinical Assistant Professor
University of Massachusetts, Amherst

Daryle Wane, APRN, BC

Assistant Professor of Nursing
Pasco-Hernando Community College
New Port Richey, Florida

Prentice
Hall

Upper Saddle River, New Jersey 07458

Library of Congress Cataloging-in-Publication Data

Fluids, electrolytes, and acid-base balance: reviews & rationales / [edited by] Mary Ann Hogan, Daryle Wayne.
    p.; cm.
Includes bibliographical references and index.
  ISBN: 0-13-030454-9 (alk. paper)
  1. Water-electrolyte imbalances—Nursing. 2. Acid-base imbalances—Nursing.
  [DNLM: 1. Water-Electrolyte Imbalance—nursing. 2. Acid-Base Equilibrium. 3. Acid-Base Imbalance—nursing. 4. Water-Electrolyte Balance.
WY 100 F646 2003] I. Hogan, Mary Ann, MSN. II. Wayne, Daryle.
  RC630.F5928 2003
  616.3′992—dc21
                        2002002383

Publisher: Julie Levin Alexander
Assistant to Publisher: Regina Bruno
Executive Editor: Maura Connor
Managing Development Editor: Marilyn Meserve
Development Editor: Jeanne Allison
Director of Production and Manufacturing: Bruce Johnson
Managing Production Editor: Patrick Walsh
Production Liaison: Danielle Newhouse
Production Editor: Jessica Balch, Pine Tree Composition
Manufacturing Buyer: Pat Brown
Design Director: Cheryl Asherman
Design Coordinator: Maria Guglielmo
Interior Designer: Jill Little
Cover Designer: Joseph DePinho
Electronic Art Creation: Precision Graphics
Marketing Manager: Nicole Benson
Assistant Editor: Yesenia Kopperman
Editorial Assistant: Sladjana Repic
Production Information Manager: Rachele Triano
Media Editor: Sarah Hayday
New Media Production Manager: Amy Peltier
New Media Project Manager: Stephen Hartner
Composition: Pine Tree Composition, Inc.
Printer/Binder: Courier/Westford

Pearson Education Ltd., *London*
Pearson Education Australia Pty. Limited, *Sydney*
Pearson Education Singapore, Pte. Ltd.
Pearson Education North Asia Ltd., *Hong Kong*
Pearson Education Canada, Ltd., *Toronto*
Pearson Educaión de Mexico, S.A. de C.V.
Pearson Education—Japan, *Tokyo*
Pearson Education Malaysia, Pte. Ltd.
Pearson Education, Upper Saddle River, New Jersey

Notice: Care has been taken to confirm the accuracy of the information presented in this book. The authors, editors, and the publisher, however, cannot accept any responsibility for errors or omissions or for the consequences for application of the information in this book and make no warranty, express or implied, with respect to its contents.

The authors and the publisher have exerted every effort to ensure that drug selections and dosages set forth in this text are in accord with current recommendations and practice at time of publication. However, in view of ongoing research, changes in government regulations, and the constant flow of information relating to drug therapy and drug reactions, the reader is urged to check the pakage inserts of all drugs for any change in indications of dosage and for added warnings and precautions. This is particularly important when the recommended agent is a new and/or infrequently employed drug.

The authors and publisher disclaim all responsibility for any liability, loss, injury, or damage incorred as a consequence, directly or indirectly, of the use and application of any of the contents of this volume.

10 9 8 7 6 5 4 3
ISBN 0-13-030454-9

Contents

Preface

INTRODUCTION

Welcome to the new Prentice Hall Reviews and Rationales Series! This 9-book series has been specifically designed to provide a clear and concentrated review of important nursing knowledge in the following content areas:

- Child Health Nursing
- Maternal-Newborn Nursing
- Mental Health Nursing
- Medical-Surgical Nursing
- Pathophysiology
- Pharmacology
- Fundamentals and Skills
- Nutrition and Diet Therapy
- Fluids, Electrolytes, & Acid-Base Balance

The books in this series have been designed for use either by current nursing students as a study aid for nursing course work or NCLEX-RN licensing exam preparation, or by practicing nurses seeking a comprehensive yet concise review of a nursing specialty or subject area.

This series is truly unique. One of its most special features is that it has been authored by a large team of nurse educators from across the United States and Canada to ensure that each chapter is written by a nurse expert in the content area under study. Prentice Hall Health representatives from across North America submitted names of nurse educators and/or clinicians who excel in their respective fields, and these authors were then invited to write a chapter in one or more books. The consulting editor for each book, who is also an expert in that specialty area, then reviewed all chapters submitted for comprehensiveness and accuracy. The series editor designed the overall series in collaboration with a core Prentice Hall team to take full advantage of Prentice Hall's cutting edge technology, and also reviewed the chapters in each book.

All books in the series are identical in their overall design for your convenience (further details follow at the end of this section). As an added value, each book comes with a comprehensive support package, including free CD-ROM, free companion website access, and a Nursing Notes card for quick clinical reference.

STUDY TIPS

Use of this review book should help simplify your study. To make the most of your valuable study time, also follow these simple but important suggestions:

- Use a weekly calendar to schedule study sessions.
  - Outline the timeframes for all of your activities (home, school, appointments, etc.) on a weekly calendar.
  - Find the "holes" in your calendar—the times in which you can plan to study. Add study sessions to the calendar at times when you can expect to be mentally alert and follow it!
- Create the optimal study environment.
  - Eliminate external sources of distraction, such as television, telephone, etc.
  - Eliminate internal sources of distraction, such as hunger, thirst, or dwelling on items or problems that cannot be worked on at the moment.
  - Take a break for 10 minutes or so after each hour of concentrated study both as a reward and an incentive to keep studying.
- Use pre-reading strategies to increase comprehension of chapter material.
  - Skim the headings in the chapter (because they identify chapter content).
  - Read the definitions of key terms, which will help you learn new words to comprehend chapter information.
  - Review all graphic aids (figures, tables, boxes) because they are often used to explain important points in the chapter.
- Read the chapter thoroughly but at a reasonable speed.
  - Comprehension and retention are actually enhanced by not reading too slowly.
  - Do take the time to reread any section that is unclear to you.
- Summarize what you have learned.
  - Use questions supplied with this book, CD-ROM, and companion website to test your recall of chapter content.
  - Review again any sections that correspond to questions you answered incorrectly or incompletely.

TEST TAKING STRATEGIES

Use the following strategies to increase your success on multiple-choice nursing tests or examinations:

- Get sufficient sleep and have something to eat before taking a test. Take deep breaths during the test as needed. Remember, the brain requires oxygen and glucose as fuel. Avoid concentrated sweets before a test, however, to avoid rapid upward and then downward surges in blood glucose levels.
- Read each question carefully, identifying the stem, the four options, and any key words or phrases in either the stem or options.
  - Key words in the stem such as "most important" indicate the need to set priorities, since more than one option is likely to contain a statement that is technically correct.
  - Remember that the presence of absolute words such as "never" or "only" in an option is more likely to make that option incorrect.

- Determine who is the client in the question; often this is the person with the health problem, but it may also be a significant other, relative, friend, or another nurse.
- Decide whether the stem is a true response stem or a false response stem. With a true response stem, the correct answer will be a true statement, and vice-versa.
- Determine what the question is really asking, sometimes referred to as the issue of the question. Evaluate all answer options in relation to this issue, and not strictly to the "correctness" of the statement in each individual option.
- Eliminate options that are obviously incorrect, then go back and reread the stem. Evaluate the remaining options against the stem once more.
- If two answers seem similar and correct, try to decide whether one of them is more global or comprehensive. If the global option includes the alternative option within it, it is likely that the more global response is the correct answer.

THE NCLEX-RN LICENSING EXAMINATION

The NCLEX-RN licensing examination is a Computer Adaptive Test (CAT) that ranges in length from 75 to 265 individual (stand-alone) test items, depending on individual performance during the examination. Upon graduation from a nursing program, successful completion of this exam is the gateway to your professional nursing practice. The blueprint for the exam is reviewed and revised every three years by the National Council of State Boards of Nursing according to the results of a job analysis study of new graduate nurses (practicing within the first six months after graduation). Each question on the exam is coded to one *Client Need Category* and one or more *Integrated Concepts and Processes.*

Client Need Categories

There are 4 categories of client needs, and each exam will contain a minimum and maximum percent of questions from each category. Each major category has subcategories within it. The *Client Need* categories according to the NCLEX-RN Test Plan effective April 2001 are as follows:

- Safe, Effective Care Environment
  - Management of Care (7–13%)
  - Safety and Infection Control (5–11%)
- Health Promotion and Maintenance
  - Growth and Development Throughout the Lifespan (7–13%)
  - Prevention and Early Detection of Disease (5–11%)
- Psychosocial Integrity
  - Coping and Adaptation (5–11%)
  - Psychosocial Adaptation (5–11%)
- Physiological Integrity
  - Basic Care and Comfort (7–13%)
  - Pharmacological and Parenteral Therapies (5–11%)
  - Reduction of Risk Potential (12–18%)
  - Physiological Adaptation (12–18%)

Integrated Concepts and Processes

The integrated concepts and processes identified on the NCLEX-RN Test Plan effective April 2001, with condensed definitions, are as follows:

- Nursing Process: a scientific problem-solving approach used in nursing practice; consisting of assessment, analysis, planning, implementation, and evaluation.

- Caring: client-nurse interaction(s) characterized by mutual respect and trust and directed toward achieving desired client outcomes.
- Communication and Documentation: verbal and/or nonverbal interactions between nurse and others (client, family, health care team); a written or electronic recording of activities or events that occur during client care.
- Cultural Awareness: knowledge and sensitivity to the client's beliefs/values and how these might impact on the client's healthcare experience.
- Self-Care: assisting clients to meet their health care needs, which may include maintaining health or restoring function.
- Teaching/Learning: facilitating client's acquisition of knowledge, skills, and attitudes that lead to behavior change.

More detailed information about this examination may be obtained by visiting the National Council of State Boards of Nursing website at http://www.ncsbn.org and viewing the *NCLEX-RN Examination Test Plan for the National Council Licensure Examination for Registered Nurses.* *

HOW TO GET THE MOST OUT OF THIS BOOK

Chapter Organization

Each chapter has the following elements to guide you during review and study:

- Chapter Objectives: describe what you will be able to know or do after learning the material covered in the chapter.

OBJECTIVES

▮ Review basic principles of growth and development.

▮ Describe major physical expectations for each developmental age group.

▮ Identify developmental milestones for various age groups.

▮ Discuss the reactions to illness and hospitalization for children at various stages of development.

- Review at a Glance: contains a glossary of key terms used in the chapter, with definitions provided up-front and available at your fingertips, to help you stay focused and make the best use of your study time.

REVIEW AT A GLANCE

anticipatory guidance *the process of understanding upcoming developmental needs and then teaching caregivers to meet those needs*

cephalocaudal development *the process by which development proceeds from the head downward through the body and towards the feet*

chronological age *age in years*

critical periods *times when an individual is especially responsive to certain environmental effects, sometimes called sensitive periods*

development *an increase in capability or function; a more complex concept that*

is a continuous, orderly series of conditions that lead to activities, new motives for activities; and eventual patterns of behavior

developmental age *age based on functional behavior and ability to adapt to the environment; does not necessarily correspond to chronological age*

- Pretest: this 10-question multiple choice test provides a sample overview of content covered in the chapter and helps you decide what areas need the most—or the least—review.

Pretest

1   The nurse discusses dental care with the parents of a 3-year-old. The nurse explains that by the age of 3, their child should have:
(1) 5 "temporary" teeth.
(2) 10 "temporary" teeth.
(3) 15 "temporary" teeth.
(4) 20 "temporary" teeth.

2   The mother of a 6-month-old infant is concerned that the infant's anterior fontanel is still open. The nurse would inform the mother that further evaluation is needed if the anterior fontanel is open after:
(1) 6 months.
(2) 10 months.
(3) 18 months.
(4) 24 months.

- Practice to Pass questions: these are open-ended questions that stimulate critical thinking and reinforce mastery of the chapter content.

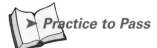

Practice to Pass

What would you explain as normal motor development for a 10-month old infant?

- NCLEX Alerts: the NCLEX icon identifies information or concepts that are likely to be tested on the NCLEX licensing examination. Be sure to learn the information flagged by this type of icon.

NCLEX!

- Case Study: found at the end of the chapter, it provides an opportunity for you to use your critical thinking and clinical reasoning skills to "put it all together;" it describes a true-to-life client case situation and asks you open-ended questions about how you would provide care for that client and/or family.

Case Study

A 6-month-old female infant is brought into the pediatric clinic for a well-baby visit. You as the pediatric nurse will be assigned to care for this family.

❶ Identify the primary growth and development expectations for a 6-month-old.

❷ What type common behavior is expected of this 6-month-old towards the nurse?

❸ What immunization(s) are recommended at this age to maintain health and wellness?

For suggested responses, see page 406.

- Posttest: a 10-question multiple-choice test at the end of the chapter provides new questions that are representative of chapter content, and provide you with feedback about mastery of that content following review and study. All pretest and posttest questions contain rationales for the correct answer, and are coded according to the phase of the nursing process used and the NCLEX category of client need (called the Test Plan). The Test plan codes are PHYS (Physiological Integrity), PSYC (Psychosocial Integrity), SECE (Safe Effective Care Environment), and HPM (Health Promotion and Maintenance).

Posttest

1. When using the otoscope to examine the ears of a 2-year-old child, the nurse should:

   (1) Pull the pinna up and back.
   (2) Pull the pinna down and back.
   (3) Hold the pinna gently but firmly in its normal position.
   (4) Hold the pinna against the skull.

2. To assess the height of an 18-month-old child who is brought to the clinic for routine examination, the nurse should:

   (1) Measure arm span to estimate adult height.
   (2) Use a tape measure.
   (3) Use a horizontal measuring board.
   (4) Have the child stand on an upright scale and use the measuring arm.

CD-ROM

For those who want to practice taking tests on a computer, the CD-ROM that accompanies the book contains the pretest and posttest questions found in all chapters of the book. In addition, it contains 10 NEW questions for each chapter to help you further evaluate your knowledge base and hone your test-taking skills. In several chapters, one of the questions will have embedded art to use in answering the question. Some of the newly developed NCLEX test items are also designed in this way, so these items will give you valuable practice with this type of question.

Companion Website (CW)

The companion website is a "virtual" reference for virtually all your needs! The CW contains the following:

- 50 NCLEX-style questions: 10 pretest, 10 posttest, 10 CD-ROM, and 20 additional new questions
- Definitions of key terms: the glossary is also stored on the companion website for ease of reference
- In Depth With NCLEX: features drawings or photos that are each accompanied by a one- to two-paragraph explanation. These are especially useful when describing something that is complex, technical (such as equipment), or difficult to mentally visualize.
- Suggested Answers to Practice to Pass and Case Study Questions: easily located on the website, these allow for timely feedback for those who answer chapter questions on the web.

Nursing Notes Clinical Reference Card

This laminated card provides a reference for frequently used facts and information related to the subject matter of the book. These are designed to be useful in the clinical setting, when quick and easy access to information is so important!

ABOUT THE FLUIDS, ELECTROLYTES, AND ACID–BASE BALANCE BOOK

Chapters in this book cover "need-to-know" information about principles of fluids, electrolytes, and acid–base balance, including focused assessments and how they affect entire body systems. Individual chapters focus on specific electrolytes (sodium, potassium, calcium, magnesium, chloride, and phosphorus), acid–base disturbances, and replacement therapies for common fluids and electrolytes imbalances. Each chapter includes definitions, etiologies, clinical manifestations, and therapeutic management of fluids, electrolytes, and acid–base problems in the context of the nursing process.

ACKNOWLEDGMENTS

This book is a monumental effort of collaboration. Without the contributions of many individuals, this first edition of *Fluids, Electrolytes, and Acid–Base Balance: Reviews and Rationales* would not have been possible. We gratefully acknowledge all the contributors who devoted their time and talents to this book. Their chapters will surely assist both students and practicing nurses alike to extend their knowledge in the area of fluid, electrolyte, and acid–base balance.

We owe a special debt of gratitude to the wonderful team at Prentice Hall Health for their enthusiasm for this project, as well as their good humor, expertise, and encouragement as the series developed. Maura Connor, Executive Editor for Nursing, was unending in her creativity, support, encouragement, and belief in the need for this series. Marilyn Meserve, Senior Managing Editor for Nursing, devoted many long hours to coordinating different facets of this project, and tirelessly and cheerfully encouraged our efforts as well. Her high standards and attention to detail contributed greatly to the final "look" of this series. Jeanne Allison, Developmental Editor, actively kept in communication with the different writers in this book and also facilitated getting the book itself into production. Editorial assistants, including Beth Ann Romph, Sladjana Repic, and others, helped to keep the project moving forward on a day-to-day basis, and we are grateful for their efforts as well. A very special thank you goes to the designers of the book and the production team, led by Danielle Newhouse, who brought our ideas and manuscript into final form.

Thank you to the team at Pine Tree Composition, led by Project Coordinator Jessica Balch, for the detail-oriented work of creating this book. We greatly appreciate their hard work, attention to detail, and spirit of collaboration. A special thanks also goes to Yesenia Kopperman, Assistant Editor for Nursing at Prentice Hall, and to Carlos Cooper, Lisa Donovan, and staff at the Pearson Education Development Group for designing and producing the *Nursing Notes* clinical reference card that accompanies this book.

Mary Ann Hogan acknowledges and gratefully thanks her husband Michael and children Mike Jr., Katie, Kristen, and Billy, who sacrificed hours of time that would have been spent with them, to bring this book to publication. Your love and support kept me energized, motivated, and at times, even sane. I love you all very much!

Daryle Wane would like to thank her husband Robert, and her children Brandon and Derek, and also her cats, for their unending support during this project. The pleasure of their company and their love kept me on track and focused to the tasks at hand. A special thank you to my parents—my mother Audrey, who inspired me to seek a profession and my father Murray, who taught me the importance of logic and is smiling from above. I love you all!

*Reference: National Council of State Boards of Nursing, Inc. *NCLEX Examination Test Plan for National Council Licensure Examination for Registered Nurses.* Effective April, 2001. Retrieved from the World Wide Web September 5, 2001 at http://www.ncsbn.org/public/resources/res/NCSBNRNTestPlan Booklet.pdf.

Contributors

Julie A. Adkins, RN, MSN, FNP
Family Nurse Practitioner
West Frankfort, Illinois
Chapter 5

Linda Wilson Covington, PhD, RN
Associate Professor of Nursing
Middle Tennessee State University
Murfreesboro, Tennessee
Chapter 6

June S. Goyne, RN, MSN, EdD(C), CEN
Associate Professor of Nursing
Columbus State University
Columbus, Georgia
Chapter 1

Ann Putnam Johnson, EdD, RN
Associate Dean, College of Applied Sciences
Associate Professor of Nursing
Western Carolina University
Cullowhee, North Carolina
Chapter 2

Kristy A. Nielson, BSN, CCRN, BS
Assistant Professor of Nursing
Western Wyoming Community College
Intensive Care Unit Staff Nursing
Memorial Hospital of Sweetwater County
Rock Springs, Wyoming
Chapter 4

Mary Catherine Rawls
Assistant Professor of Nursing
Castleton State College
Castleton, Vermont
Chapter 7

Lynn Rhyne, MN, RN
Assistant Professor of Nursing
Coastal Georgia Community College
Brunswick, Georgia
Chapter 3 & Chapter 8

Bernadette VanDeusen, MSN, RN
Associate Professor of Nursing
Ohlone College
Fremont, California
Chapter 9

Reviewers

Kathy M. Ketchum, RN, PhD
Assistant Professor
Southern Illinois University-Edwardsville
Edwardsville, Illinois

Karen Whitman, RN, MS CCPN
Major, US Army Nurse Corps
Head Nurse, Medical and Pediatric ICU
Walter Reed Army Medical Center
Washington, DC

Student Consultants

Alisa Beaulieu
Santa Fe Community College
Gainesville, Florida

Alison Cody
Germanna Community College
Locust Grove, Virginia

Daniel Dale
Valdosta State University
Valdosta, Georgia

Stephanie Hornby
George Mason University
Fairfax, Virgina

Amy Jeter
Ohio University-Chillicothe
Chillicothe, Ohio

Joan Lawrence
Auburn University
Auburn, Alabama

Lisa Marie Mays
Boise State University
Boise, Idaho

Shawn Shaughnessy
Santa Fe Community College
Gainesville, Florida

Phyllis Thieken
Ohio University-Chillicothe
Chillicothe, Ohio

Jenefer Thomas
Boise State University
Boise, Idaho

Gyleen Vickerman
Boise State University
Boise, Idaho

Carolyn Wilkinson
Auburn University
Auburn, Alabama

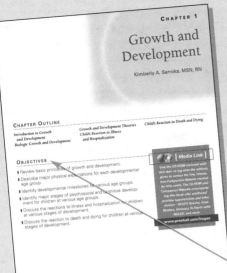

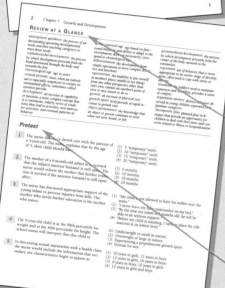

A Guide To
Prentice Hall's Reviews and Rationales Series

Each chapter has the following **feature elements** to guide you during review and study.

Chapter **Objectives** describe what you will be able to know or do after learning the material covered in the chapter.

Review at a Glance contains a glossary of key terms used in the chapter, with definitions provided up-front and available at your fingertips, to help you stay focused and make the best use of your study time.

The **Pretest** is a 10-question multiple choice test providing a sample overview of content covered in the chapter and helps you decide what areas need the most – or the least – review.

The **Practice to Pass** questions are open-ended questions that stimulate critical thinking and reinforce mastery of the chapter content.

NCLEX The NCLEX icon identifies information or concepts that are likely to be tested on the NCLEX licensing examination.

A detailed **Outline Review** of core content is given to provide both a comprehensive overview and review.

The **Case Study**, found at the end of the chapter, provides an opportunity for you to use your critical thinking and clinical reasoning skills to "put it all together." It describes a true-to-life client case situation and asks you open-ended questions about how you would provide care for that client and/or family.

The **Posttest** is a 10-question multiple-choice test at the end of the chapter providing new questions that are representative of chapter content. This posttest provides you with feedback about mastery of that content following review and study.

Answers and Rationales For all questions, answers and rationales for each correct answer are provided.

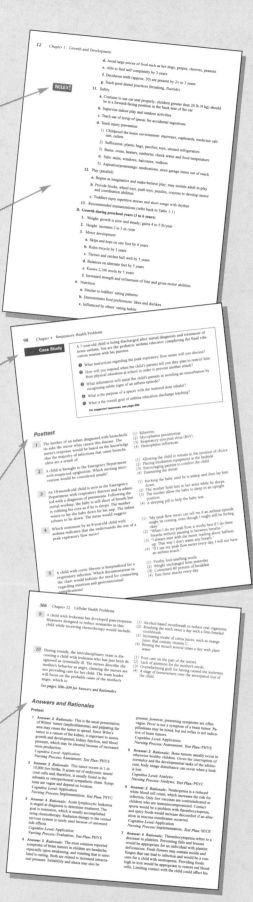

CHAPTER 1

Fluid Balance and Imbalances

June S. Goyne, RN, MSN, EdD(C), CEN

CHAPTER OUTLINE

Overview of Fluid Movement   *Fluid Volume Deficit (FVD)*   *Fluid Volume Excess (FVE)*

OBJECTIVES

▌ Review concepts of fluid movement.

▌ Review assessment data and diagnostic testing indicated to determine fluid volume deficit (dehydration) and fluid volume excess (overload).

▌ Identify clinical presentations of clients exhibiting fluid volume deficit or fluid volume excess.

▌ Identify priority nursing diagnoses for clients experiencing fluid imbalance.

▌ Discuss therapeutic management of clients exhibiting fluid volume deficit and fluid volume excess.

▌ Discuss nursing management of clients exhibiting fluid imbalances.

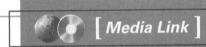

[Media Link]

Use the CD-ROM enclosed with this text, or log onto the address given to access the free, interactive Companion Website created for this series. The CD-ROM and Companion Website accompanying this book offer additional practice opportunities and information—NCLEX Review, Case Studies, Glossary, In Depth with NCLEX, and more.

www.prenhall.com/hogan

REVIEW AT A GLANCE

albumin *a major plasma protein produced by the liver*

aldosterone *hormone produced and released by the adrenal gland that causes the kidney to reabsorb sodium into the blood (which causes more water to be reabsorbed by osmosis) and excrete potassium into the urine, resulting in concentrated urine and lower urine output*

antidiuretic hormone (ADH) *hormone produced by hypothalamus and stored/released by posterior pituitary that causes the kidney to retain more water in the blood, thus increasing body water, resulting in concentrated urine and lower urine output*

colloids *large solute particles, such as protein, in solution that exert a pulling force for water*

colloid osmotic pressure *the pulling force for water created by colloids in solution*

diffusion *the movement of particles in a solution from an area of higher concentration to an area of lower concentration in order to equalize the concentration*

electrolyte *a substance that, when dissolved in water, separates into charged particles (ions)*

extracellular fluid (ECF) *the fluid space that lies outside of the cells; composed of two spaces, the interstitial (tissue) spaces around the cells and the vascular space inside blood vessels*

filtration *the movement of fluid and solute through a semipermeable membrane due to hydrostatic and osmotic forces*

free water *a hypotonic solution that provides more water than electrolytes, diluting the ECF, making it hypotonic; water then shifts by osmosis from the ECF to the*

ICF *until osmotic equilibrium is reached in both spaces; this rehydrates the ICF as well as the ECF*

hemoconcentration *condition in which the plasma is more concentrated than normal (higher osmolality than normal)*

hemodilution *condition in which the plasma is more dilute than normal (lower osmolality than normal)*

hydrostatic pressure *the pushing force of a fluid against the walls of the space it occupies*

hypertonic *having an osmolality higher than normal plasma; hypertonic intravenous solutions make the ECF hypertonic, thus water shifts by osmosis from the ICF to the ECF; therapeutically, this shifts excess cell water to vessels, where the kidneys can eliminate it in the urine; uncontrolled administration of hypertonic intravenous fluids can result in cell dehydration and vascular volume overload*

hypotonic *having an osmolality lower than normal plasma; hypotonic intravenous solutions dilute ECF, making it hypotonic; water then shifts by osmosis from the ECF into the ICF until osmotic equilibrium is achieved; therapeutically, this replaces water primarily inside cells; excess administration of hypotonic intravenous fluids can result in cell overhydration and water intoxication*

interstitial fluid *the fluid space that lies around the cells (cells "float" in interstitial fluid); the interstitial space and vascular space make up the extracellular fluid (ECF)*

intracellular fluid (ICF) *the fluid space that lies inside of the cells*

isotonic *having the same osmolality as normal plasma; isotonic intravenous solutions provide equal amounts of water and solute, thus not changing the concentra-*

tion *of the ECF; osmosis does not shift water into or out of the cells; therapeutically, this type of fluid replaces ECF water losses*

oncotic pressure *the pulling force a solution has for water due to its protein content*

osmolality *the concentration of solute (particles) per kilogram of water, which creates the pulling power of that solution for water*

osmolarity *the concentration of solute (particles) per liter of solution, which creates the pulling power of that solution for water*

osmosis *the pulling of water through a semipermeable membrane from an area of lower concentration (fewer particles, more water) to an area of higher concentration (more particles, less water) in order to equalize concentration on both sides*

osmotic pressure *the pulling force a solution has for water; a solution's osmotic pressure is determined by its osmolality (concentration)—the higher the osmolality, the higher the osmotic pressure (force with which it will pull water in from other areas)*

semi-permeable membrane *a membrane that allows some particles to pass through freely and not others (e.g., cell walls and capillary membranes)*

specific gravity *a measure of the concentration of a solution using solute-solvent ratio; specific gravity of water (no solute) is 1.000; urine specific gravity is normally 1.010–1.030, and is used to indirectly reflect serum osmolality*

vascular space *the space within the blood vessels, usually discussed in terms of its blood volume carrying capacity*

Pretest

1 Which of the following clients is at highest risk for developing fluid volume deficit?

(1) A 76-year-old client who has an NG tube to low suction following colon cancer surgery
(2) A thin 55-year-old client who smokes and takes glucocorticoids for chronic lung disease
(3) A 1-year-old child being treated in the clinic for a runny nose and ear infection
(4) A 30-year-old client jogging in 50-degree weather

2 Which of the following statements should not be included in an education program for the elderly about prevention of dehydration during hot weather?

(1) "Observe your urine and immediately drink more fluid if it starts getting darker."
(2) "Keep a variety of fluids in your home and drink them frequently throughout the day."
(3) "Popsicles, gelatin, and ice cream provide fluid intake as well as liquids you drink."
(4) "Use your thirst as a guide to the amount of fluid you should be drinking."

3 An adult client in the clinic complains of a cough, fever, nausea, and vomiting for three days. Examination reveals dry tongue and oral mucosa and concentrated urine. The client also reports feeling weak and dizzy. Which vital sign measurement would provide the best indicator of current fluid status?

(1) Temperature
(2) Respiratory rate and depth
(3) BP and pulse in lying and standing positions
(4) Pulse oximetry reading at rest

4 An intravenous (IV) infusion of normal saline is being initiated for a 10-month-old infant diagnosed with fluid volume deficit. The order states to deliver a 200 mL bolus, then reduce the fluid rate to 30 mL/hour. How should the nurse implement this therapy?

(1) Control the fluid infusion rate using an infusion pump, checking it often.
(2) Ask the mother to notify the nurse when 200 mL of fluid has infused.
(3) Calculate and set the gravity drip rate and monitor the infusion every hour.
(4) Teach the mother to slow the rate and call the nurse once 200 mL is infused.

5 A 40-year-old client is hospitalized for gastrointestinal (GI) bleeding. Orders include nasogastric tube (NGT) placement with irrigations until the returns are clear. Which fluid should be used for the NG irrigations?

(1) 3% saline
(2) D_5W
(3) Normal saline
(4) Plain water

6 A 70-year-old client with a past medical history of hypertension and myocardial infarction is in the hospital following stomach surgery. Vital signs have been stable and an IV of $D_5\frac{1}{2}NS$ is infusing at 100 mL/hour. The client now complains of trouble breathing, has a moist cough, and pulse oximetry reading has fallen to 92%. What action should the nurse take first?

(1) Measure blood pressure and heart rate.
(2) Assess legs and arms for pitting edema.
(3) Telephone and notify the physician.
(4) Slow the intravenous rate to 10 to 20 mL/hour.

7 A 45-year-old client diagnosed with fluid volume overload due to acute kidney dysfunction is placed on a 1,000 mL fluid restriction per 24-hour period. The client asks the nurse, "Why there is such a severe fluid restriction when I already have dry lips and mouth?" Which response by the nurse is best?

(1) "The doctor ordered the fluid restriction, so you must comply with those orders."
(2) "Your kidneys are not able to eliminate extra fluid right now, so fluid intake has to be limited to protect your heart and lungs from being overloaded with fluid."
(3) "You probably drank too much fluid before you got sick, so you can't compare your usual intake to your limitations now that your kidneys are not working."
(4) "Too much fluid will cause your heart to fail and your lungs to fill with water, which could be fatal."

8 Which of the following is the best indicator of an excessive response to diuretic therapy?

(1) Elevated blood urea nitrogen (BUN) and hematocrit (HCT) and an 8-pound weight loss in 24 hours
(2) Elevated BUN and HCT and an 8-pound weight gain in 24 hours
(3) Decreased BUN and HCT and an 8-pound weight loss in 24 hours
(4) Decreased BUN and HCT and an 8-pound weight gain in 24 hours

9 A client is receiving an intravenous (IV) infusion of 0.0225% NS intravenously at 50 mL/hour. During such an infusion, what is especially important to monitor to detect complications of therapy?

(1) Urine output and concentration
(2) Legs and arms for edema
(3) Tongue and mouth for dryness
(4) Mental status and orientation

10 When an adult is receiving an intravenous (IV) infusion of 3% saline, what are the monitoring priorities for the early detection of complications of therapy?

(1) Neurological status, lung sounds, and serum sodium levels
(2) Heart rate, blood pressure, and daily weights
(3) Serum glucose levels and urine specific gravity
(4) Pulse oximetry and peripheral edema in legs

See pages 34–35 for Answers and Rationales.

I. Overview of Fluid Movement

A. Fluid transport issues

1. Body fluid spaces (see Figure 1-1)

   a. Intracellular fluid (ICF): fluid within the cells; two-thirds of body fluid is ICF

   b. Extracellular fluid (ECF): fluid outside of the cells; made up of two components, the **interstitial fluid** (fluid surrounding the cells) and fluid within the **vascular space** (the blood vessels)

   c. Fluid constantly moves among the intracellular, interstitial, and vascular spaces to maintain body fluid balance

Figure 1-1

Body fluid spaces.

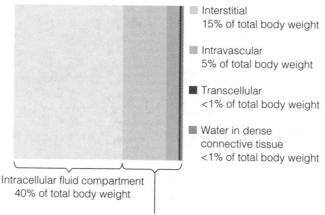

Total body fluids = 60% of body weight

Interstitial
15% of total body weight

Intravascular
5% of total body weight

Transcellular
<1% of total body weight

Water in dense connective tissue
<1% of total body weight

Intracellular fluid compartment
40% of total body weight

Extracellular fluid compartment
20% of total body weight

1) ICF is the most stable and is fairly resistant to major fluid shifts

2) Vascular fluid is the least stable; it is quickly lost or gained in response to fluid intake or losses

3) Interstitial fluid is the reserve fluid, replacing fluid either in the blood vessels or cells, depending on the need

2. **Osmosis** (see Figure 1-2)

   a. Water moves through a **semipermeable membrane** (membrane that allows water and small particles, but not large particles, to easily pass through) from an area of lower concentration (fewer particles, more water) to an area of higher concentration (more particles, less water) until concentrations are equalized on both sides of the membrane

   b. Osmosis is a major force in body fluid movement and intravenous (IV) fluid therapy

      1) Cell membranes and capillary membranes are semipermeable

      2) Water moves into and out of the cells and capillaries by osmosis

3. Osmolality and osmotic pressure

   a. Osmolality and osmolarity are both terms that refer to the concentration of a solution, which creates its **osmotic pressure** (the pulling power of a solution for water)

      1) **Osmolality** is the concentration of solute (particles) per kilogram of water, while **osmolarity** is the concentration of solute (particles) per liter of a solution (the solvent does not have to be water)

      2) Because body fluid solvent is water and one liter of water weighs one kilogram, the terms can be used interchangeably in discussing human fluid physiology; the term osmolality will be used here

      3) The higher the osmolality (concentration) of a solution, the greater its pulling power for water

   b. Serum osmolality is the concentration of particles (major particles are sodium and protein) in the plasma

      1) Normal serum osmolality is 275 to 295 mOsm/L

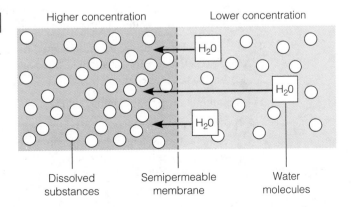

Figure 1-2

Osmosis.

Higher concentration   Lower concentration

H_2O

H_2O

H_2O

Dissolved substances   Semipermeable membrane   Water molecules

2) Serum osmolality can be estimated

a) Sodium is the major solute in plasma contributing to its osmolality (estimated serum osmolality = 2 times the serum sodium level)

b) Urea (BUN) and glucose are both large particles that increase serum osmolality, when present in excess amounts in the blood

c) When either or both are elevated, the serum osmolality will be higher than 2 times the sodium level, so the following formula will be more accurate:

$$\text{Serum osmolality} = 2 \times \text{serum sodium} + \frac{\text{BUN}}{3} + \frac{\text{glucose}}{18}$$

c. The term **isotonic** is defined as having the same osmolality as normal plasma

1) Isotonic IV fluids have the same osmolality as normal plasma; no osmotic pressure difference is created, so the fluids remain primarily in the ECF

2) Isotonic IV fluids are used to replace extracellular fluid losses and to expand vascular volume quickly

3) Isotonic intravenous fluids include:

a) Normal saline (NS; 0.9% NaCl): sodium and chloride in water with same osmolality as normal plasma; NS provides no calories or **free water** (water without solute)

b) Ringer's solution: contains sodium, potassium, calcium, and potassium in similar concentrations to plasma, but no dextrose, magnesium, or bicarbonate; Ringer's solution provides no calories or free water

c) Lactated Ringer's solution (LR): contains sodium, chloride, potassium, calcium, and lactate in concentrations similar to normal plasma; LR provides no dextrose, magnesium, or free water

d. The term **hypotonic** is defined as having a lower osmolality than normal plasma

1) Hypotonic IV fluids have a lower osmolality than normal plasma

2) Water is pulled out of vessels into the cells, resulting in decreased vascular volume and increased cell water

3) Hypotonic IV fluids are used to prevent and treat cellular dehydration by providing free water to the cells

4) Hypotonic IV fluids are contraindicated in acute brain injuries because cerebral cells are very sensitive to free water, absorbing it rapidly and leading to cellular edema

5) Hypotonic intravenous fluids include:

a) 5% dextrose in water (D_5W): although 5% dextrose (D_5W) is isotonic in the IV bag, it has a hypotonic effect in the body; the dextrose is quickly metabolized once infused intravenously, leaving free water that shifts by osmosis from vessels into cells; for each liter of D_5W, roughly ⅔ enters cells and ⅓ remains in extracellular space

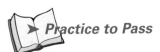

b) 0.45% saline (½ NS) and 0.225 saline (¼ NS): these fluids provide free water to cells as well as small amounts of sodium and chloride; approximately ½ of each liter infused moves into cells and ½ remains in extracellular space

c) Maintenance fluids: saline mixed with dextrose and water

   i) 5% dextrose in 0.45 saline (D_5½ NS) and 5% dextrose in 0.225% saline (D_5¼ NS): both are hypertonic in the IV bag, but because of rapid dextrose metabolism, both also have a degree of hypotonic effect, providing some water to cells; are composed of hypotonic saline solutions combined with dextrose to provide calories and are often used as maintenance fluids; the dextrose content does not meet daily nutritional caloric requirements, but it does help prevent ketosis associated with starvation

   ii) 5% dextrose in 0.9% saline (D_5NS) is also hypertonic in the bag, but provides some free water and calories to cells, dextrose is mixed with NS and provides less free water and more extracellular water than D_5½NS or D_5¼NS

e. The term **hypertonic** is defined as having a higher osmolality than normal plasma

   1) Hypertonic IV fluids have a higher osmolality than normal plasma, causing water to be pulled from the cells into the vessels, resulting in increased vascular volume and decreased cell water

   2) Hypertonic solutions are used to treat very specific problems and are administered in carefully controlled, limited doses in order to avoid vascular volume overload and cell dehydration; they are also used to pull excess fluid from cells and to promote osmotic diuresis

   3) Hypertonic IV solutions

      a) Include saline solutions greater than 0.9% (3% saline and 5% saline); used infrequently

      b) Clinical indication for hypertonic saline use is when the serum sodium is dangerously low (115 mg/dL or less); it is given with great caution in carefully controlled, limited doses using an IV infusion pump

      c) Note: clients receiving hypertonic saline solutions require frequent monitoring of vital signs, neurological status, lung sounds, urine output, and serum sodium levels to avoid hypernatremia and vascular volume overload

      d) Dextrose solutions greater than 5% (such as 10% dextrose and 50% dextrose) are also considered hypertonic solutions; these are used on a limited basis to treat clients with hypoglycemia

      e) Hypertonic dextrose solutions are given in controlled settings by IV push or IV infusion pump; 50% dextrose is used as part of a hypoglycemic treatment protocol or in a code situation; a 10% dextrose solution is used to treat newborns as part of a hypoglycemic treatment protocol

Figure 1-3

Diffusion.

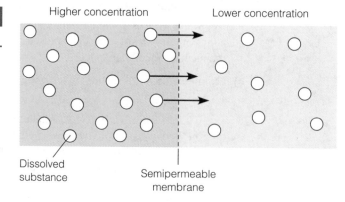

Higher concentration   Lower concentration

Dissolved substance

Semipermeable membrane

NCLEX!

  f) **Colloid** volume expanders (Albumin, Dextran, Hetastarch)

    i) A colloid is a large solute particle, such as protein in solution, that normally does not pass through cell and capillary membranes

    ii) Colloid volume expanders pull fluid from tissue into the vessels by osmosis, increasing vascular volume

NCLEX!

  g) Osmotic diuretics (such as mannitol [Osmitrol]) pull fluid from third spaces, tissues, and cells into vessels to be eliminated by kidneys

4. **Diffusion** (see Figure 1-3)

  a. Particles move from an area of higher concentration (more particles, less water) to an area of lower concentration (fewer particles, more water) until concentrations are equalized; some particles easily diffuse through semipermeable membranes and other do not

  b. Electrolytes (e.g., sodium, potassium, chloride, calcium, magnesium, and phosphate) are small particles that tend to move through semipermeable membranes easily

  c. Urea, glucose, and **albumin** (a plasma protein produced by the liver) are large particles that do not pass through semipermeable membranes easily

B. Capillary fluid movement (see Figure 1-4)

1. **Hydrostatic pressure**

  a. Hydrostatic pressure is the pushing force of a fluid against the walls of the space it occupies

Figure 1-4

Capillary filtration dynamics.

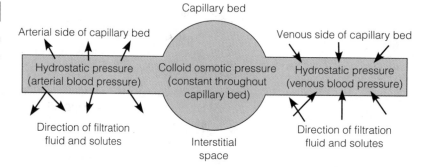

Capillary bed

Arterial side of capillary bed

Venous side of capillary bed

Hydrostatic pressure (arterial blood pressure)

Colloid osmotic pressure (constant throughout capillary bed)

Hydrostatic pressure (venous blood pressure)

Direction of filtration fluid and solutes

Interstitial space

Direction of filtration fluid and solutes

    b. Hydrostatic pressure in blood vessels is generated by the heart's pumping action and varies within the vascular system

  2. Oncotic pressure

    a. Oncotic pressure (also called **colloid osmotic pressure** or **COP**) is the pulling force exerted by colloids in a solution

    b. Albumin is important in maintaining normal serum oncotic pressure (pulling force for water) and adequate vascular fluid volume

    c. Since plasma proteins do not normally cross the vessel wall, the plasma protein concentration remains the same in arteries, veins, and throughout the capillaries

  3. Starling's Law of the Capillaries

    a. Filtration (net fluid movement into or out of the capillary) is determined by the difference between the forces favoring filtration and those opposing it (like a tug of war—pushing and pulling)

    b. Interstitial hydrostatic pressure (pushing water into capillary) and interstitial oncotic pressure (pulling water out of capillary) are very low and are essentially equal, thus normally exert little influence on fluid movement into or out of capillaries

    c. Capillary hydrostatic pressure (pushing water out of capillary) and capillary oncotic pressure (pulling water into capillary) are not the same, and fluid movement is seen in the capillary bed

      1) At the arterial end of the capillary, capillary hydrostatic pressure (pushing water out of capillary) exceeds capillary oncotic pressure (pulling water into capillary), thus net fluid movement is from the capillary into tissue, carrying nutrients with it

      2) At the venous end of the capillary, capillary hydrostatic pressure (pushing water out of capillary) is less than capillary oncotic pressure (pulling water into capillaries), thus net fluid movement is into the capillary from the tissue, carrying wastes with it

  C. Chemical regulation of fluid balance

    1. Antidiuretic hormone (ADH) (see Figure 1-5)

      a. ADH is a hormone synthesized by the hypothalamus and secreted by the posterior pituitary, which regulates water

      b. ADH is released and inhibited in a feedback loop

        1) ADH release is triggered by a drop in BP or blood volume or by a rise in blood osmolality, causing the kidneys to reabsorb more water in the blood (resulting in higher vascular volume and low output of concentrated urine)

        2) ADH release is inhibited by a rise in BP or blood volume or by a drop in blood osmolality, causing the kidneys to excrete more water in the urine (resulting in lower vascular volume and high output of dilute urine)

Figure 1-5

ADH regulation of water.

Prolonged fever
Prolonged vomiting
Prolonged diarrhea
Excessive perspiration
Severe blood loss
Severe burns
Septic shock
Other pathologic vasodilation

↓ Blood pressure
↓ Blood volume
↑ Blood osmolality

 Osmoreceptors in hypothalamus stimulate posterior pituitary to secrete ADH

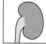 ADH stimulates renal tubules to ↑ reabsorption of H_2O

Scant, concentrated urine
↑ Blood pressure
↑ Blood volume
↓ Blood osmolality

2. **Aldosterone** (see Figure 1-6)

   a. Aldosterone is a hormone produced by the adrenal gland that conserves sodium in the body by causing the kidneys to retain sodium and excrete potassium in its place

   b. Water follows sodium due to osmosis, thus aldosterone has an indirect effect on water

   c. Aldosterone is released and inhibited in a feedback loop as part of the renin-angiotensin-aldosterone system (refer again to Figure 1-6)

      1) Aldosterone release is triggered by a drop in BP, blood volume, *or* serum sodium, or a rise in serum potassium

         a) Aldosterone causes the kidneys to reabsorb more sodium into the blood, increasing serum sodium levels; water follows sodium into the blood by osmosis, raising vascular volume

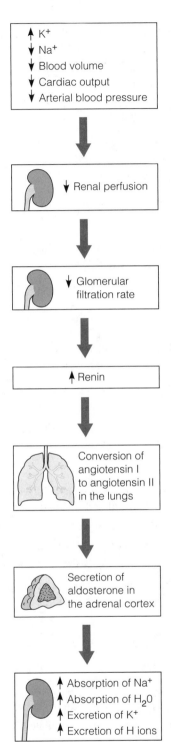

Figure 1-6

Aldosterone regulation of sodium and water.

↑ K+
↓ Na+
↓ Blood volume
↓ Cardiac output
↓ Arterial blood pressure

↓ Renal perfusion

↓ Glomerular filtration rate

↑ Renin

Conversion of angiotensin I to angiotensin II in the lungs

Secretion of aldosterone in the adrenal cortex

↑ Absorption of Na+
↑ Absorption of H$_2$0
↑ Excretion of K+
↑ Excretion of H ions

b) As more sodium is retained in the blood, the kidney must excrete more potassium in the urine to maintain a balance of positive ions in the blood, this mechanism lowers serum potassium levels

2) Aldosterone release is inhibited by a rise in BP, blood volume, *or* serum sodium, or a drop in serum potassium

a) Decreasing aldosterone levels cause the kidneys to excrete more sodium in the urine, decreasing serum sodium levels; water follows sodium, thereby lowering vascular volume

b) As more sodium is excreted in the urine, the kidneys must retain more potassium in the blood to maintain positive ion balance in the blood, this mechanism raises serum potassium levels

3. Glucocorticoids (cortisol)

a. Cortisol is a glucocorticoid hormone produced and released by the adrenal gland when the body is stressed

b. Glucocorticoids promote renal retention of sodium and water

4. Atrial natriuretic peptide (ANP)

a. ANP is a cardiac hormone found in the atria of the heart that is released when atria are stretched by high blood volume or high BP

b. ANP works in the following ways to lower blood volume and BP:

1) Causes vasodilation by direct effect on blood vessels and suppression of renin-angiotensin system

2) Decreases aldosterone release by adrenal glands, causing increased urinary excretion of sodium and water

3) Decreases ADH release by pituitary gland, causing increased urinary excretion of water

4) Increases glomerular filtration rate, increasing rate of urine production and water excretion

5. Thirst mechanism

a. Thirst normally occurs with even small fluid losses or small increases in serum osmolality; it is stimulated by thirst receptors in the hypothalamus that can detect as little as 1 mOsm/L change in plasma concentration

b. Thirst also stimulates ADH and aldosterone release, which promotes reabsorption of water

c. The thirst mechanism is depressed in older people (> 60 years old), including the healthy elderly living in the community and people living with debilitating illnesses

II. Fluid Volume Deficit (FVD)

A. Etiology and pathophysiology

1. Isotonic fluid loss

a. Fluid and solute are lost in proportional amounts, thus serum osmolality remains normal and no osmotic force is created

b. Intracellular water is not disturbed and fluid losses are primarily ECF (especially the vascular volume), which can quickly lead to shock

c. Causes

1) Hemorrhage results in loss of fluid, electrolytes, proteins, and blood cells in proportional amounts, often resulting in inadequate vascular volume

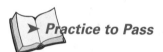

Practice to Pass

An adult client has 3% saline infusing intravenously. What nursing observations and measures should be implemented to protect client safety? Why?

NCLEX!

2) Gastrointestinal losses (vomiting, continuous NG suction, diarrhea, drainage from fistulas and tubes) contain abundant electrolytes; thus GI fluid and electrolytes tend to be lost in fairly proportional amounts

3) Fever, environmental heat, and diaphoresis result in profuse sweating, which causes water and sodium loss from the skin in fairly equal proportions

4) Burns (especially large burns) initially damage skin and capillary membranes, allowing fluid, electrolytes, and proteins to escape into the burned tissue area, which often results in inadequate vascular volume

5) Diuretics can cause excessive loss of fluid and electrolytes in fairly proportional amounts

6) Third space fluid shifts occur when fluid moves from the vascular space into physiologically useless extracellular spaces (where it is unavailable as reserve fluid or to transport nutrients)

d. Isotonic fluid loss is primarily an extracellular fluid loss that requires extracellular fluid replacement, with emphasis on the vascular volume

2. Hypertonic dehydration

a. More water is lost than solute (primarily sodium) creating a fluid volume deficit and a relative solute excess

b. Solute (sodium or glucose more commonly) can also be gained in excess of water, creating a similar imbalance

c. Serum osmolality is elevated, resulting in hypertonic extracellular fluid that pulls fluid into vessels from cells by osmosis and causes the cells to shrink and become dehydrated

d. Causes of hypertonic dehydration

1) Inadequate fluid intake

a) Clients who are unable to respond to thirst independently (infants, elderly, disabled, and bedridden), who have nausea, anorexia, or dysphagia, or who are NPO without IV fluid replacement are at risk to develop fluid volume deficit

b) Decreased water intake results in increased ECF solute concentration, which leads to cellular dehydration

c) A client can go several weeks to months without food, but only two to three days without water

2) Severe or prolonged isotonic fluid losses

a) May occur in conditions such as vomiting and diarrhea and eventually result in loss of more water than solute

b) ECF becomes hypertonic as compensatory mechanisms are exhausted, and the body has no more water to conserve through the kidneys

c) The hypertonic ECF then begins to draw water from the cells, dehydrating them as well

3) Watery diarrhea causes loss of more water than electrolytes

4) Diabetes insipidus (DI) is caused by insufficient ADH production or release, which leads to massive, uncontrolled diuresis of very dilute urine (as much as 30 liters per day) and can quickly lead to shock and death

   a) Brain injury that damages or puts pressure on the hypothalamus or pituitary often causes DI

   b) Once acute DI develops, parenteral administration of vasopressin (pharmacologic form of ADH) is indicated to stop the massive fluid loss

5) Increased solute intake (e.g., salt, sugar, protein) without a proportional intake of water increases plasma osmolality, resulting in water being pulled from cells, increasing ECF and causing cellular dehydration; increasing ECF is dangerous for clients with heart or kidney problems, and the resulting osmotic diuresis actually makes the cellular dehydration worse; conditions that can cause hypertonic dehydration include:

   a) Highly concentrated enteral or parenteral feedings (increased glucose)

   b) Improperly prepared infant formulas (too concentrated)

   c) Hyperglycemia and/or diabetic ketoacidosis (excess glucose and ketones in the blood)

   d) Increased sodium ingestion (e.g., seawater ingestion, salt tablets)

   e) Excess osmotic diuretic use

   e. Fluid loss is both extracellular and intracellular

3. Third spacing

   a. Third spaces are extracellular body spaces in which fluid is not normally present in large amounts, but in which fluid can accumulate

   b. Fluid that accumulates in third spaces is physiologically useless because it is not available for use as reserve fluid or to transport nutrients

   c. Common locations for third space fluid to accumulate include:

   1) Tissue spaces (edema)

   2) Abdomen (ascites)

   3) Pleural spaces (pleural effusion)

   4) Pericardial space (pericardial effusion)

   d. Causes of third spacing

   1) Injury or inflammation (e.g., massive trauma, crush injuries, burns, sepsis, cancer, intestinal obstruction, abdominal surgery) increase capillary permeability, allowing fluid, electrolytes, and proteins to leak from vessels

   2) Malnutrition or liver dysfunction (e.g., starvation, cirrhosis, chronic alcoholism) prevent the liver from producing albumin, thus lowering capillary oncotic pressure

3) High vascular hydrostatic pressure (e.g., heart failure, renal failure, or other forms of vascular fluid overload) pushes abnormal volumes of fluid from vessels

B. Dehydration concepts

1. Isotonic dehydration involves equal losses of all fluid components and is the most commonly seen type of fluid volume deficit

2. Hypotonic dehydration involves greater losses of electrolytes, leading to a decreased plasma osmolality; fluid shifting occurs as ECF volume decreases

3. Hypertonic dehydration involves greater losses of ECF volume than electrolytes, leading to an increased plasma osmolality; fluid shifting occurs as the body tries to compensate to restore balance

C. Assessment

1. Clinical manifestations of dehydration

   a. Thirst (an early sign), unreliable as an indicator in the elderly and in the young who cannot express needs

   b. Concentrated urine and low urine volume

      1) Minimum normal urine output in children is 1 to 2 mL/kg/hour

      2) Minimum normal urine output in the average adult is 30 mL/hour (240 mL/8 hours)

      3) Concentrated, dark urine with high **specific gravity** (concentration of a solution, for urine normally 1.010 to 1.030) that is > 1.035

      4) Note: if diabetes insipidus is causing the fluid volume deficit, urine will be pale, dilute, and high in volume

   c. Dry skin with decreased turgor and elasticity and dry mucous membranes

      1) Skin "tenting" occurs as tissues stick together because of interstitial fluid loss

      2) Skin of older clients loses elasticity with aging (elastin decreases), so tenting is not a reliable sign in the elderly

      3) Test elderly skin on sternum, forehead, inner thigh, or top of hip bone rather than arms or legs

      4) Skin of infant is very elastic, even when there is a fluid volume deficit, thus tenting is not a reliable sign in infants

      5) Check tenting in infants over abdomen or inner thighs, but rely on other signs (heart rate, tongue and mucous membranes, urine output, mental status, and behavior)

      6) Breathing and environmental conditions can cause dry lips when oral mucosa is actually moist; keep this in mind when assessing mucous membranes

      7) Dry tongue with longitudinal furrows is a reliable sign in all age groups

      8) Decreased tearing and dry conjunctiva

    d. Sunken eyeballs; sunken or depressed fontanels in infants < 18 months old

    e. Flat neck veins and poor peripheral vein filling

        1) Flat neck veins even with head of bed < 45 degrees (normally some distention seen due to gravity when lying down flat)

        2) Delayed or absence of hand vein filling when hand is placed lower than heart (normally fill within 3 to 5 seconds)

    f. Hypotension (late sign in infants and young children)

        1) Postural hypotension

            a) Rise in pulse rate > 10 to 15 beats per minute and/or fall in systolic BP > 10 to 15 mm Hg after rising from lying to standing position

            b) Indicates vascular volume has fallen enough that the body cannot maintain adequate BP when standing; the greater the fall in BP and/or rise in heart rate, the greater the fluid volume deficit

        2) Frank hypotension (low BP even when lying down)

        3) Complaints of weakness, dizziness, light-headedness

        4) Syncope when rising from lying position

    g. Other signs of decreased cardiac output

        1) Tachycardia (early sign, especially in infants and young children)

        2) Weak, thready pulses

        3) Cool extremities with delayed capillary refill

    h. Tachypnea (usually without dyspnea)

    i. Low grade fever (higher fever can occur in severe dehydration)

    j. Mental status changes (e.g., irritability, restlessness, lethargy, confusion, drowsiness)

        1) This is often the first sign noticed in the elderly and is often the first sign causing alarm in parents of infants and small children

        2) Changes in mental status are a serious sign of significant fluid loss; if the fluid loss if severe, the client can progress to seizures and coma

    k. Acute weight loss (an important sign in infants and young children)

        1) 1 L water = 1 kg (2.2 pounds)

        2) Considered a more accurate reflection of fluid balance than intake and output because of the difficulty in keeping accurate records

        3) Note: exception occurs in weight changes with significant third space fluid shifts as weight gain is often seen; clients with third spacing may initially have signs/symptoms of hypervolemia but the primary problem is fluid volume deficit

        4) 2% body weight loss = mild fluid deficit (may only see thirst; ~1 to 2 L fluid loss in adult)

5) 5% body weight loss = moderate fluid deficit (signs and symptoms appear; ~3 to 5 L fluid loss in adult)

6) 8% body weight loss = severe fluid deficit (frank hypotension and delirium; ~5 to 10 L fluid loss in adult)

7) > 15% body weight loss can be fatal (anuria, coma; > 10 L fluid loss in adult)

2. Diagnostic and laboratory findings

a. Normal or high hematocrit (HCT) and blood urea nitrogen (BUN) because of **hemoconcentration** (plasma is more concentrated than normal, thus the number of red blood cells and urea particles per liter of plasma is higher); *note:* if hemorrhage is the cause of the fluid volume deficit, red blood cells are being lost in proportion to plasma, thus HCT will be low

b. High urine specific gravity (> 1.030) as kidneys conserve water while continuing to excrete solute (unless the cause is diabetes insipidus, in which specific gravity will be low [< 1.010])

c. In hypertonic dehydration, lab values will also reflect increased plasma concentration

1) Serum osmolality elevated > 300 mOsm/kg

2) Serum sodium elevated (hypernatremia) > 150 mEq/L

3) Serum glucose elevated (if that is the cause of the dehydration) > 120 mg/dL

3. Identification of risk factors (predisposing to fluid volume deficit)

a. Age, gender, and body fat

1) Infants and young children

   a) Total body water percentage is higher (infant 80%, premature infant 90%, adult 60%); thus infants require more water for size than older children and adults

   b) ECF, which is more easily lost, equals 40% of an infant's body water (compared to 20% of an adult's); infants may exchange 50% of their ECF daily, compared to 18% in an adult

   c) Kidneys are immature up to age 2 years, thus cannot conserve or excrete water or sodium in response to imbalances as efficiently as adults, making them less able to handle large amounts of solute-free water or concentrated fluids

   d) Body surface area is relatively larger, thus infants lose more fluid through the skin for their size than adults

   e) Higher metabolic rate of infants requires more water for size than adults and produces more heat, which results in more water loss

   f) Fever tends to be higher and last longer in acute illnesses of infants and children, which increases fluid loss with acute illness

   g) Children 2 to 12 years of age have less stable regulatory responses to fluid imbalances than adults

2) Elderly

   a) After age 60, only 45 to 50% of body weight is water (compared to 60% in younger adult), thus small water losses have a greater impact

   b) Skeletal muscle mass (which holds more water than fat) declines and percentage of body fat rises with aging

   c) Kidneys lose function and cannot concentrate or dilute urine as efficiently, thus cannot compensate as well for imbalance or excrete heavy solute loads (such as those from tube feedings)

   d) Diminished thirst mechanism is seen with aging

   e) Decreased pancreatic functioning and glucose tolerance with aging increases risk of hyperglycemia and resulting osmotic diuresis

3) Women and obese individuals have a higher percentage of body fat, which holds less water than muscle; thus they have a lower percentage of body water for their weight

b. Acute illness

1) Surgery can result in blood and fluid loss

2) Gastroenteritis causing nausea, vomiting, and/or diarrhea or nasogastric suctioning lead to fluid and electrolyte loss

3) Burns: the larger the burn surface area, the greater the fluid loss

4) Brain injury from stroke, trauma, or tumor can cause cerebral edema, which can put pressure on the hypothalamus and/or pituitary, altering ADH release; problems with ADH regulation can lead to the client developing syndrome of inappropriate ADH secretion (SIADH) or diabetes insipidus (DI), which is more commonly seen

c. Chronic illness

1) Liver disease reduces the production of albumin, which affects the ability to maintain adequate circulating vascular volume

2) Renal disease limits ability to regulate fluid or electrolytes via urine output

3) Diabetes mellitus increases risk for hyperglycemia and hypertonic dehydration

4) Cancer can predispose to fluid shifts; chemotherapy often causes nausea and vomiting with loss of fluid and lack of intake

d. Environmental factors

1) Vigorous exercise increases metabolism, ventilation, and sweating, causing both an increased demand for fluid as well as increased fluid losses

2) Heat injuries: exposure to hot, humid environments can increase sweat production to as much as 2 L/hour; body fluid weight loss > 7% is associated with failure of body cooling mechanisms, leading to heat injuries

NCLEX**!**

e. Diet and lifestyle

    1) Difficulty chewing or swallowing can lead to inadequate intake of oral fluids and food (which is also a major source of fluid intake)

    2) Malnutrition, starvation, and low protein intake will affect volume status

    3) Excess alcohol consumption causes liver damage and/or malnutrition leading to altered volume status

f. Medications

NCLEX**!**

    1) Diuretics can predispose to excess fluid loss

    2) Chemotherapy can cause nausea, vomiting, and poor oral intake of fluids and food

D. Priority nursing diagnoses

NCLEX**!**

  1. Fluid volume deficit related to excessive fluid losses and/or decreased fluid intake

NCLEX**!**

  2. Risk for hypovolemic shock related to fluid loss

NCLEX**!**

  3. Risk for injury related to altered sensorium and/or dizziness

  4. Altered comfort related to signs and symptoms of fluid deficit

  5. Risk for impaired skin integrity related to skin and mucous membrane dryness

  6. Knowledge deficit related to risk factors and therapeutic interventions

E. Therapeutic management

  1. Oral replacement therapies

NCLEX**!**

    a. Fluids can be replaced orally if the deficit is mild, thirst is intact, and client can drink

      1) Commercial oral rehydration solutions (ORSs) provide fluids, glucose, and electrolytes in a concentration that is quickly absorbed even if vomiting and diarrhea are present; these include such brand names as Pedialyte, Gastrolyte, Oralyte, Rehydralyte, and Resol; client should drink small amounts frequently

      2) Infants and young children may only tolerate a few teaspoonfuls every few minutes, but will absorb a significant amount each hour, even if vomiting; for small children, freeze fluids into flavored ice pops, which are often better received than liquids; as fluids are replaced, begin alternating with low sodium fluids such as water, breast milk, lactose-free formula, or $\frac{1}{2}$-strength lactose formula

      3) Adults should sip frequent, small amounts of ORS, progressing to a variety of oral fluids

NCLEX**!**

    b. During initial rehydration, avoid fluids such as sodas, fruit juice, and sports drinks because their high sugar content (hypertonic) can worsen diarrhea and promote fluid loss; avoid salty fluids that can make diarrhea worse; avoid caffeine because it is a mild diuretic and may worsen fluid loss

c. Early reintroduction of regular diet has been shown to decrease the number of diarrhea stools and shorten the duration of gastroenteritis; BRAT diet (bananas, rice, applesauce, and toast) may be utilized briefly during the acute phase although it provides inadequate electrolytes, protein, or calories for the long term

2. Parenteral replacement therapies

a. Parenteral therapy for isotonic fluid losses

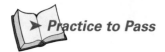

Practice to Pass

A 23-year-old client is admitted to the Emergency Department with multiple fractures of the legs and pelvis. BP is 86/40, heart rate 120, respirations 30, skin is cool and pale, and peripheral pulses are weak and thready. What intravenous fluids should be given immediately? Why?

1) Initially, expand ECF volume with isotonic IV fluids until adequate circulating blood volume and renal perfusion are achieved

   a) Fluid challenges (large amounts of IV fluids infused rapidly, often in 30 minutes or less) may be used

   b) Infuse a 1 to 2 liter bolus of isotonic fluid (e.g., NS) for adults, with up to 2 or 3 additional boluses to achieve response to therapy (improving urine output, blood pressure, heart rate, and mental status)

   c) Infuse a 20–30 mL/kg bolus of isotonic fluid (e.g., NS) for infants and young children, with up to 2 or 3 further boluses to achieve response to therapy (improving urine output, heart rate, respiratory rate, and mental status)

   d) Blood transfusion should be considered to replace lost red blood cells for clients experiencing severe hypovolemia due to hemorrhage

2) Once initial parenteral rehydration is accomplished for mild to moderate fluid losses, oral rehydration can be continued at home

3) If dehydration is severe, IV rehydration may continue with maintenance IV fluids (usually saline and dextrose combination fluids such as $D_5\frac{1}{2}NS$ or D_5NS)

4) If the cause of the fluid volume deficit is third spacing, osmotic diuretics can be used to mobilize some of the fluid back into the blood vessels for elimination by the kidneys; however, due to the nature of the disease processes that often cause third space fluid shifts, this is usually only a temporary measure; large third space fluid collections may need to be physically removed (paracentesis for ascites; thoracentesis for pleural effusion) and the vascular space rehydrated with IV fluids

b. Parenteral therapy for hypertonic dehydration

1) If hypovolemia and impending shock are present, isotonic fluids are given first to achieve adequate circulation and renal perfusion

2) Cellular dehydration is corrected with IV solutions having a hypotonic effect (provide free water to cells); be alert—hypotonic fluids must be given slowly to prevent rehydrating brain cells too rapidly, which could result in cerebral edema and brain injury

3) If hypervolemia is present (as with excess sodium intake), a diuretic may be given with hypotonic fluid infusions (to provide free water to cells while preventing vascular volume overload)

3. Monitoring of client during therapy

   a. Vital signs for changes in heart rate, BP, and respiratory rate

   b. Mental status and behavior for improvement in mentation (less lethargic, more alert, less confused, appropriate behavior for situation); lack of improvement or worsening mental status could indicate too rapid infusion of hypotonic fluids

   c. Monitor urine concentration and output for improvement; adequate urine output of normal color and concentration (in healthy kidneys) is a good indicator of adequate vascular volume

   d. Monitor IV infusion rate to avoid administration of excess fluid, especially in those with cardiac or renal dysfunction, the elderly, infants, and young children (who are all at increased risk for fluid volume overload); use infusion pumps in this population to prevent fluid overload

   e. Monitor intake, output, and daily weights (same scale, same time of day, same clothing for consistency)

F. **Planning and implementation**

   1. Monitor specific assessment parameters related to the management of FVD

   2. Assist with rehydration and promote return to adequate oral intake

   a. Provide indicated oral fluids in frequent, small amounts; keep fluids fresh and place within easy reach

   b. Remind elderly to drink something each hour due to decreased thirst mechanism

   c. Chill, warm, or freeze the indicated fluids to enhance intake based on client's preference

   d. Clients with altered mobility may require assistance in drinking fluids

   e. When using an infusion pump, check it frequently to ensure it is delivering fluid according to programmed settings

   3. Provide comfort measures

   a. Provide oral hygiene frequently, including brushing teeth and rinsing mouth, to promote comfort

   1) A rinse of equal parts peroxide and water can help deodorize the mouth

   2) Avoid glycerin and lemon or alcohol-based commercial mouthwash, which can be drying

   3) Avoid sucking on hard candy or chewing gum, both of which can further dry oral mucous membranes

   b. Apply a lip moisturizer

   c. Apply skin moisturizer to dry skin to prevent cracking and breakdown

   4. Listen to client's concerns, answer questions, and implement teaching

   a. Explain and answer questions in simple terms that foster client understanding

b. Focus on client's concerns and demonstrate respect for client's feelings

c. Offer reassurance and emotional support

5. Provide measures to prevent fluid volume deficits and dehydration

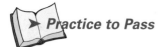

a. Provide additional plain water boluses periodically during enteral feedings

1) Note: 1 mL of water is recommended for each kCal of formula

2) If one can of formula has 380 kCal in 240 mL of fluid, an additional 140 mL of fluid is needed to achieve the recommended total fluid intake

3) However, watch for signs of water toxicity and hyponatremia, which can result if water boluses are excessive; check serum sodium levels periodically

6. Implement measures to control nausea, vomiting, diarrhea, and high fever as these may cause further complications

7. Recognize acutely ill clients at risk for inadequate fluid intake and initiate measures to provide adequate fluids by the oral, enteral, or parenteral routes

G. Medication therapy

1. Antiemetics are used to prevent fluid losses due to nausea and vomiting (e.g., promethazine [Phenergan])

2. Antidiarrheals are used to prevent fluid losses from the GI tract (e.g., loperamide [Imodium])

3. ADH: vasopressin (Pitressin) is used to correct diabetes insipidus

4. Antipyretics are used to control fever and minimize fluid losses (e.g., acetaminophen [Tylenol] or ibuprofen [Motrin])

H. Client education

1. Awareness of predisposing factors

a. Explain the nature of the client's condition and the causes for it

b. Explain risk factors and help identify those relevant to client (e.g., age, gender, body size, physical activities, illnesses, medications, diet, and lifestyle)

c. Explain early signs of impending fluid volume deficit and importance of initiating ORS in small, frequent amounts early to decrease nausea and replace electrolytes

d. Explain importance of contacting a physician if illness lasts more than 24 hours, if client is elderly or very young, or if client has a chronic illness (such as diabetes, heart disease, kidney disease, or liver problems)

2. Explain measures to help prevent fluid deficit and dehydration

a. Elderly should drink a variety of fluids frequently throughout the day even if not thirsty, especially in hot humid weather, since thirst is not a reliable indicator because of diminished thirst mechanism

b. Foods that are liquid at room temperature provide fluid intake (frozen ice pops, ice cream, gelatin) for those at risk

NCLEX!

    c. Drink cool water prior to exercise, 5–6 oz every 15 minutes during exercise, and following exercise

        1) If exercise is prolonged (> 1 hour for average person) or vigorous or if it occurs in a hot, humid climate, drink solutions for hydration that contain both water, carbohydrate, and electrolytes (e.g., sports drinks)

        2) Avoid highly salty fluids or salt tablets, which can raise sodium levels and draw fluid from cells, worsening dehydration

  3. Provide dietary education

NCLEX!

    a. Commercial oral rehydration solutions are recommended for vomiting and diarrhea, especially in children; they do not contain large amounts of sugar that can make diarrhea and dehydration worse but do contain needed electrolytes

NCLEX!

    b. During diarrhea, avoid ingesting salty fluids (e.g., salty broth) as well as those high in sugar (gelatin, soda, and fruit juice) because the high solute content can worsen diarrhea and dehydration

NCLEX!

    c. Avoid caffeine because it acts as a mild diuretic, increasing fluid loss

NCLEX!

    d. Recommend early progression to a soft, easily digestible, regular diet; limiting intake to a BRAT diet exclusively has fallen out of favor, especially in acute diarrhea, because it contains few electrolytes and is low in energy and protein; recommend use of ORSs that are rich in electrolytes to provide needed nutritional value

I. Evaluation

  1. Adequate fluid volume reflected by:

NCLEX!

    a. Adequate urine output and concentration

    b. Stable heart rate and blood pressure (lying and standing) within individual norms

    c. Skin and mucous membranes moist with normal turgor and elasticity; fontanels soft

    d. Return to usual mental state and behavior

    f. HCT, BUN, serum osmolality, and serum electrolytes within normal range during first 48 to 72 hours

  2. Free of injury

    a. No signs of injury from falls (e.g., bruises, abrasions, bumps)

    b. No reported episodes of falls with injury

  3. Skin and mucous membranes intact

    a. Absence of cracks, fissures, or ulcers

    b. Mouth and oral mucosa moist

  4. Verbalizes adequate knowledge of condition as well as therapeutic and preventive measures

    a. Verbalizes understanding of risk factors and preventive measures

    b. Verbalizes understanding of followup care

▶ *Practice to Pass*

A young mother phones the clinic and reports that her 8-month-old infant awakened about 6 hours ago with fever, vomiting, and diarrhea. She has taken him off food and formula and has been giving him plain water to drink. What advice should you give her and why?

III. Fluid Volume Excess (FVE)

A. Etiology and pathophysiology

1. Isotonic fluid excess (hypervolemia and edema)

   a. Fluid and solute (primarily sodium) are gained or retained in proportional amounts, leading to an overall gain in extracellular fluid volume without a change in serum osmolality

   b. Excess vascular fluid volume results in the development of hypervolemia

   c. Excess tissue (interstitial) fluid volume results in the development of edema, which can occur throughout the body or can be situated in a specific body tissue or organ

   d. Causes of isotonic FVE

      1) Renal failure leads to decreased excretion of water and sodium

      2) Heart failure leads to stasis of blood in the circulation and venous congestion, as well as decreased renal blood flow leading to decreased renal excretion of fluid and sodium

      3) Excess fluid intake (isotonic IV solutions infused in excess or too rapidly) exceeding the heart and kidneys' ability to compensate results in vascular overload (hypervolemia)

      4) High corticosteroid levels due to therapy, stress response, or disease results in sodium and water retention

      5) High aldosterone levels (stress response, adrenal dysfunction, liver damage, and metabolic problems) result in sodium and water retention

2. Hypotonic fluid excess (water intoxication)

   a. More fluid is gained than solute (primarily sodium), creating FVE and a relative deficit of sodium

   b. Serum osmolality falls, resulting in hypotonic ECF that gets pulled into the cells by osmosis, causing cells to swell; cerebral cells absorb free water more readily than other cells, thus are very sensitive to hypotonic ECF

   c. Causes of hypotonic FVE

      1) Repeated plain water enemas or repeated plain water NG tube or bladder irrigations (the free water from the enemas or irrigations can be drawn into cells, while the expelled water washes out electrolytes)

      2) Overuse of hypotonic IV fluids or infusing hypotonic fluids too rapidly, causing too much free water to be drawn into the cells too quickly

      3) Overzealous plain water intake to replace isotonic fluid and electrolyte losses (water is replaced but not electrolytes, especially sodium)

      4) In young children and infants, a common cause is ingestion of inappropriately prepared formula and/or excess water

         a) Parents who run low on formula or can't afford to buy enough may mix it half strength, which provides excess free water to infants

b) Using a water bottle frequently as a pacifier to calm infants may result in excess ingestion of water

5) SIADH, the excess production or release of ADH, causes kidneys to retain large amounts of water without sodium

a) This creates hypotonic extracellular fluid, which is drawn into cells by osmosis; urine is highly concentrated and urine volume is low

b) Stress, surgery, anesthesia, opioid analgesics, pain, and tumors of the lung and brain are associated with increased ADH release

6) Psychogenic polydipsia is the compulsive drinking of excess amounts of water associated with certain psychiatric disorders, such as acute schizophrenia

7) Severe or prolonged isotonic fluid volume excess in a person with a healthy heart and kidneys is usually compensated through increasing urinary output; clients who have existing disease states (heart failure, renal failure, diabetes) will have difficulty handling excess fluid administration

B. Mechanisms of edema formation

1. Increased capillary hydrostatic pressure disrupts the normal filtration of fluid into and out of capillaries (refer back to Figure 1-4)

   a. The increased pushing pressure inside the capillary forces more fluid out of the arterial end of the capillary and draws less fluid back into the venous end of the capillary, resulting in excess fluid accumulation (edema) in the tissues

   b. Hypertension and vascular fluid volume overload (hypervolemia) are causes of edema

2. Decreased capillary oncotic pressure also disrupts the normal movement of fluid into and out of capillaries

   a. Weaker pulling pressure within the capillary allows more fluid to be pushed out of the arterial end of the capillary and draws less fluid back into the venous end of the capillary, resulting in excess fluid accumulation (edema) in the tissues

   b. Causes of low capillary oncotic pressure

      1) Injury or inflammation (e.g., trauma, burns, sepsis, bacterial infections, allergic reactions, cancer, intestinal obstruction), which increases capillary permeability, allowing fluid and proteins to leak from vessels

      2) Malnutrition or liver dysfunction (e.g., starvation, cirrhosis, chronic alcoholism) prevents the liver from producing albumin, decreasing capillary oncotic pressure (which normally helps keep adequate fluid inside vessels)

3. Lymphatic obstruction or surgical removal of lymph nodes impairs lymph drainage and the normal flow of lymph fluid from body tissues to the venous system, creating local edema in the area distal to the obstruction or node removal

4. Sodium excess (e.g., due to renal failure, decreased renal perfusion, excess aldosterone, or excess corticosteroids) causes water retention that elevates blood pressure, increasing hydrostatic pressure within capillaries; this forces more fluid into tissues, resulting in edema

C. Assessment

1. Clinical manifestations of FVE

   a. Peripheral edema

   1) Edema tends to follow gravity; thus it is often seen in the legs, ankles, feet, and hands of ambulatory clients and on the sacrum and back of clients confined to bed

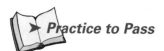

Practice to Pass

A young mother who comes to the clinic with her 2-month-old infant for a well-baby visit tells the nurse that she has been mixing the formula half-strength because it is so expensive. What fluid imbalance does this predispose the infant to develop? Why? How should the nurse respond to the mother?

   2) Edema can develop from local obstruction of veins, as when legs and feet swell after sitting for long periods; this usually resolves with walking and/or leg elevation

   3) Edema that is present in the legs and feet even after elevating them for a period of time (e.g., upon awakening in the morning) and in the face as puffiness, especially around the eyes (periorbital edema and puffy eyelids), is more indicative of generalized edema related to fluid overload associated with a heart or kidney problem

   4) Edematous skin is often tight and shiny due to decreased circulation in swollen tissue

   5) Edema severity can be estimated on a scale from 1+ (minimal) to 4+ (severe)

   6) Pitting edema occurs when a finger pressed into the edematous area leaves an imprint that does not resolve immediately when the finger is removed

   b. Tense or bulging fontanels in children under 18 months old

   c. High central venous pressure with venous engorgement

   1) Distended neck veins when head of bed is elevated to 45 degrees or higher (normally veins are flat due the effect of gravity)

   2) Delayed or absent hand vein emptying when hand is raised above heart (normally 3 to 5 seconds); engorged veins are evident

   3) Gallop heart rhythm in adults (S_3 heart sound) is evident when ventricles become overdistended due to venous congestion

   4) Hepatomegaly and splenomegaly are signs of venous congestion

   d. Pulmonary edema because of increasing extravascular fluid retention

   1) Tachypnea and dyspnea, irritated cough (often early sign of fluid in alveoli)

   2) Hacking cough that eventually becomes moist and productive (clear to white sputum); a late sign of fluid in the alveoli and larger airways

   3) Labored breathing (seen as intercostal and substernal retractions, nasal flaring, and expiratory grunting in infants)

4) Wet lung sounds (moist crackles) on auscultation (first appear in bases bilaterally and progress upward as the lung water increases)

5) Decreased O_2 saturation due to inadequate or mismatched ventilation and perfusion as a result of FVE

6) Wet lung sounds (moist crackles) on auscultation

7) Cyanosis (a late sign of hypoxemia)

8) Note: acute pulmonary edema is a life-threatening medical emergency caused by large amounts of fluid pooling in the alveoli and airways; respiratory signs and symptoms will be severe and immediate action is required to prevent death

e. Vital signs (reflect normal or increased cardiac output)

1) Normal heart rate

2) Full or bounding peripheral pulses

3) Warm extremities

4) Brisk capillary refill

f. Third space fluid accumulations: may be present as fluid is forced from vessels into spaces that normally do not contain much fluid (ascites, pleural effusion, pericardial effusion)

g. Acute, rapid weight gain

h. Urine output and concentration

1) In the client with functioning heart and kidneys, the body will maintain homeostasis by increasing urine output, leading to polyuria

2) Decreased urine output associated with fluid retention is seen in clients with impaired cardiac or renal function

i. A weight gain of 3 pounds or more can occur over 2 to 5 days

1) 2% body weight gain = mild fluid excess

2) 5% body weight gain = moderate fluid excess

3) 8% body weight gain = severe fluid excess

2. Diagnostic and laboratory findings

a. HCT and BUN are decreased due to **hemodilution** (plasma has more water than normal, thus is more dilute); the percentage of RBCs and urea particles per liter of plasma is lower than normal in dilute plasma even though the actual number of cells and particles has not dropped; once extra fluid is removed, HCT and BUN return to normal

b. In hypotonic fluid volume excess (water intoxication):

1) Serum osmolality (concentration) is low (< 275 mOsm/kg)

2) Serum sodium is very low (< 125 mEq/L)

c. Chest X-ray may show pleural effusions

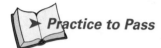

A 62-year-old client is receiving IV therapy of $D_5\frac{1}{2}NS$ at 150 mL/hour following gallbladder surgery. The client has a past medical history of mild hypertension and coronary artery disease. The client awakens at 1 A.M. complaining of trouble breathing and is sitting straight up in bed coughing up small amounts of clear mucus. What is the priority nursing action and why? What followup actions are needed and why?

    d. Arterial blood gases

        1) Low pO_2 indicates hypoxemia, which usually occurs before pCO_2 is affected (carbon dioxide diffuses more easily than oxygen)

        2) Low pCO_2 (hyperventilation) is often present in early phases of compensation, but will be low (hypoventilation) in later phases when compensation is failing

        3) As pulmonary edema progresses to hypoventilation and respiratory failure, respiratory acidosis causes the pH to drop

  3. Identification of risk factors predisposing to fluid volume excess

    a. Age

        1) Due to decreased heart and kidney function elderly clients are not able to compensate as easily for fluid volume excess

        2) Infants (up to age 2 years) have immature kidneys and cannot dilute urine well to eliminate excess fluid as efficiently as adults

        3) Children 2 to 12 years of age have less stable regulatory responses to fluid imbalances

    b. Acute illness

        1) Surgery stimulates the stress response, which increases release of cortisol, ADH, and aldosterone, promoting water and sodium retention

        2) Clients with medical problems (acute or preexisting) receiving IV fluids are prone to develop fluid imbalances leading to FVE

    c. Chronic illness

        1) Cardiovascular disease reduces the pumping strength of the heart and results in diminished blood flow to the kidneys, which causes sodium and water retention, leading to fluid volume excess

        2) Renal disease can lead to the abnormal retention of water, sodium, potassium, and other electrolytes

    d. Medications: long-term glucocorticoid therapy predisposes to sodium and fluid retention

D. Priority nursing diagnoses

  1. Fluid volume excess related to excessive fluid or sodium intake and/or retention

  2. Risk for pulmonary edema related to hypervolemia

  3. Altered comfort related to signs and symptoms of fluid excess

  4. Risk for impaired skin integrity related to edema

  5. Knowledge deficit related to risk factors and therapeutic interventions

E. Therapeutic management

  1. Restrict fluid intake

    a. Fluid intake by all routes my may be limited, sometimes as low as 1,000 to 1,500 mL per 24-hour period

1) Sodium-restricted diets help decrease water retention

2) Level of sodium restriction commonly varies from mild (4 to 5 g sodium per day) to moderate (2 g per day) to enhance compliance

3) Stricter (0.5 g sodium per day) restrictions are reserved for very severe conditions

b. IV access is often maintained with a "saline lock" device to avoid administering any excess IV fluids

2. Promote excretion

a. Diuretics promote the excretion of water through urine

1) Loop diuretics are commonly used (e.g., furosemide, [Lasix])

2) Potassium-sparing diuretics may also be used (e.g., spironolactone [Aldactone])

3) Thiazide diuretics may also be used (e.g., thiazide [Diuril])

b. Medications such as digoxin (Lanoxin), low-dose beta blocking agents, and angiotensin converting enzyme (ACE) inhibitors used to treat congestive heart failure may be beneficial in promoting urinary excretion by improving cardiac efficiency

c. Protein intake may be increased in clients who are malnourished and have low serum proteins to increase capillary oncotic pressure, thus pulling fluid out of tissues into vessels where it can be eliminated by the kidneys

3. Monitoring during therapy

a. Monitor respiratory status, looking for signs of worsening gas exchange, such as increased respiratory effort, falling O_2 saturation (SaO_2), and lung crackles

b. Note: pulse oximetry values below 95% are considered low in people with healthy lungs; trend the ABG results, remaining alert for decreasing PaO_2 and increasing $PaCO_2$

c. Monitor for improving or worsening venous engorgement

d. Monitor fluid intake and output carefully, looking for improved urine output in response to therapy

e. Monitor daily weights (same time, same clothing, same scale) looking for acute weight gain

f. Assess for peripheral edema, especially in the mornings before the client arises or after client has been reclining with feet elevated for some time (to differentiate dependent, or stasis, edema from the more generalized edema related to heart, kidney, or liver problems)

g. Observe for signs of developing or worsening water intoxication (hypotonic fluid volume excess), often associated with neurological changes

h. Monitor for overcorrection, in which signs of fluid volume deficit begin to appear

i. Monitor lab values for normalizing BUN, HCT, serum sodium, and arterial blood gases; watch for electrolyte imbalances (low sodium, low or high potassium) due to drug therapy

F. Planning and implementation

1. Monitor assessment parameters, observe response to therapy, note any sign of improvement, and watch for signs of hypovolemia due to overcorrection

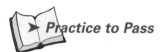

2. Restrict fluids as ordered

   a. Teach clients to measure items that are liquid at room temperature and include them in fluid intake totals

   b. Involve client in dividing fluid allowances over 24-hour period; plan for more fluids during times for meals and taking oral medications

   c. Use an infusion pump to help prevent inadvertent administration of excess fluid

   d. Provide mouth care and use measures to moisten mouth regularly to decrease thirst; ice chips can be soothing, but count as fluid intake (1 cup ice chips = ½ cup water), so calculate them into the allowed fluid intake

   e. Encourage cold fluids, which tend to decrease thirst better than warm ones; avoid or limit sweet or salty foods to minimize thirst

3. Measure fluid losses/gains

   a. Measure intake and output, noting color and concentration of urine

   b. Weigh daily and monitor patterns of weight loss/gain (remember: a change of 2.2 lbs [1 Kg] is equivalent to a 1 L water loss or gain)

4. Institute measures to prevent fluid volume excess

   a. Irrigate NG tube and bladder with normal saline rather than plain water

   b. Avoid repeated plain tap water enemas

   c. Mix infant formula according to package directions; do not use a water bottle as a pacifier for infants

5. Remain alert for acute pulmonary edema, an emergency requiring prompt action

   a. Anxious client with labored breathing

   b. Moist crackles on auscultation, bilaterally from bases into upper lung fields

   c. Productive cough with frothy, clear sputum

   d. SaO_2 below 95%; blood gases likely reveal low pO_2 (hypoxia); if impending respiratory failure, high pCO_2 (hypercarbia and respiratory acidosis)

   e. Prompt action: stop or limit any ongoing fluid intake; assess client (e.g., vital signs, lung sounds, pulse oximetry, mental status); implement actions to increase gas exchange (e.g., high Fowler's position, supplemental oxygen); and notify physician as soon as possible

G. Medication therapy

1. Diuretic therapy

   a. Loop diuretics and thiazide diuretics cause potassium and sodium loss while potassium sparing diuretics can cause hyperkalemia

   b. Monitor electrolytes during diuretic therapy

Practice to Pass

A 2-month-old infant is being treated for gastroenteritis and dehydration. The infant has received normal saline boluses and has just been switched to $D_5\frac{1}{4}NS$ at 40 mL/hour. What monitoring and nursing measures should be implemented at this time? Why?

      c. Give diuretics in the morning to avoid sleep disruption; if ordered BID, administer second dose by midafternoon

  2. Treat underlying disease processes that place client at risk for developing FVE, such as congestive heart failure, or treatment with low-dose beta-blocking agents and/or ACE inhibitors

  3. Evaluate client for potential fluid and electrolyte imbalances as a consequence of corrective therapy

H. Client education

  1. Teach clients risk factors for development of FVE

  2. Teach adults to weigh themselves daily and report a gain of more than 2 pounds per week

  3. Teach clients with peripheral edema to elevate extremities and change position frequently

  4. Dietary education

      a. Teach clients about sodium-restricted diet, including rationale, limitations, and dietary choices (see Table 1-1)

         1) Suggest use of alternative seasonings, such as natural sodium-free herbs and spices

         2) Clients taking potassium-sparing diuretics and/or ACE inhibitors (which cause potassium retention) should not use salt substitutes because most contain potassium

      b. Teach clients to avoid adding salt while cooking or at the table

      c. Teach clients to assess sodium content by reading food/OTC drug labels

      d. Consult dietitian for more detailed dietary information regarding sodium and fluid restrictions

Table 1-1	High Sodium Foods	Low Sodium Foods
Sodium Restricted Diets	Canned, processed, and pickled foods are *higher* in sodium content. • Foods prepared in brine (e.g., pickles, olives, sauerkraut) • Salty or smoked meats (e.g., bologna, hotdogs, ham, lunch meats, sausage) • Salty or smoked fish (e.g.,anchovies, herring, sardines, smoked salmon) • Salty snacks (e.g., potato chips, popcorn, nuts, crackers, pretzels) • Salty seasonings (e.g., seasoned salts, soy sauce, Worcestershire sauce, barbecue sauces) • Processed cheeses • Canned and instant soups • Canned vegetables and fruits	Fresh foods are *lower* in sodium content. • Fresh meat and fish • "No added salt" snack items • Sodium-free spices and flavorings • Soups made with fresh items • Fresh fruits and vegetables • Low-sodium canned products

I. Evaluation

NCLEX!

1. The client will regain fluid volume balance

   a. Peripheral edema is resolved; in the pediatric client fontanels are soft

   b. Unlabored breathing; lungs clear to auscultation; chest x-ray shows no infiltrates or effusion

   c. Vital signs return to baseline

   d. Level of consciousness and orientation return to baseline

   e. HCT, BUN, serum osmolality, and serum electrolytes return to client's baseline

   f. Weight returns to baseline

2. Resolution of underlying cause of fluid volume excess

3. Client/family verbalize understanding of risk factors, prevention, and followup care for fluid volume excess

---

Case Study

A 9-month-old infant enters the Emergency Department. The mother reports fever, vomiting, and diarrhea for the past two days. You are the nurse caring for them.

❶ What questions will you ask the mother about the child initially?

❷ What assessment findings will alert you to a serious fluid imbalance?

❸ If intravenous fluids are ordered, what are the priorities of care and monitoring during the intravenous infusion?

❹ What rehydration instructions should be given to the mother in preparation for discharge?

❺ When the mother asks about the BRAT diet her friends have told her to follow until the diarrhea is gone, how would you respond?

For suggested responses, see page 230.

Posttest

1. A 78-year-old client is admitted with fluid volume deficit and urinary tract infection. After rapid IV infusion of 750 mL NS, the client begins to cough and asks for the head of the bed to be raised to ease breathing. The nurse assesses jugular vein distention (JVD) and increased respiratory rate. What should the nurse suspect is happening to this client?

   (1) Fluid volume deficit is worsening
   (2) Hypervolemia is developing
   (3) Hypotonic water intoxication is beginning
   (4) Ascites is causing respiratory compromise

2 The nurse is helping a client who was recently placed on a low-sodium diet to choose foods for lunch. Which lunch menu would be best for this client?

(1) Grilled chicken sandwich on white bread, apple, salad, and iced tea
(2) Bologna sandwich on wheat bread, canned fruit cocktail, salad, and a soda
(3) Canned ham and bean soup, fresh fruit salad, pickles, and a diet soda
(4) Fast food cheeseburger, grapes, fresh pineapple, and tomato juice

3 A 28-year-old client is admitted with severe bleeding from a fractured femur. Which intravenous fluid does the nurse anticipate using as the most appropriate to replace potential fluid losses?

(1) Normal saline
(2) 3% saline
(3) 5% dextrose in water
(4) 5% dextrose in 0.225 saline

4 A 54-year-old client with liver failure due to cirrhosis comes to the clinic complaining of a swollen abdomen and dizziness upon standing. The client is pale with weak radial pulses, delayed hand vein filling, and distended abdomen. Which nursing diagnosis is most appropriate?

(1) Fluid volume excess related to third space fluid shifts
(2) Fluid volume deficit related to third space fluid shifts
(3) Fluid volume excess related to hormonal disturbances
(4) Fluid volume deficit related to hormonal disturbances

5 The nurse making rounds discovers D_5W infusing at 75 mL/hour. The order for the client states, "NS at 75 mL/hour." What is the best action for the nurse to take first?

(1) Complete the infusion of D_5W to avoid waste and then ensure the next bag is correct.
(2) Slow the infusion and contact the physician for current orders.
(3) Immediately change the infusion to the ordered solution.
(4) Complete an unusual occurrence report and submit it to the supervisor.

6 A 17-year-old client who sustained a head injury in a motorcycle collision two days ago is responsive only to pain. Which intravenous fluid order would the nurse question because it could increase the risk of complications?

(1) Ringer's solution
(2) 5% dextrose in water
(3) Normal saline
(4) Lactated Ringer's solution

7 A young mother brings her 10-month-old baby into the clinic. The mother is extremely distressed about the infant's 3-day history of severe diarrhea and development of sunken fontanels. The mother fears the infant may develop "brain damage." Which response by the nurse would be most appropriate at this time?

(1) "It is temporary. That happens when babies lose fluid, but it will return to normal without harm."
(2) "Don't worry. That happens because of hypovolemia and extracellular fluid loss."
(3) "That's nothing. We see it all the time in kids who have lost a lot of fluid."
(4) "When did you notice this? Why didn't you bring the baby in sooner?"

8 Which of the following findings would indicate to the nurse that fluid volume balance in a client with fluid volume excess has not yet been achieved?

(1) S_3 heart sounds and moist lung crackles resolving
(2) Return to coherent conversation and appropriate behavior
(3) Urine output increasing and specific gravity decreasing
(4) Skin tenting decreasing and conjunctiva of eyes moist

9   During intershift report, the nurse is told that a
    client who has suffered a stroke has also developed
    diabetes insipidus. The nurse concludes this client
    is now at risk for:

(1) Severe fluid volume deficit due to excess urine
     output.
(2) Severe fluid volume excess due to inadequate urine
     output.
(3) Hyperglycemia due to poor insulin production.
(4) Hypoglycemia due to excess insulin production.

10 A father telephones the clinic nurse asking what he
    should do for his 3-year-old son who developed
    fever, vomiting, and diarrhea today. What dietary
    advice would be best?

(1) "Have him drink as much water as you can get him to
     drink."
(2) "Give him small sips of commercial oral rehydration
     fluids frequently."
(3) "Provide frequent sips of fruit juice and commercial
     sports drinks."
(4) "Have him eat only bananas, rice, applesauce, and
     toast (BRAT diet)."

See pages 35–36 for Answers and Rationales.

Answers and Rationales

Pretest

1   **Answer: 1** *Rationale:* Infants and the elderly can't
    compensate as well for fluid losses. Clients with NG
    suction (loss of fluid and electrolytes in fairly propor-
    tional amounts) are at greater risk for fluid volume
    deficit. The elderly client with NG suction has both
    risk factors, while the child's age is the only risk fac-
    tor. The client taking glucocorticoids is predisposed
    to sodium and fluid retention rather than fluid loss.
    The 30-year-old jogger is a young adult in a moderate
    climate, which lowers the risk from exertion alone.
    Cognitive Level: Analysis
    Nursing Process: Analysis; *Test Plan:* PHYS

2   **Answer: 4** *Rationale:* With aging, the thirst mecha-
    nism becomes less effective. Significant fluid can be
    lost before thirst is triggered, so the elderly should not
    rely solely on thirst to indicate when they need to
    drink fluids. All of the other choices should be in-
    cluded in this type of education program.
    Cognitive Level: Application
    Nursing Process: Implementation; *Test Plan:* HPM

3   **Answer: 3** *Rationale:* The client has symptoms of
    fluid volume deficit and hypovolemia. The presence
    of postural hypotension when rising from a lying po-
    sition indicates the presence of significant
    hypovolemia. The other vital signs are important but
    do not directly reflect circulating fluid volume.
    Cognitive Level: Analysis
    Nursing Process: Assessment; *Test Plan:* PHYS

4   **Answer: 1** *Rationale:* An infusion pump should be
    used to control IV fluid rates on infants receiving IV
    fluids to avoid accidental fluid overload. Infusing by
    gravity and monitoring only every hour does not pro-
    tect from this risk, since the bolus may be completed
    in less than half an hour. Placing responsibility for
    monitoring IV infusions on the mother is not ethical,
    safe, or legally advisable.
    Cognitive Level: Analysis
    Nursing Process: Implementation; *Test Plan:* SECE

5   **Answer: 3** *Rationale:* Normal saline is an isotonic
    fluid that prevents fluid shifts into or out of the GI
    tract. Option 1 (3% saline) is hypertonic and could
    pull water from the GI tract, resulting in water loss.
    D_5W and plain water are hypotonic and could be
    pulled into GI tissue as well as wash electrolytes out
    of the GI tract, resulting in water intoxication.
    Cognitive Level: Application
    Nursing Process: Implementation; *Test Plan:* SECE

6   **Answer: 4** *Rationale:* A moist cough, dyspnea, and
    falling pulse oximetry reading in a client with a his-
    tory of heart disease are signs of developing pul-
    monary edema secondary to fluid volume overload.
    The first action should be to reduce IV fluid intake to
    prevent more fluid from accumulating in the lungs,
    then further assessment can be done, emergency ac-
    tions taken, and the physician contacted.
    Cognitive Level: Analysis
    Nursing Process: Implementation; *Test Plan:* SECE

7   **Answer: 2** *Rationale:* Option 2 provides accurate
    information in simple terms without unduly alarming

the client. Option 4 is technically correct but is stated in an abrupt and alarming manner. Option 1 offers no explanation to facilitate understanding. Option 3 assigns the client blame for the current condition without providing a clear explanation for the fluid restriction.
Cognitive Level: Application
Nursing Process: Implementation; *Test Plan:* PSYC

8 **Answer: 1** *Rationale:* An excess response to diuretic therapy results in an excess loss of water and electrolytes in the urine, leaving the blood hemoconcentrated and causes a high BUN and HCT. The water loss results in an acute weight loss. Weight gain indicates ineffective response to diuretic therapy.
Cognitive Level: Analysis
Nursing Process: Assessment; *Test Plan:* PHYS

9 **Answer: 4** *Rationale:* ¼ NS (0.225% saline) is a hypotonic solution that provides free water to the cells. Cerebral cells are especially sensitive to fluid gains from hypotonic fluids. If infused too rapidly, the cerebral cells will be the first to gain fluid too quickly, resulting in neurological changes. Monitoring the client for urine output, edema, and oral cavity dryness are important, but this reflects a response to IV therapy rather than detection of a complication.
Cognitive Level: Analysis
Nursing Process: Assessment; *Test Plan:* PHYS

10 **Answer: 1** *Rationale:* 3% saline is very hypertonic and, if infused too rapidly, will increase serum sodium and osmolality, causing high volumes of water to be pulled into vessels from cells. This results in cellular dehydration and vascular volume overload. Serum sodium levels, neurological status, and lung function should be closely monitored. Although daily weights are important, they do not provide information leading to early detection of complications of therapy. Vital signs, serum glucose levels, urine specific gravity, oxygen saturation, and peripheral edema provide later indications of complications of therapy.
Cognitive Level: Analysis
Nursing Process: Evaluation; *Test Plan:* SECE

Posttest

1 **Answer: 2** *Rationale:* The elderly have less cardiac and renal reserve to compensate for acute fluid imbalances, and thus are more susceptible to overcorrection when being treated for them. JVD, tachypnea, cough, and dyspnea indicate that this client has received too much IV fluid at too rapid a rate. Elderly clients cannot tolerate rapid rehydration due to decreased cardiac and renal function.
Cognitive Level: Analysis
Nursing Process: Analysis; *Test Plan:* PHYS

2 **Answer: 1** *Rationale:* Processed and canned foods (bologna, soup, tomato juice), sodas, and pickled foods are high in sodium. Fresh foods (grilled chicken, fruit, vegetables) are lower in sodium.
Cognitive Level: Application
Nursing Process: Implementation; *Test Plan:* PHYS

3 **Answer: 1** *Rationale:* Acute bleeding results in isotonic fluid loss and can quickly lead to shock and vascular collapse. The priority is to expand vascular volume and restore circulation using isotonic intravenous fluid. Hypertonic (3% saline) and hypotonic solutions (D_5W, $D_5¼NS$) are not indicated.
Cognitive Level: Application
Nursing Process: Implementation; *Test Plan:* SECE

4 **Answer: 2** *Rationale:* The failing liver does not make enough albumin to keep capillary oncotic pressure at normal levels, thus excess fluid is lost from vessels into the peritoneum, causing ascites and vascular fluid volume deficit. Orthostatic hypotension, weak peripheral pulses, and delayed hand vein filling are all signs of low circulating fluid volume.
Cognitive Level: Analysis
Nursing Process: Analysis; *Test Plan:* PHYS

5 **Answer: 3** *Rationale:* The nurse's immediate responsibility is to ensure compliance with currently ordered intravenous fluids. Although an unusual occurrence report should be filed, it is not the first priority.
Cognitive Level: Analysis
Nursing Process: Implementation; *Test Plan:* SECE

6 **Answer: 2** *Rationale:* 5% dextrose in water (D_5W) has a hypotonic effect once dextrose is metabolized, providing free water to cells, which would worsen this client's cerebral edema. The other fluids listed are isotonic and would primarily remain in the extracellular spaces.
Cognitive Level: Analysis
Nursing Process: Implementation; *Test Plan:* PHYS

7 **Answer: 1** *Rationale:* The mother needs a simple explanation and reassurance that the baby will return to normal. Sunken fontanels are a sign of fluid volume deficit, but this finding resolves when fluid balance is restored. Option 2 is accurate, but is too technical and offers no reassurance. The others offer no reassurance, and option 4 is accusatory.
Cognitive Level: Application
Nursing Process: Implementation; *Test Plan:* PSYC

8 **Answer: 1** *Rationale:* S_3 heart sounds and moist lung crackles are signs associated with fluid overload, not deficit. Option 2 indicates resolution. Options 3 and 4 show resolving signs of fluid volume deficit and dehydration.
Cognitive Level: Analysis
Nursing Process: Evaluation; *Test Plan:* PHYS

9 **Answer: 1** *Rationale:* Diabetes insipidus is a condition caused by insufficient production and/or release of ADH. Inadequate ADH leads to increased excretion of dilute urine. Changes in glucose levels and insulin production are associated with diabetes mellitus.
Cognitive Level: Analysis
Nursing Process: Analysis; *Test Plan:* PHYS

10 **Answer: 2** *Rationale:* Commercial oral rehydration fluids, such as Pedialyte or Rehydralyte, are balanced water, carbohydrate, and electrolyte solutions that replace both fluids and electrolytes lost in diarrhea. They also do not have a high osmolality, caffeine, or excess sodium, which can all worsen diarrhea and fluid loss. Replacing diarrhea losses with only water could lead to electrolyte imbalances. Fruit juice and sports drinks are too high in sugar, which can worsen diarrhea and fluid loss. Solid foods, including the BRAT diet, are not appropriate while the client is vomiting.
Cognitive Level: Application
Nursing Process: Implementation; *Test Plan:* PHYS

References

Gulanick, M., Klopp, A., Lalanes, S., Gradishar, D., & Puzas, M. (1998). *Nursing care plans: Nursing diagnosis and intervention* (4th ed.). St. Louis: Mosby, pp. 84–85.

Haas, L. (2000). Nursing management of endocrine problems. In S. Lewis, M. Heitkemper, & S. Dirksen (Eds.), *Medical-surgical nursing: Assessment and management of clinical problems* (5th ed.). St. Louis: Mosby, pp. 1406–1448.

Horne, M. & Bond, E. (2000). Nursing management of fluid, electrolyte, and acid-base imbalances. In S. Lewis, M. Heitkemper, & S. Dirksen (Eds.), *Medical-surgical nursing: Assessment and management of clinical problems* (5th ed.). St. Louis: Mosby, pp. 323–351.

House-Fancher, M. & Martinez, L. (2000). Nursing management of congestive heart failure and cardiac surgery. In S. Lewis, M. Heitkemper, & S. Dirksen (Eds.), *Medical-surgical nursing: Assessment and management of clinical problems* (5th ed.). St. Louis: Mosby, pp. 887–917.

Huether, S. E. (1998). The cellular environment: Fluids, electrolytes, acids and bases. In K. McCance & S. Huether (Eds.), *Pathophysiology: The biological basis for disease in adults and children*. St. Louis: Mosby, pp. 82–113.

Koran, Z. & Newberry, L. (1998). Vascular access and fluid replacement. In L. Newberry (Ed.), *Sheehy's emergency nursing:*

Principles and practice (4th ed.). St. Louis: Mosby, pp. 147–174.

Kozier, B., Erb, G., Berman, A., & Burke, K. (2000). *Fundamentals of nursing: Concepts, process and practice* (6th ed.). Upper Saddle River, NJ: Prentice-Hall, Inc.

LeMone, P. & Burke, K. (2000). *Medical surgical nursing: Critical thinking in client care* (2nd ed.). Upper Saddle River, NJ: Prentice-Hall, Inc.

Monahan, F. D. & Neighbors, M. (1998). *Medical-surgical nursing: Foundations for clinical practice* (2nd ed.). Philadelphia: W. B. Saunders, pp. 82–83.

Potter, P. & Perry, A. (2001). Fluid, electrolytes, and acid-base balances. In P. Potter & A. Perry (Eds.), *Fundamentals of nursing* (5th ed). St. Louis: Mosby, pp. 1191–1249.

White, B. (2001). Clients with fluid imbalances: Promoting positive outcomes. In J. Black, J. Hawks, & A. Keene (Eds.), *Medical surgical nursing: Clinical management for positive outcomes* (6th ed.). Philadelphia: W. B. Saunders, pp. 215–231.

Wong, D., Hockenberry-Eaton, M., Wilson, D., Winkelstein, M., Ahmann, E., & DiVito-Thomas, P. (1999). *Whaley & Wong's nursing care of infants and children* (6th ed.). St. Louis: Mosby, pp. 1290–1291, 1301–1302, 1321–1322.

Sodium Balance and Imbalances

Ann Putnam Johnson, EdD, RN

CHAPTER OUTLINE

OBJECTIVES

▋ Review basic functions of sodium in the body.

▋ Discuss the pathophysiology and etiology of sodium imbalances.

▋ Discuss specific assessment findings in sodium imbalances.

▋ Identify priority nursing diagnoses for a client experiencing a sodium imbalance.

▋ Discuss therapeutic management of sodium imbalances.

▋ Discuss nursing management of a client who is experiencing a sodium imbalance.

[Media Link]

Use the CD-ROM enclosed with this text, or log onto the address given to access the free, interactive Companion Website created for this series. The CD-ROM and Companion Website accompanying this book offer additional practice opportunities and information—NCLEX Review, Case Studies, Glossary, In Depth with NCLEX, and more.

www.prenhall.com/hogan

REVIEW AT A GLANCE

anion *an ion with a negative charge*

cation *an ion with a positive charge*

cerebral demyelination *an adverse outcome of hyponatremia that causes demyelination of the pons in the brain and leads to dysphagia, delirium, coma, and even death*

chloride *anion found in the ECF that is linked to sodium, bicarbonate, and water in the body and participates in osmotic pressure regulation and acid-base balance*

diabetes insipidus (DI) *endocrine disturbance whereby ADH is either not secreted (central DI) or there is kidney failure (nephrogenic DI) that leads to an*

increased dilute urine, hypernatremia, and thirst

dilutional hyponatremia *a term used to describe hyponatremia where the serum sodium level is diluted by excess fluid*

euvolemia *normal fluid volume in the body*

hypernatremia *serum sodium level above 145 mEq/L*

hyperosmolar *osmotic pressure greater than normal plasma pressure*

hypervolemia *increase in the circulating volume (intravascular fluid)*

hyponatremia *serum sodium level below 135 mEq/L; also called dilutional hyponatremia or water intoxication*

hypovolemia *low circulating blood volume*

syndrome of inappropriate antidiuretic hormone secretion (SIADH) *excessive release of ADH hormone that causes fluid and electrolyte imbalances resulting in fluid retention, increased ECF volume, hyponatremia, and concentrated urine*

water intoxication *another term to describe hyponatremia where the serum sodium level is diluted by excess fluid*

Pretest

1   A client has just finished an hour of strenuous exercise. Which of the following laboratory results would the nurse expect?

(1) Increased hemoglobin
(2) Decreased creatinine
(3) Decreased osmolality
(4) Increased osmolality

2   Which of the following serum electrolyte imbalances would the nurse assess for in a client admitted with a high fever and severe dehydration?

(1) Hypercalcemia and hypophosphatemia
(2) Hypokalemia and hyponatremia
(3) Hypernatremia and hyperchloremia
(4) Hypophosphatemia and hypocalcemia

3   Which of the following clients would be most at risk to develop a sodium imbalance?

(1) An adult client taking corticosteroid therapy
(2) An elderly client who drinks 8 glasses (8 ounces each) of water each day
(3) A diabetic client who is under glycemic control
(4) A teenager who is drinking Gatorade during exercise workouts

4   The nurse is monitoring IV fluid therapy for a client with hyponatremia. The nurse knows that which of the following types of solutions exerts the same osmotic pressure as the fluid on the other side of the cell membrane and thus maintains equilibrium and minimizes fluid shifts?

(1) Hypertonic
(2) Hyperosmolar
(3) Hypotonic
(4) Isotonic

5   Which of the following interventions is not warranted in planning care for a client admitted with hypernatremia?

(1) Monitoring intake and output
(2) Observing for possible increase in temperature
(3) Observing and preparing for possible seizures
(4) Restricting fluids to 1,200 mL per day

6   Which of the following interventions is not warranted in planning care for a client admitted with hyponatremia?

(1) Assessing for symptoms of nausea and malaise
(2) Encouraging the intake of low-sodium liquids
(3) Monitoring neurological status
(4) Restricting tap water intake

7 A 70-year-old client is admitted with nausea, vomiting, and hyponatremia. The nurse would write which of the following in the care plan about weighing this client?

(1) Obtain a physician order to measure daily weight.
(2) Rotate the scales used on a daily basis.
(3) Weigh the client at the same time each day.
(4) Weigh the client without clothing.

8 Lab chemistry results reveal a client's serum sodium is within normal range. Based on this finding, how would the nurse estimate the client's serum (plasma) osmolality?

(1) Less than 136 mOsm/kg
(2) 270 to 290 mOsm/kg
(3) Greater than 408 mOsm/kg
(4) 350 to 544 mOsm/kg

9 A client with abnormal sodium loss is receiving a regular diet. To encourage foods high in sodium the nurse would provide:

(1) An American cheese and ham sandwich.
(2) Chicken salad on lettuce.
(3) Tossed salad with vinegar dressing.
(4) White fish and plain baked potato.

10 Which of the following interventions should be utilized in a client who is experiencing hyponatremia in a hypervolemic state?

(1) Use normal saline IV to correct extracellular fluid deficit.
(2) Restrict additional fluids.
(3) Remove sources of salt excess.
(4) Replace deficit with free water.

See pages 56–57 for Answers and Rationales.

I. Overview of Sodium Regulation

A. Sodium balance and function: major extracellular fluid (ECF) *cation* (positively charged ion), making up about 99% of the body's sodium level; the remaining 1% is in the intracellular fluid (ICF) and is responsible for water balance and determination of plasma osmolality; the movement of *chloride* (major *anion*—negatively charged ion—in the ECF) is also closely associated with the movement of sodium

1. Serum levels

   a. Normal ECF range is 135 to 145 mEq/L; normal intracellular level is 10 mEq/L

   b. Sodium works with chloride in the body to affect electrolyte changes; they may occur at the same time or independently

   c. The effect of serum sodium levels has a profound effect on cellular fluid dynamics

   d. Serum sodium levels are used to monitor electrolyte, water, and acid-base balance in the body

2. Determinant of plasma osmolality

   a. Sodium is the major determinant of plasma osmolality

   b. Osmolality determines the movement of water between the ECF and the ICF; water will move from a lower concentration of solute (hypotonic) to a higher concentration of solute (hypertonic)

   c. Osmolality of the ECF and ICF are roughly equal (isotonic) at 270 to 290 mOsm/kg water

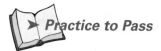

Practice to Pass

What methods can the nurse utilize to get an estimate of a client's plasma osmolality?

   d. Osmotic force helps to move water across the cell membrane to equalize osmotic pressure; water follows sodium, so a sodium imbalance is usually accompanied by an associated imbalance in water

   e. Plasma osmolality can be roughly estimated by doubling the plasma sodium value

   f. Formula used to determine serum osmolality:

$$2 \text{ X serum Na} + \frac{\text{BUN}}{3} + \frac{\text{glucose}}{18} = \text{serum osmolality}$$

   g. Free water (pure water) is available to all body compartments and helps to maintain osmotic balance

3. Functions in the body

   a. Determines plasma osmolality and regulates water balance and distribution

   b. Helps maintain electrolyte balance by exchanging for potassium and attracting chloride

   c. Assists with acid-base balance by combining with bicarbonate and chloride to alter pH

   d. Promotes neuromuscular response and stimulates conduction of nerve impulses and muscle fiber impulse transmission through the sodium-potassium pump

4. System interactions

   a. The primary regulator of sodium concentration is in the kidney (renal tubules)

   b. In addition, the posterior pituitary and adrenal glands of the endocrine system help to regulate sodium levels by hormonal control

     1) Aldosterone (a mineralocorticoid) and cortisone increase serum sodium by increasing tubular reabsorption

     2) Antidiuretic hormone (ADH) increases sodium and water renal tubular reabsorption

   c. The movement and regulation of sodium is also affected by the sodium-potassium pump, which is located in the cell membrane; ATP helps to actively move sodium from the cell into the ECF; the process of diffusion offsets the continual movement

NCLEX!

   d. The cerebral cells are very sensitive to changes in serum sodium levels and exhibit adaptive changes to sodium imbalances

     1) In acute situations where there is a dramatic change in sodium levels, the brain tries to adapt to maintain fluid balance

     2) It is important to recognize both the acuity and severity of onset in managing the care of clients who exhibit severe sodium disturbances

NCLEX!

   e. Since the brain utilizes an adaptive response to sodium imbalances, the restoration of normal sodium levels can be especially problematic; too rapid a correction can cause further fluid and cellular shifting, which can further compromise the client's condition

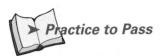

Practice to Pass

Where does the chief regulation of sodium occur?

NCLEX!

f. Sodium imbalances can exist in different volume states: **euvolemia** (normal volume), **hypovolemia** (low volume) and **hypervolemia** (increased volume)

B. Sources of sodium

1. Cellular level

   a. A greater amount of sodium is found in bones than in the ECF, but it is not involved in electrolyte exchange

   b. Sodium is found in all body fluids including blood, bile, gastric and intestinal secretions, pancreatic fluid, and saliva

   c. Sodium is found normally in body perspiration

2. Dietary level

   a. Most Americans eat more sodium (average of 4 to 6 grams on a daily basis) than is needed; safe minimum levels have been established for infants and children, adults, and pregnant and lactating women; 500 mg is the minimally safe recommended sodium intake for an adult client (refer to current findings of the National Research Council-National Academy of Sciences for further information)

   b. The primary dietary source of sodium is found in table salt (NaCl); table salt contains approximately 40% sodium

   c. Sodium is found in a variety of foods in the Western diet such as cheese, eggs, fish, milk, poultry, shellfish, and processed foods

   d. Hidden sources of sodium in the diet are found in processed foods, preservatives, seasonings, and flavorings; in addition, hidden sources of sodium are found in medications; although this may not be considered a dietary form, it still contributes to the overall dietary intake (refer to Box 2-1 for hidden sources of sodium)

II. *Hyponatremia:* serum level of sodium below 135 mEq/L

   A. Etiology and pathophysiology

   1. Cellular level transport

      a. Sodium deficit is usually associated with hypervolemia (increased volume) states and can also be referred to as **dilutional hyponatremia** or **water intoxication** (excess fluid that dilutes serum sodium)

Box 2-1

Hidden Sources of Sodium

The following items should be evaluated for their hidden sodium content:

- Processed foods: contain increased amounts of sodium used in the processing and preserving process
- Medications: such as OTC cold products, cough syrups, antacids, and Alka-Seltzer®
- Canned food items: often contain increased amounts of sodium
- Seasonings: such as MSG (monosodium glutamate)
- Baking products: such as baking powder and baking soda

b. Sodium deficit can also occur in euvolemia (normal volume) and hypovolemia (low volume) states (see Table 2-1 for a summary of this disorder)

c. Water will shift from the ECF (area of lower volume of solutes) to the ICF (area of higher volume of solutes) in an attempt to restore equilibrium, resulting in decreased circulating plasma volume and an increased intracellular fluid volume

d. In response to low sodium levels, the body responds by using the following compensatory mechanisms:

1) Decreased circulating plasma volume leads to activation of pressure receptors in the cardiac atria and thoracic veins in an attempt to increase plasma volume; ADH hormone responds to changes in ECV and plasma osmolality

2) Renal sodium excretion is decreased in order to prevent further sodium depletion

3) Hormonal response of aldosterone helps to promote sodium retention and potassium excretion

e. Cellular response results in cellular swelling/edema (see Figure 2-1a)

f. Cerebral cell response

1) Osmotic force of water in the brain cells leads to the development of cerebral edema in hyponatremic disorders

2) If hyponatremia is severe (acuity and severity of onset), **cerebral demyelination** can occur; this is a serious complication whereby the pons is severely affected, leading to mutism, dysphagia, delirium, coma, and possibly death

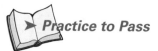

Practice to Pass

What happens to the fluid balance of the body when the sodium level is decreased?

Table 2-1	**Euvolemic State**	**Hypervolemic State**	**Hypovolemic State**
Hyponatremia in Various Fluid Volume States	***Description*** Decrease in fluids in both the intravascular and interstitial space Results in a normal serum osmolality Use of sodium free solutions that dilute the ECF	High glucose states that pull water from cells leading to cellular dehydration as seen in diabetic ketoacidosis (DKA) Fluid loss from ECF greater than solute loss leading to increased serum osmolality	Glucose in isotonic solutions is oxidized leading to cellular swelling Loss of solute from ECF is greater than excess of water resulting in a decreased serum osmolality
	Clinical presentations SIADH, medications, hypothyroidism, psychiatric disorders	Congestive heart failure (CHF), cirrhosis, nephrotic syndrome, and renal failure	GI fluid loss, diuretic therapy, osmotic diuresis, adrenal insufficiency, burns, and sweating, hypotonic dehydration
	Treatment Water restriction, correction of underlying cause, treat SIADH with demeclocycline (unlabeled use), and increase dietary salt intake	Water restriction, treat existing disease states, loop diuretics, and restrict dietary salt intake	NS to correct ECF deficits, increase dietary salt intake; hypertonic saline to raise Na level

Figure 2-1

Cellular dynamics in response to sodium levels. A. Hyponatremia (cells edematous), B. Hypernatremia (cells shrink).

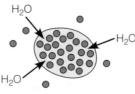

Cell swells as water is pulled in from ECF

A Hyponatremia: Na less than 135 mEq/L

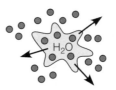

Cell shrinks as water is pulled out into ECF

B Hypernatremia: Na greater than 145 mEq/L

2. Predisposing clinical conditions

   a. Conditions that cause loss of body fluids

      1) Renal losses through excretion, diuretic administration, and renal disease (salt-wasting nephropathy)

      2) Gastrointestinal (GI) losses through vomiting, diarrhea, suctioning, tap water enemas (TWE), GI surgery, and bulimia

      3) Skin losses through perspiration, environmental conditions, burns, and tissue destruction

   b. Conditions that increase extracellular water

      1) Hormone regulation response of ADH and aldosterone, leading to fluid shifting and water gain

      2) Disease states that add to increased volume such as congestive heart failure (CHF), cirrhosis, and nephrotic syndrome

      3) Disease states such as psychiatric disorders that involve compulsive water drinking

      4) Disease states such as tumors, **syndrome of inappropriate antidiuretic hormone secretion** or **SIADH,** and adrenal insufficiency affect hormonal response leading to increased secretion (refer to Box 2-2 for additional information on SIADH)

      5) Hyperglycemic states such as diabetic ketoacidosis (DKA) that cause cellular dehydration

      6) Medications can promote the development of hyponatremia (refer to Table 2-2 for a listing of medications that affect serum sodium levels)

      7) Prolonged or excessive use of hypotonic fluid administration can lead to the development of hyponatremia

   c. Conditions that lead to inadequate dietary intake of sodium

      1) Prolonged use of fluids without sodium replacement by individuals can result in the development of hyponatremia

      2) The presence of anorexia and other eating disorders can lead to inadequate intake of sodium in the diet

Box 2-2 **Syndrome of Inappropriate Antidiuretic Hormone Secretion (SIADH)**	• Increased ADH secretion occurs due to malignancies, CNS disorders, pulmonary disorders, medications, and in postoperative states. • Plasma osmolality is decreased, urine sodium is high, and urine osmolality is increased. • Hyponatremia is present. • Clients present with significant fluid retention, GI symptoms, and neurological symptoms related to fluid retention. • Free water restriction is used to treat this clinical condition. • Demeclocycline (blocks ADH secretion) is used if fluid restriction alone does not correct the disturbance. Lithium also blocks ADH secretion but it is not commonly used as it can reach toxic levels in the body and cause additional complications. • Clients can be placed on a high-salt, high-protein diet to restore normal sodium level and allow the kidneys to excrete more urine (increased solute load). • It is important to identify and correct the underlying cause of the problem. • It is important when restoring normal sodium balance that the correction is done per protocol so as not to cause further complications.

C. Assessment

1. Clinical manifestations

   a. Common signs are related to the shift of water into the cells and to sodium's role in nerve impulse transmission and muscle contraction

      1) Cardiovascular: bounding pulse, tachycardia, hypotension (with decreased ECV), hypertension (with increased ECV)

      2) Integument: pale, dry skin and dry mucous membranes (with decreased ECV), edema and weight gain (with increased ECV)

      3) Renal: thirst, renal failure

      4) Neuromuscular: weakness, headache, confusion, seizures

      5) Gastrointestinal: vomiting, diarrhea

Table 2-2 **Medications That Can Affect Sodium Levels**	**Increase Sodium Levels**	**Decrease Sodium Levels**
	Corticosteroids (Cortisone, Prednisone)	Diuretics
	Hypertonic saline solutions	Lithium
	Sodium bicarbonate, sodium phosphate, and sodium salicylate	Antineoplastic agents* (Cisplatin, Vincristine)
	Antibiotics* (Penicillin Na, Ticarcillin)	Psychotropic medications* (Elavil, Mellaril)
	Amphotericin B	Antidiabetic agents* (Diabenase, Orinase)
	Demeclocycline (Declomycin)	CNS depressants* (Morphine, barbiturates)
	Lactulose	Motrin
	Darvon	Nicotine
		Oxytocin (Pitocin)

*For these medications please refer to a drug textbook for specific names as there are many different types of drugs in each category.

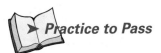

Practice to Pass

The pathophysiologic effects of hyponatremia are most evident in which areas of the body?

b. Common symptoms are related to the water shift from the vascular space into the cells and sodium's role in nerve impulse transmission and muscle contraction

1) Neuromuscular: lethargy, agitation, dizziness

2) Gastrointestinal: abdominal cramps, anorexia, nausea

2. Diagnostic and laboratory findings

   a. Plasma levels and urinary levels

      1) Plasma level less than 135 mEq/L

      2) Change in urine sodium level reflects the cause of the deficit

      3) Urine sodium levels > 20 mEq/L correlate to renal etiology or SIADH

      4) Urine sodium levels < 10 mEq/L correlate with edema etiology (CHF, cirrhosis and nephrotic syndrome)

   b. Associated electrolyte and other levels

      1) Serum osmolality < 270 mOsm/kg

      2) Serum chloride may be decreased

      3) Urine specific gravity < 1.010 (except in SIADH)

      4) Decreased blood urea nitrogen (BUN) and hematocrit (HCT)

   c. Trending of results

      1) Identify primary cause of mechanism for sodium deficit

      2) Confirm compensatory response to sodium loss

      3) Determine client fluid balance status and response to treatment measures

3. Identification of risk factors

   a. Aging and gender variables

      1) Very young and elderly clients are more likely to be prone to sodium deficit

      2) There is an increased risk for development of acute hyponatremia in female clients

   b. Medications

      1) Obtain pertinent client history of medications that can alter sodium levels (refer again to Table 2-2 for a listing of medications that cause sodium deficit)

      2) Treatment measures that include intravenous solutions (such as D_5W), hypotonic fluids, irrigations, and tap water enema (TWE) as part of the therapeutic plan of care can lead to the development of hyponatremia

      3) Clients undergoing operative procedures involving irrigations may develop hyponatremia (such as TURP syndrome and endometrial ablation)

NCLEX!

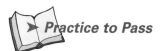

   c. Dietary

   1) Prolonged NPO status

   2) Overcorrection with nonelectrolyte solutions, causing free water accumulation

D. Priority nursing diagnoses: Risk for fluid volume excess, Risk for sensory/perceptual alterations, Risk for injury, Risk for altered oral mucous membranes, Altered mental status, and Risk for impaired skin integrity

E. Therapeutic management: treatment focuses on restoring normal levels, preventing complications, and treating underlying problems

   1. Replacement therapies

   a. Encourage inclusion of high-sodium foods in the diet

   b. Referral to a dietician for assistance in meal planning and including adequate sources of sodium in the diet (refer to Box 2-3 for sodium food sources)

   c. If a client has hyponatremia with normal fluid volume (euvolemic), then use water restriction and treat the underlying cause to correct the deficit

   d. If a client has hyponatremia with hypovolemic volume, treat with normal saline (NS) or Lactated Ringer's (LR) solution to correct ECF deficit

   e. If a client has hyponatremia with hypertonic dehydration, treat with fluid restriction and treat the underlying cause to correct the deficit

   f. If a client requires irrigation as a part of therapy, use of appropriate solutions (isotonic saline) should prevent further fluid shifting and sodium deficit

   g. A client with acute hyponatremia can be treated with 3% hypertonic saline (refer to physician order, pharmacy, and hospital protocols for rate of infusion) and loop diuretics to promote water excretion if indicated by the clinical picture

   h. Loop diuretics, salt and fluid restrictions, and even dialysis may have to be utilized if the clinical picture dictates

   2. Continued monitoring of client

   a. Monitor laboratory results

   b. Keep accurate intake and output records

NCLEX!

NCLEX!

NCLEX!

Box 2-3	The following foods are considered adequate sources of sodium:
Sodium Food Sources	• Processed food products (highest sources of sodium in the diet) • Ham, bacon, and pork products (high sodium levels) • Dill pickles, corned beef, and products that are "pickled" in brine solutions • Potato chips • Anchovies, mackerel, and other saltwater fish products

c. Obtain daily weights

d. Monitor for central nervous system changes such as confusion, lethargy, and seizures and maintain safe environment

e. Monitor and document routes of fluid loss

3. Restoration of balance

a. Depending on acuity and severity of deficit, the client may present as asymptomatic or symptomatic; it is important to look both at the laboratory values and correlate them with the client's overall physical condition in order to maintain sodium and fluid balance

b. If client's sodium deficit is acute and symptomatic, prompt management should be initiated

1) Follow physician order, pharmacy, and hospital protocol for rate of infusion and length of therapy

2) It is critical to raise sodium levels per established protocols as cerebral cell adaptation can cause further complications

3) A target goal of 120 to 125 mEq/L should be aimed for and sodium levels should be raised no more than 25 mEq/L in the first 48 hours with a rate not to exceed 1 to 2 mEq/L/hr

c. It is important to identify and treat the underlying cause in order to prevent reoccurrence of deficit and restore sodium and fluid balance

F. Planning and implementation

1. Monitor pertinent client assessment data for potential effects related to hyponatremia and for response to treatment

a. Monitor for confusion, changes in the level of consciousness, and seizures

b. As the clinical condition progresses, signs and symptoms may become more acute, ranging from anorexia, nausea, and lethargy in the early phase to disorientation, agitation, focal neurological deficits, coma, and seizures in the advanced phase

2. Protect the client from injury and maintain a safe environment if client experiences neurological changes due to hyponatremia

3. Employ dietary interventions to promote normal sodium levels

a. Encourage use of high-sodium foods in the diet

b. Give appropriate amounts of fluids in the diet to prevent dehydration

4. Provide replacement therapy as ordered by physician paying attention to baseline laboratory results, client's response, and therapeutic benefits

a. Keep accurate fluid intake and output records looking at shift and 24-hour totals to determine fluid balance

b. Depending on acuity and severity, hourly monitoring may be indicated

c. Weigh client daily, at same time using same scale and in similar clothing

d. A weight loss of > 0.5 pounds in 24 hours is considered to be due to fluid loss

G. Medication therapy

1. Oral replacement therapy

   a. Salt tablets can be used to correct sodium deficits

   b. There are numerous medications that contain sodium (refer again to Table 2-2 for medications that can affect sodium levels)

   c. Depending on the nature of volume status, diuretic therapy may either be restricted (no thiazide diuretics) or utilized (loop diuretics) to promote fluid loss in order to maintain sodium balance

2. Parenteral replacement therapy

   a. LR or 0.9% sodium chloride (NS) can be used to treat hyponatremia with isotonic dehydration

   b. 3% or 5% hypertonic saline can be used to treat clients with a more severe deficit

3. Dietary therapy

   a. Foods high in sodium include items such as bacon, cheese, and table salt

   b. The use of processed foods and foods containing preservatives adds sodium to the diet

H. Client education

NCLEX!

1. Awareness of predisposing factors

   a. Elderly and very young clients are at risk for hyponatremia due to potential fluid volume disturbances

   b. Teach clients to recognize environmental conditions (heat and humidity) that may increase sodium and fluid loss and to use appropriate oral replacement therapies to prevent further electrolyte depletion

NCLEX!

2. Dietary education

   a. Provide a list of foods that are high in sodium during client education

   b. Collaborate with dietician

3. Teach clients to observe for early signs and symptoms of hyponatremia such as abdominal cramps, muscle weakness, and nausea

4. Teach clients and family members to observe for changes in mental status, especially if the client already has contributory medical conditions such as cardiac, renal, and endocrine problems that might exacerbate hyponatremia

I. Evaluation

1. Serum sodium level returns to a normal range (135–145 mEq/L)

2. Client is alert and oriented to time, place, and person

3. Client is free of any signs or symptoms of hyponatremia

4. Client is euvolemic

5. Vital signs are within normal limits

6. Mucous membranes are moist and intact

7. Client remains free from injury

III. *Hypernatremia:* serum sodium level above 145 mEq/L

    A. Etiology and pathophysiology

        1. Cellular level transport

            a. Sodium excess always exists in a **hyperosmolar** (osmotic pressure greater than normal plasma pressure) state

            b. Sodium excess can exist in hypovolemic, euvolemic, and hypervolemic states (see Table 2-3 for summary of this disorder)

            c. To restore equilibrium between the ECF and the ICF, water will shift from the ICF to the ECF, which results in cellular shrinkage/dehydration (refer back to Figure 2-1b)

            d. Cerebral cells adapt to high sodium levels by shrinking as the osmotic pressure drives fluid out of the cells leading to a decreased brain volume

            e. High serum sodium levels lead to an increase in neurological activity

            f. In response to high sodium levels, the body utilizes the thirst mechanism

        2. Predisposing clinical conditions

            a. Clients who have disturbances in water regulation such as decreased intake, increased insensible loss, or watery diarrhea are prone to develop hypernatremia

            b. Clients who experience water loss due to fever, hyperventilation, diuretic therapy, and burns are prone to develop hypernatremia

            c. Clients who have increased sodium intake either due to dietary intake or infusion of sodium fluids are prone to develop hypernatremia

NCLEX!

Table 2-3	**Euvolemic State**	**Hypervolemic State**	**Hypovolemic State**
Hypernatremia in Various Fluid Volume States	*Description* Decrease in water that leads to elevation of serum sodium levels. Does not present with contracted volume unless there is a severe water loss	Greater gain of sodium in relation to fluids that leads to elevation of serum sodium levels	Greater loss of water than sodium leading to elevation of serum sodium levels
	Clinical presentations Increased fluid loss via skin or lungs (hyperventilation)	Seen with administration of hypertonic saline solutions or $NaHCO_3$, in primary hyperaldosteronism or hypertonic dehydration	Renal losses with osmotic diuresis, insensible loss with sweating and/or fever, GI losses with diarrhea. Young and elderly clients are prone to develop
	Treatment Free water replacement either orally or by fluid-hydrating solutions	Remove sodium source, administer diuretics, and replace water	NS to correct intravascular volume deficit, then hypotonic fluids can be used to restore Na level

Note: All hypernatremic states are hyperosmolar.

    d. Clients who have renal losses or disease/hormonal states such as Cushing's syndrome (increased cortisol production) or **diabetes insipidus** or **DI** (a defect in ADH secretion causing sodium retention and increased secretion of a dilute urine) are prone to develop hypernatremia (refer to Box 2-4 for more information on DI)

    e. Clients who experience near-drowning in salt water are at risk for developing hypernatremia

C. Assessment

    1. Clinical manifestations

        a. Common signs are related to the water shift from the cells (cellular dehydration) into the vascular space and sodium's role in nerve impulse transmission and muscle contraction

            1) Cardiovascular: tachycardia, hypertension, decreased cardiac contractility

            2) Integument: dry and sticky mucous membranes, rough, dry tongue, flushed skin

            3) Renal: thirst, increased urine output

            4) Neuromuscular: twitching, tremor and hyperreflexia, agitation and central nervous system irritability, seizures, coma

            5) Gastrointestinal: watery diarrhea, nausea

        b. Common symptoms are primarily related to the shift of water from the cells into the vascular space and brain cell shrinkage

---

Box 2-4

Diabetes Insipidus (DI)

- DI is characterized by decreased secretion of ADH or failure to respond to ADH secretion due to malignancies, excessive water intake, medications (demeclocycline and lithium), and genetic defects.
- DI can be further classified as central (insufficient production) or nephrogenic (related to decreased renal sensitivity).
- Plasma osmolality is increased, urine osmolality and specific gravity are decreased.
- Hypernatremia is present.
- Clients present with polyuria (increased dilute urine) and polydipsia (increased thirst).
- Treatment for central DI consists of desmopressin acetate (DDAVP) administration.
- Treatment for nephrogenic DI consists of a low-salt diet and thiazide diuretics to increase sodium excretion.
- Monitoring of I & O is critical to clients with this disorder.
- Complications of treatment: therapy can lead to water intoxication so client must be closely monitored by looking at labs/diagnostics and performing frequent physical assessment.
- Continued monitoring of fluid status upon discharge is necessary for clients who experience this type of disorder so as to prevent further recurrences.
- Correction of underlying disorder and recognition of clients at risk in the clinical setting will lead to better client outcomes.

1) Neuromuscular: agitation, hallucinations

2) Gastrointestinal: nausea, thirst

c. Clients whose levels rise slowly may be asymptomatic for some time

2. Diagnostic and laboratory findings

a. Plasma levels and urinary levels

1) Plasma levels greater than 145 mEq/L

2) May see increased urine output

b. Associated electrolyte and other levels

1) Chloride may be elevated

2) Serum osmolality greater than 290 mOsm/kg

3) Urinary specific gravity (SG) greater than 1.015 unless diabetes insipidus is present, leading to dilute urine with SG of less than 1.005

4) Increased BUN and HCT

c. Trending of results

1) Identify primary cause of sodium excess

2) Confirm compensatory response to sodium excess

3) Determine client fluid balance status and response to treatment measures

NCLEX!

3. Identification of risk factors

a. Aging variables

1) Very young clients can be at risk for fluid deprivation due to poor nutritional care or having an activity level that overlooks hydration (so busy playing that they don't eat or drink enough)

2) Elderly clients are at risk due to decreased thirst mechanism and renal concentrating ability

b. Medications

1) Obtain pertinent client history of medications as certain medications are hidden sodium sources and the client may not be aware of this (refer again to Table 2-2 for a listing of medications that can affect sodium levels)

2) OTC medications with high sodium content such as Alka-Seltzer®, cough syrups, and aspirin may contribute to increased sodium levels

3) Treatment measures that include the use of sodium such as sodium bicarbonate administration during a code, use of hypertonic saline solutions, and saline-induced abortions can contribute to increased sodium levels

4) Clients who receive medical treatment with cortisone therapy, loop diuretics, or who experience saltwater ingestion can have increased sodium levels

    c. Dietary

        1) Diet that contains large amount of salt

        2) Use of salt as a flavoring agent in the diet can contribute to increased sodium levels as the diet normally contains adequate salt

D. Priority nursing diagnoses: Risk for injury, Risk for fluid volume deficit, Impaired physical mobility, Risk for sensory/perceptual alterations, Risk for altered mucous membranes

E. Therapeutic management: treatment focuses on restoring normal levels, preventing complications, and treating underlying problems

  1. Decrease sodium intake

    a. Restrict sodium use in the diet; restrictions vary depending on severity of clinical condition and may be set at 3 grams, 2 grams, 1 gram, or 500 mg/day

    b. Adhere to sodium restrictions in treatment plan

    c. Refer client to a dietician to evaluate dietary intake for hidden sodium sources

  2. Promote sodium excretion

    a. If a client has hypernatremia with normal fluid volume (euvolemic), then use water replacement and treat the underlying cause to promote sodium loss

    b. If a client has hypernatremia with hypovolemia, treat with NS initially to correct the intravascular deficit

    c. If a client has hypernatremia with hypervolemia, remove source of sodium excess, administer diuretics, and replace water as needed

  3. Continued monitoring of client

    a. Monitor laboratory results

    b. Keep accurate intake and output records, monitoring for trends

    c. Obtain daily weights at the same time using same equipment and similar clothing in order to accurately trend results

    d. Monitor for central nervous system/neurological changes such as agitation, hallucinations, and seizures and maintain a safe environment

NCLEX!

NCLEX!

  4. Restoration of balance

    a. With hypernatremia, it is important to use a gradual reduction to restore serum sodium levels to normal, as cerebral cells are both adaptive and sensitive to changes in sodium levels

    b. The usual protocol with chronic hypernatremia is to correct 50% of calculated water deficit in the first 12 to 24 hours with the remainder being corrected in 1 to 2 days; follow physician order, and pharmacy and hospital protocols as directed when correcting hypernatremia in the clinical setting

    c. It is important to look at the volume status of the client before and during attempts to restore sodium balance in order to prevent further complications

    d. If the client has hypernatremia as a result of solute excess, then the use of diuretics with water replacement may be warranted

    e. It is important to identify and treat the underlying cause in order to prevent occurrence of excess and to restore sodium and fluid balance

F. Planning and implementation

  1. Monitor pertinent client assessment data for potential effects related to hypernatremia and for response to treatment

    a. Serum sodium levels and plasma osmolality

    b. Urine sodium levels and urine osmolality

    c. Monitor neurological status closely as client is likely to have CNS irritability, possibly leading to seizures

  2. Maintain safe environment as a result of CNS irritability and risk of seizure activity; initiate seizure precautions

  3. Dietary interventions to decrease sodium levels

    a. Place client on a salt restricted diet (refer to Box 2-5)

    b. Refer client to a dietician as needed to assist with dietary measures

  4. Provide therapy as ordered by physician, paying attention to baseline labs, client's response, and therapeutic benefits

  5. Assess intake and output

    a. Keep accurate fluid intake and output records looking at shift and 24-hour totals to determine fluid balance

    b. Depending on acuity and severity, hourly monitoring may be indicated

    c. Weigh client on daily basis using the same equipment and similar clothing

    d. Weight gain can be a consequence of fluid retention from hypernatremia, which could lead to further clinical compromise

NCLEX!

NCLEX!

▶ *Practice to Pass*

In caring for a client with hypernatremia, what should the nurse do to help ensure client safety?

Box 2-5

Sodium-Restricted Diet Instructions

The following interventions should be employed when following a sodium-restricted diet:

- Do not routinely add salt to foods prior to tasting.
- The physician should order the amount of sodium restriction as there can be confusion between following a low-sodium diet and a sodium-restricted diet. A restricted diet can range from a severe restriction (500 mg) to a mild restriction (3,000–4,000 mg).
- Limit or avoid use of bottled or canned sauce products, as they are usually higher in sodium than homemade preparations.
- Use pure herbs, seasonings, and wine in cooking preparation, as many "seasoned" products and cooking wine contain sodium.
- When eating outside the home at restaurants, have food items prepared without salt.
- Eat freshly prepared bakery products; commercially prepared and frozen products contain more sodium due to processing and use of preservative agents.
- Be aware that artificial sweeteners used in soft drinks and other products can contain additional sodium. Limit your intake of such products.
- There are a wide range of "low-sodium" and "sodium-free" products available. Learn to read and interpret nutrition labels so as to make wise food selections.

G. Medication therapy

1. Diuretic therapy

   a. Loop diuretics can be used to treat sodium excess

   b. Thiazide diuretics can be used in the treatment of diabetes insipidus

2. Parenteral administration of fluids

   a. NS to correct intravascular volume deficit

   b. D_5W solution can be used once volume deficit has been restored

3. Dietary restrictions

   a. Limit sodium intake

   b. Use low-sodium foods and fluids

H. Client education

1. Awareness of predisposing factors

   a. Elderly clients are also at risk for hypernatremia due to limited mobility, multiple medication profile, and restricted access to fluids

   b. Teach clients potential signs and symptoms of hypernatremia and have them report problems to their healthcare provider

NCLEX!

2. Dietary education (refer again to Box 2-5)

   a. Teach clients about the daily sodium requirement needed in the diet along with proper fluid management; the majority of individuals ingest a daily intake above the needed RDA

   b. Teach clients about the sodium content of foods and the sources of hidden sodium in the diet

   c. Teach client to follow a low-sodium diet after discharge

   d. Teach client to read all labels for sodium content prior to ingestion

NCLEX!

   e. Teach client to use herbs, lemon juice, spices, and vinegar instead of salt or salt substitutes to season foods

   f. Teach clients not to routinely salt their food prior to tasting

I. Evaluation

1. Serum sodium level returns to normal range (between 135 and 145 mEq/L)

2. Client is free of any signs or symptoms of hypernatremia

3. Client is alert and oriented to time, place, and person

4. Client is euvolemic

5. Vital signs are within normal limits

6. Client remains free from injury

| **Case Study** | A 45-year-old construction company owner was brought from work to the Emergency Department reporting dizziness, nausea, weakness, abdominal cramps, and headache. During the admission assessment, the following information was obtained: |

- Onset of symptoms occurred three days ago but were mild until today when client stated that he "almost fell off a building at work."
- Previously diagnosed with hypertension (HTN) six weeks ago.
- Has been following a low-sodium diet and has been taking hydrochlorothiazide as directed since being diagnosed six weeks ago.

❶ What does the initial data provided by the client suggest?

❷ What questions will you ask of the client prior to performing your physical examination?

❸ What data do you expect your physical assessment to reveal?

❹ What do you expect the laboratory tests to reveal?

❺ What discharge teaching would be important to perform?

For suggested responses, see pages 230–231.

Posttest

1 Which of the following client laboratory results is reflective of hypernatremia?

(1) Serum osmolality of 245 mOsm/kg
(2) Serum sodium of 150 mEq/L
(3) Urine specific gravity below 1.003
(4) Potassium level of 5.5 mEq/L

2 A client receiving treatment for hypernatremia is being monitored for signs and symptoms of complications of therapy. The nurse knows that one of the primary risks when treating hypernatremia is:

(1) Cellular dehydration.
(2) Cerebral edema.
(3) RBC destruction.
(4) Renal shutdown.

3 A 55-year-old client is semiconscious, restless, and exhibits tremors and muscle weakness. Physical examination reveals a dry, swollen tongue, body temperature of 99.8°F, and urine specific gravity of 1.030. The nurse knows that the serum sodium value for this client is most likely to be which of the following?

(1) 115 mEq/L
(2) 125 mEq/L
(3) 135 mEq/L
(4) 155 mEq/L

4 A 58-year-old client was brought to the hospital following a near-drowning experience in the Atlantic Ocean. In providing care to this client, the nurse knows that it is important to monitor for:

(1) Hypernatremia.
(2) Hyponatremia.
(3) Hypocalcemia.
(4) Hypercalcemia.

5 Which of the following should be restricted when caring for an adult client diagnosed with hyponatremia?

(1) Water
(2) Sodium
(3) Potassium
(4) Chloride

6 Which of the following manifestations should the nurse assess for when developing a plan of care for a client with hypernatremia?

(1) Muscle weakness
(2) Moist mucous membranes
(3) Serum sodium level of 140 mEq/L
(4) Thirst

7 When providing care to clients with syndrome of inappropriate antidiuretic hormone (SIADH), water intake should be:

(1) Encouraged.
(2) Restricted.
(3) Given according to the client's preference.
(4) Given via intravenous fluids only.

8 A client with a diagnosis of bipolar disorder has been drinking copious amounts of water and voiding frequently. The patient is experiencing bounding pulse and confusion and is reporting headache. The nurse checks laboratory test results for which of the following?

(1) Low platelet count
(2) Low sodium level
(3) High serum osmolality
(4) High urine specific gravity

9 An 85-year-old client with a feeding tube has been experiencing severe watery diarrhea. The client is lethargic with decreased skin turgor, pulse rate of 110, and hyperactive reflexes. Nursing interventions would include:

(1) Monitoring and recording intake, output, and daily weights.
(2) Administering salt tablets and monitoring hypertonic parenteral solutions.
(3) Administering sedatives and analgesics.
(4) Restricting fluid intake.

10 The nurse who is caring for a client with hyponatremia would conclude that which of the following client factors probably contributed to this electrolyte imbalance?

(1) Osmotic diuretic therapy
(2) Diaphoresis
(3) Fluid retention
(4) Use of salt pills during exercise

See pages 57–58 for Answers and Rationales.

Answers and Rationales

Pretest

1 **Answer: 4** *Rationale:* When a person experiences a loss of body fluids, such as that seen with perspiration during strenuous exercise, the extracellular fluid volume is decreased and the osmolality is increased. Hemoglobin levels do not increase in response to an hour of strenuous exercise. Creatinine levels are usually stable in response to exercise.
Cognitive Level: Application
Nursing Process: Analysis; *Test Plan:* PHYS

2 **Answer: 3** *Rationale:* The combination of high fever and severe dehydration leads to insensible water loss. This indicates a loss of pure water and does not contain electrolytes. Therefore, excessive amounts of insensible water loss result in a hypertonic dehydration that leads to a state of hypernatremia and hyperchloremia. Calcium levels usually decrease in the presence of dehydration and fever. Phosphate levels usually increase in the presence of dehydration and fever. Potassium levels can usually remain normal in the serum and are increased in the urine.
Cognitive Level: Application
Nursing Process: Analysis; *Test Plan:* PHYS

3 **Answer: 1** *Rationale:* The use of corticosteroids can lead to the development of hypernatremia as they cause sodium to be retained and potassium to be excreted. The elderly client drinking 8 glasses of water each day is within a normal range of fluid intake and is not at risk for developing sodium imbalances. The diabetic client whose blood glucose is within normal range is not at risk for developing sodium imbalances. The teenager who is using Gatorade as an oral replacement therapy to compensate for fluid and electrolyte loss during exercise is not at risk for developing sodium imbalances.
Cognitive Level: Analysis
Nursing Process: Assessment; *Test Plan:* PHYS

4 **Answer: 4** *Rationale:* There are minimal shifts between isotonic fluids due to equal osmotic pressure. Hypertonic solutions will cause cellular dehydration to occur. Hyperosmolar refers to osmotic pressure greater than normal plasma pressure and is associated with hypertonic solutions. Hypotonic solutions will cause cellular swelling to occur.
Cognitive Level: Comprehension
Nursing Process: Analysis; *Test Plan:* PHYS

5 **Answer: 4** *Rationale:* Clients with hypernatremia have an increased need for fluids, not a decreased need. Clients with hypernatremia should have their I & O monitored, temperature recorded, and level of consciousness assessed for potential development of neurological complications such as seizures.
Cognitive Level: Application
Nursing Process: Implementation; *Test Plan:* SECE

6 **Answer: 2** *Rationale:* The client with hyponatremia needs an increase in sodium consumption; therefore, restriction of sodium intake is not advised. A client with hyponatremia needs to have neurological status monitored along with assessing for signs and symptoms consistent with hyponatremia such as nausea and malaise. It is important to prevent further fluid/serum dilution by restricting tap water intake.
Cognitive Level: Application
Nursing Process: Implementation; *Test Plan:* PHYS

7 **Answer: 3** *Rationale:* The correct use of consistent equipment will provide the most objective baseline for client weights. Therefore it is important to weigh the client at the same time each day to provide the most accurate results. Daily weights do not require a physician order and can be incorporated in a nursing plan of care. Weighing a client in the clinical setting without clothing is not usually indicated, although it is helpful for the client to wear the same type of clothing.
Cognitive Level: Application
Nursing Process: Planning; *Test Plan:* HPM

8 **Answer: 2** *Rationale:* The serum osmolality can be roughly estimated by doubling the serum sodium level. The normal range for serum sodium is 135 to 145 mEq/L. Using a rough determination would make the plasma osmolality fall in the range of 270 to 290 mOsm/kg. Option 1 reflects a greatly decreased plasma osmolality that would not correlate with a normal serum sodium level. Options 3 and 4 reflect an elevated plasma osmolality that would correlate with an increased sodium level.
Cognitive Level: Application
Nursing Process: Analysis; *Test Plan:* SECE

9 **Answer: 1** *Rationale:* Processed foods such as cheese are higher in sodium content. Ham is high in sodium because it is cured as a preservative process. The addition of these types of foods will supply extra sodium in the diet. The other options are lower in sodium content.
Cognitive Level: Application
Nursing Process: Implementation; *Test Plan:* PHYS

10 **Answer: 2** *Rationale:* The hyponatremia is due to an excess of water, which is diluting the amount of sodium present in the plasma. Clients who are experiencing hyponatremia with a hypervolemic state are in fluid volume excess (FVE). It is important to restrict additional fluids as this can further increase the sodium deficit. In addition, the client already is an FVE state, which can lead to development of further disturbances of fluid balance. Option 1 is incorrect, as the client does not require additional fluids at this time. Removing excess salt and replacement of free water would be indicated in a client experiencing hypernatremia.
Cognitive Level: Application
Nursing Process: Planning; *Test Plan:* PHYS

Posttest

1 **Answer: 2** *Rationale:* Hypernatremia reflects a state of sodium excess; therefore, the level will be > 145 mEq/L. Option 1 reflects a decreased serum osmolality, which is inconsistent with hypernatremia, as all hypernatremic states are hyperosmolar. Option 3 reflects a decreased urine specific gravity, whereas an increased urine specific gravity is associated with hypernatremia. Option 4 reflects a slightly elevated potassium level, which is not associated with hypernatremia.
Cognitive Level: Application
Nursing Process: Analysis; *Test Plan:* PHYS

2 **Answer: 2** *Rationale:* Too rapid a correction of hypernatremia can lead to changes in vascular tone, which can affect vessels and cause increased fluid entry into the brain, thereby causing cerebral edema. Option 1 reflects cellular dehydration, which is caused by hypernatremia. Options 3 and 4 are not viewed as risks when treating hypernatremia.
Cognitive Level: Comprehension
Nursing Process: Assessment; *Test Plan:* PHYS

3 **Answer: 4** *Rationale:* This client has signs and symptoms of hypernatremia and the serum sodium level would be > 145 mEq/L. Options 1 and 2 reflect decreased serum sodium levels and are considered to be hyponatremic. Option 3 reflects a normal serum sodium level.
Cognitive Level: Application
Nursing Process: Analysis; *Test Plan:* PHYS

4 **Answer: 1** *Rationale:* Near drowning in saltwater often results in hypernatremia due to the high sodium level in sea/saltwater. Hyponatremia and disturbances in calcium levels are not seen in this clinical situation.
Cognitive Level: Application
Nursing Process: Assessment; *Test Plan:* HPM

5 **Answer: 1** *Rationale:* In hyponatremia, water is already present in an excessive amount compared to the amount of sodium present. This can result in water intoxication or dilutional hyponatremia; therefore, water restriction is a primary cornerstone of therapy. The other electrolytes (sodium, potassium, and chloride) should not be restricted but rather should be included in the treatment plan so as to prevent further electrolyte imbalances from occurring.
Cognitive Level: Application
Nursing Process: Implementation; *Test Plan:* SECE

6 **Answer: 4** *Rationale:* Thirst is a primary indicator of sodium excess (hypernatremia) and should be assessed for in a plan of care for a client with hypernatremia. Muscle weakness is not reflective of hypernatremia but is more likely to be found with sodium deficit. Moist mucous membranes are not associated with sodium imbalances and reflect a normal parameter. A serum sodium level of 140 mEq/L is within normal range.
Cognitive Level: Application
Nursing Process: Assessment; *Test Plan:* HPM

7 **Answer: 2** *Rationale:* In SIADH, the antidiuretic hormone is present in excess amounts. This causes excessive water reabsorption. Water must be restricted to avoid water intoxication. Giving additional fluids would only further serve to increase fluid levels and increase sodium deficit. While it is important to consider a client's preference in fluid selection, fluid restriction is the major priority. Administering fluids only via the intravenous route is not the preferred method. While fluid therapy can be given IV, it is important to allow the client to take PO fluids even if they are on a restricted basis.
Cognitive Level: Application
Nursing Process: Implementation; *Test Plan:* PHYS

8 **Answer: 2** *Rationale:* The client has exhibited behavior that could indicate a sodium and water imbalance and is actually exhibiting signs of hyponatremia. The nurse would check the electrolyte levels, expecting to find a low sodium level. Monitoring the CBC for a platelet level is not indicated, as there is no correlation between sodium levels and platelet activity. The client's serum osmolality and urine specific gravity are expected to be low due to water intoxication.
Cognitive Level: Application
Nursing Process: Assessment; *Test Plan:* SECE

9 **Answer: 1** *Rationale:* The client is exhibiting signs of hypernatremia and dehydration. The most appropriate nursing intervention is to measure and record intake and output and daily weight. Administering salt tablets would further contribute to the client's hypernatremic state. Administering sedatives and analgesics is not warranted, as the client is not complaining of pain at the present time. A pain assessment profile would be needed to assess the need for pain management. Restricting fluid intake could further contribute to the client's state of hypernatremia with fluid volume deficit (hypertonic dehydration) as the client already has extensive fluid loss due to diarrhea, elevated pulse rate, and decreased skin turgor.
Cognitive Level: Analysis
Nursing Process: Implementation; *Test Plan:* SECE

10 **Answer: 3** *Rationale:* Fluid retention can result in hyponatremia through dilutional effect. Options 1 and 2 could lead to hypernatremia. Option 4 could lead to hypernatremia if the client did not also drink fluids during exercise.
Cognitive Level: Application
Nursing Process: Assessment; *Test Plan:* PHYS

References

DeLaune, S. & Ladner, P. (1998). *Fundamentals of nursing: Standards and practice.* Albany, NY: Delmar, pp. 1030–1033, 1037–1042.

Hansen, M. (1998). *Pathophysiology: Foundations of disease and clinical intervention.* Philadelphia: W. B. Saunders, pp. 179–182.

Ignatavicius, D., Workman, M., & Mishler, M. (1999). *Medical-surgical nursing across the health care continuum* (3rd ed.). Philadelphia: W. B. Saunders, pp. 220–222, 250–254.

Kee, J. L. & Paulanka B. L. (2000). *Fluids and electrolytes with clinical applications: A programmed approach* (6th ed.). Albany, NY: Delmar, pp. 128–153.

Kidd, P. & Wagner, K. (2001). *High acuity nursing* (3rd ed.). Upper Saddle River, NJ: Prentice-Hall, Inc., pp. 64–65.

Kozier, B., Erb, G., Berman, A., & Burke, K. (2000). *Fundamentals of nursing: Concepts, process, and practice* (6th ed.). Upper Saddle River, NJ: Prentice-Hall, Inc., p. 1301–1339.

LeMone, P. & Burke, K. (2000). *Medical surgical nursing: Critical thinking in client care* (2nd ed.). Upper Saddle River, NJ: Prentice-Hall, Inc., pp. 119–126.

Malarkey, L. & McMorrow, M. (2000). *Nurse's manual of laboratory tests and diagnostic procedures* (2nd ed.). Philadelphia: W. B. Saunders, pp. 99–102.

Metheny, N. (2000). *Fluid and electrolyte balance: Nursing considerations* (4th ed.). Philadelphia: Lippincott, pp. 51–89, 226–269, 353–388.

Smeltzer, S. & Bare, B. (2000). *Brunner and Suddarth's textbook of medical-surgical nursing* (9th ed.). Philadelphia: Lippincott, pp. 213–218.

CHAPTER 3

Potassium Balance and Imbalances

Lynn Rhyne, MN, RN

CHAPTER OUTLINE

Overview of Potassium Regulation   *Hypokalemia*   *Hyperkalemia*

OBJECTIVES

▌ Review basic functions of potassium in the body.

▌ Discuss the pathophysiology and etiology of potassium imbalances.

▌ Discuss specific assessment findings in potassium imbalances.

▌ Identify priority nursing diagnoses for a client experiencing a potassium imbalance.

▌ Discuss therapeutic management of potassium imbalances.

▌ Discuss nursing management of a client who is experiencing a potassium imbalance.

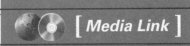

[*Media Link*]

Use the CD-ROM enclosed with this text, or log onto the address given to access the free, interactive Companion Website created for this series. The CD-ROM and Companion Website accompanying this book offer additional practice opportunities and information—NCLEX Review, Case Studies, Glossary, In Depth with NCLEX, and more.

www.prenhall.com/hogan

REVIEW AT A GLANCE

actual hyperkalemia *potassium level in the extracellular fluid is elevated*

actual hypokalemia *the actual loss of potassium or lack of adequate intake of potassium*

hyperkalemia *serum potassium level above the laboratory normal value (usually 5.0 mEq/L)*

hypokalemia *serum level of potassium falls below 3.5 mEq/L*

relative hyperkalemia *movement of potassium from the intracellular fluid to the extracellular fluid, leading to elevated serum potassium levels without a true body increase of potassium*

relative hypokalemia *movement of potassium from the extracellular fluid to the intracellular fluid, leading to lowered serum potassium levels without a true decrease of potassium in the body*

sodium-potassium pump *controls the concentration of potassium by removing three sodium ions from the cell for every two potassium ions that return to the cell; fueled by the breakdown of ATP and responsible for causing muscle cells to generate action potentials and transmit impulses*

Pretest

1 Which of the following potassium levels would be of greatest concern in a client who is taking furosemide (Lasix)?

(1) 5.4 mEq/L
(2) 6.2 mEq/L
(3) 4.3 mEq/L
(4) 3.2 mEq/L

2 Which of the following statements made by the nurse is correct when performing client education regarding oral potassium supplementation?

(1) "When you take your potassium pill, if you can't swallow it, you can crush it up and put it in orange juice."
(2) "Potassium should only be taken in the morning on an empty stomach."
(3) "Take your potassium tablet after you have eaten breakfast."
(4) "You can continue to use salt substitute while you are taking your potassium supplement."

3 Which of the following clients would be most likely to develop hyperkalemia?

(1) A client with chronic renal failure.
(2) A client just diagnosed with cirrhosis.
(3) A client with intestinal and nasogastric suctioning.
(4) A client who has had diarrhea for the last four days.

4 A client in renal failure has an abnormally high potassium level. Which of the following is a priority nursing intervention?

(1) Obtain an electrocardiogram (ECG).
(2) Evaluate level of consciousness.
(3) Measure urinary output.
(4) Draw arterial blood gases.

5 The nurse should include diet teaching regarding adding potassium-rich foods if which of the following diuretics is ordered?

(1) Hydrochlorothiazide (HCTZ)
(2) Spironolactone (Aldactone)
(3) Maxizide (Triamterene with hydrochlorothiazide)
(4) Midamor (Amiloride)

6 The nurse anticipates using which of the following as the most effective route to administer sodium polystyrene sulfonate (Kayexalate) ordered for a client who has a serum potassium level of 6.0 mEq/L?

(1) Intravenous (IV)
(2) Rectal
(3) Oral
(4) Subcutaneous (SC)

7   A client with hypokalemia must be assessed carefully for which of the following that can occur because of this electrolyte imbalance?

(1) Perforated bowel
(2) Paralytic ileus
(3) Renal failure
(4) Diabetes

8   What is the expected result when calcium gluconate is given intravenously to a client with hyperkalemia?

(1) Increased excretion of potassium in the urine
(2) Increased excretion of potassium via the stools
(3) Reversing the effects of the potassium on the heart's conduction system
(4) Pulling potassium back into the intracellular fluid to reduce the serum potassium

9   Which of the following statements by a client indicates a need for further instruction regarding treatment for hypokalemia?

(1) "I will eat more bananas and cantaloupes for breakfast."
(2) "I will eat more bran flakes to increase my potassium level."
(3) "I will take my potassium in the morning after breakfast so it doesn't upset my stomach."
(4) "I will tell my doctor if I start having any of the symptoms on the list you gave me."

10   Which of the following is the best response by the nurse to the daughter of a 46-year-old client who was admitted with hypokalemia and is complaining of being dizzy upon standing?

(1) "Your mother has just stayed in bed too long and when she stands up she will get dizzy."
(2) "The level of your mother's potassium is making her dizzy."
(3) "Your mother is probably dizzy because her heart is not pumping as effectively, making her blood pressure low."
(4) "Your mother is dizzy because her nervous system isn't functioning correctly; once her potassium level goes up she will improve."

See pages 81–82 for Answers and Rationales.

I. Overview of Potassium Regulation

A. Potassium balance and function: major cation of the intracellular fluid (ICF); 98% of the body's potassium store is located in ICF; the remaining 2% is in the extracellular fluid (ECF), i.e., the intravascular and interstitial spaces outside the cells; responsible for neuromuscular function

1. Serum levels

   a. Normal serum concentration ranges from 3.5 to 5.0 mEq/L

   b. Even small changes in potassium level have a profound effect on the body and are poorly tolerated

2. Role in acid-base balance

   a. Hydrogen and potassium ions shift back and forth between the ICF and ECF to maintain the pH

   b. Hydrogen ions move out of cells in alkalotic states to help correct the high pH and potassium ions move in to maintain an electrically stable state; the reverse happens in acidosis

3. Functions in the body

    a. ECF potassium (K^+) is responsible for maintaining action potentials in excitable cells of muscles, neurons, and other tissues

    b. ECF K^+ assists in controlling cardiac rate and rhythm, conduction of nerve impulses, skeletal muscle contraction, and function of smooth muscles and endocrine tissues

    c. Intracellular K^+ has a role in cellular metabolism and functions in the regulation of protein and glycogen synthesis

    d. Due to the fact that K^+ is the primary intracellular cation, it has some control over intracellular osmolarity and volume via the sodium-potassium ion exchange mechanism

4. System interactions

    a. The primary control of ECF K^+ concentration is the **sodium-potassium pump,** contained within the cell membrane of all the cells in the body

    b. The sodium-potassium pump controls the concentration of potassium by removing three sodium ions from the cell for every two potassium ions that return to the cell

    c. The pump is fueled by the breakdown of ATP and is responsible for causing muscle cells to generate action potentials and transmit impulses

B. Sources of potassium

1. Cellular level: factors that affect the movement of potassium in and out of the cells contribute to the level of potassium in the ICF and the ECF

    a. The kidneys eliminate approximately 90% of potassium

    b. The remaining amount is excreted through stool and perspiration

    c. Cellular release can lead to additional potassium circulating in the body and may be due to disease processes and/or medications

2. Dietary levels

    a. Adequate intake is approximately 40–60 mEq daily

    b. Western diets consist of adequate intake of potassium daily in the form of fruits, dried fruits, and vegetables

    c. Many salt substitutes contain potassium

    d. Intake can also occur when parenteral fluid with potassium is infused

    e. Excessive intake of black licorice can lead to decreased K^+ levels due to the effect of glyceric acid (aldosterone effect)

II. *Hypokalemia:* serum level of potassium below 3.5 mEq/L; Table 3-1 provides a condensed overview of this electrolyte imbalance

A. Etiology and pathophysiology

1. Cellular level transport

    a. The amount of potassium in the ECF is so small that minute changes in the K^+ level can lead to major alterations in membrane excitability in muscle and neural cells, making them less responsive to stimuli

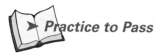

► *Practice to Pass*

A client asks the nurse why potassium levels are so important in the body. How will the nurse respond?

Table 3-1	Etiology	Manifestations	Nursing Interventions
Overview of Hypokalemia	Inadequate intake Use of potassium-wasting diuretics Excessive loss of GI fluid Heat induced diaphoresis Starvation High glucose levels leading to diuresis Increased secretion of aldosterone as seen in adrenal adenomas, cirrhosis, nephrosis, heart failure, and hypertensive crisis Diabetes insipidus	Weak, thready pulse Pedal pulses difficult to palpate ECG changes—ST segment depression, flattened T wave, appearance of U wave, ventricular dysrhythmias (especially PVCs), heart block Enhanced effect of digoxin leading to toxicity at therapeutic levels Decreased breath sounds Shallow respiratory pattern Dyspnea Polyuria; difficulty in concentrating urine Decreased deep tendon reflexes Muscle weakness Anxiety Lethargy Depression Confusion Paresthesias Weakness Leg cramps Abdominal distention Hypoactive bowel sounds Vomiting Nausea Constipation Paralytic ileus	Monitor vital signs, especially blood pressure; orthostatic hypotension common Monitor serum potassium levels Assess heart rate and rhythm Assess ECG changes Assess respiratory rate, depth, and pattern Assess for signs of hypokalemia if client taking diuretics Protect from injury Monitor serum magnesium and calcium levels Monitor intake and output Check for signs of metabolic alkalosis Give potassium supplements as ordered Use an infusion pump when administering parenteral potassium and assess IV site frequently for infiltration, phlebitis, and tissue necrosis Assess mental status and cognition Client education (as described in Box 3-1)

b. Rapid changes in ECF potassium cannot be compensated for quickly and can result in profound changes in body function

c. If this decrease is not corrected very quickly, death can occur from cardiac and respiratory arrest

d. Relative hypokalemia occurs when potassium moves from the ECF to the ICF (the total body level of potassium remains unchanged), leading to abnormal distribution of potassium

1) Alkalosis causes K^+ to migrate into the cell as hydrogen ions move out to correct the high pH

2) Increased secretion of insulin causes K^+ to move into skeletal muscles and hepatic cells when there is increased secretion of insulin

3) Tissue repair causes shifting of K^+ concentration

4) Water intoxication causes dilution of serum potassium

2. Predisposing clinical conditions: **actual hypokalemia** is the actual loss of potassium or lack of adequate intake of potassium

   a. Increased secretion of aldosterone leads to the excretion of K^+ from the renal tubules and is seen in clients with:

      1) Adrenal adenomas

      2) Cirrhosis

      3) Nephrosis

      4) Heart failure and hypertensive crisis

      5) Cushing's syndrome

      6) Diabetes insipidus

   b. Excessive loss of potassium by use of certain medications, such as loop diuretics (such as furosemide [Lasix]), thiazide diuretics (such as hydrochlorothiazide [Hydrodiuril]), corticosteroids, cardiac glycosides (digoxin [Lanoxin]), penicillin derivatives (such as ampicillin, sodium penicillin, carbenicillin), amphotericin B, gentamicin (Garamycin), theophylline (Theo-Dur), cisplatin (Platinol), and tocolytic agents (such as Terbutaline); refer to Table 3-2 for a summary of medication classes that affect potassium levels

   c. Gastrointestinal loss by vomiting, diarrhea, prolonged nasogastric suctioning, newly created ileostomy, villous adenoma on the intestinal tract, laxative abuse, or enema administration

   d. Heat induced diaphoresis

   e. Renal disease affecting the reabsorption of potassium seen in the diuretic phase of renal failure

   f. Hemodialysis and peritoneal dialysis

   g. Altered intake

      1) Potassium-restricted diets

      2) NPO status without sufficient IV replacement therapy

      3) Starvation, malnutrition, alcoholism, and anorexia

Table 3-2	Increase Potassium Levels	Decrease Potassium Levels
Common Medications That Affect Potassium Levels	Potassium chloride and salts Angiotensin converting enzyme (ACE) inhibitors* Heparin Barbiturates, sedatives, heroin, and amphetamines Nonsteroidal anti-inflammatory drugs (NSAIDs)* Beta blockers and alpha agonists* Cyclophosphamide Potassium-sparing diuretics*	Laxatives, enemas, and Kayexalate Corticosteroids (Cortisone, Prednisone) Cardiac glycosides (digoxin) Antibiotics* Insulin and glucose Beta$_2$ agonists (terbutaline, estrogen, albuterol) Potassium-wasting diuretics*

*For these medications, please refer to a drug textbook for specific names because there are many different types of drugs in each category.

4) High glucose levels, which increase osmotic pressure and lead to diuresis

5) Large ingestion of black licorice (causes aldosterone effects)

B. Clinical manifestations: rarely develop before potassium level falls below 3.0 mEq/L unless the rate of fall is rapid

1. Common signs

    a. Cardiovascular

    1) Variable pulse rate

    2) Weak, thready pulse

    3) Pedal pulses difficult to palpate

    4) ECG changes (see Figure 3-1): ST segment depression, flattened T wave, appearance of U wave, ventricular dysrhythmias (especially premature ventricular contractions [PVCs]), heart block

    5) Digitalis toxicity is potentiated

    b. Respiratory

    1) Decreased breath sounds

    2) Shallow respiratory pattern

    3) Dyspnea

    c. Renal

    1) Polyuria and nocturia

    2) Decreased specific gravity

    3) Myoglobin in urine due to breakdown of muscle fibers, leading to rhabdomyolysis (seen in clients with severe hypokalemia)

    d. Neuromuscular

    1) Deep tendon hyporeflexia

    2) Muscle weakness, paresthesias, and soft flabby muscles

    3) Fatigue and lethargy, which can proceed to depression and coma in clients with severe hypokalemia

    e. Gastrointestinal

    1) Abdominal distention

    2) Hypoactive or absent bowel sounds

    3) Vomiting and/or diarrhea

    4) Paralytic ileus

2. Common symptoms

    a. Neuromuscular

    1) Anxiety

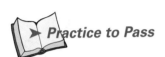

Practice to Pass

Why is an understanding of actual versus relative hypokalemia important to client safety?

NCLEX!

Figure 3-1

Electrocardiogram (ECG) changes caused by altered potassium levels. A. Normal ECG, B. Changes resulting from hyperkalemia, C. Changes resulting from hypokaleima.

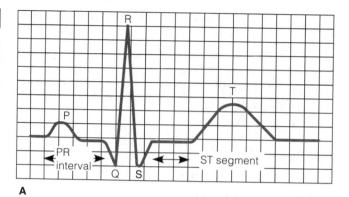

A

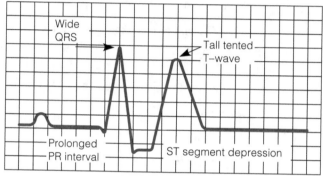

B

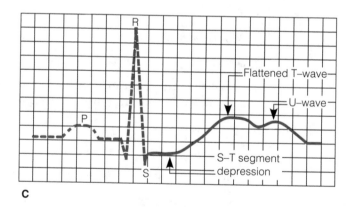

C

2) Lethargy

3) Depression

4) Confusion, can progress to coma

5) Paresthesias

6) Weakness

7) Leg cramps

b. Gastrointestinal

1) Nausea

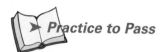

> **Practice to Pass**

How are you going to ensure client safety when that client has hypokalemia?

2) Diarrhea or constipation (from decreased peristalsis)

3) Polydipsia

C. Assessment

1. Monitoring expectations

   a. Serum potassium levels

   b. ECG changes

   c. Electrolyte levels

   d. Intake and output

      1) Diuresis can lead to excessive loss of potassium

      2) One liter of urine contains about 40 mEq of potassium

2. Identification of risk factors

   a. Assess for factors that increase the risk of hypokalemia such as:

      1) Age: aging decreases the kidneys ability to concentrate urine leading to diuresis

      2) The elderly are also more likely to be taking medications that can alter potassium levels

   b. Medications

      1) Obtain pertinent client history of medications that can alter potassium levels (refer back to Table 3-2)

      2) Examine both prescription and over-the-counter medications and supplements that the client is taking for possible interactions

   c. Dietary

      1) Obtain pertinent client history regarding food intake

      2) Determine whether the client is taking nutritional supplements and check for potential interactions

D. Diagnostic and laboratory findings

1. Plasma levels

   a. Hypokalemia is confirmed by a serum level less than 3.5 mEq/L (or the normal value indicated by a particular laboratory)

   b. Trending of serum K^+ levels is necessary in order to establish a baseline and monitor response to therapy

2. Associated electrolyte levels

   a. Elevated pH and bicarbonate levels (alkalosis)

   b. Elevated serum glucose levels (increased insulin secretion and increased osmotic pressure)

   c. Decreased serum chloride levels

   d. Decreased magnesium levels (because hypomagnesemia can potentiate hypokalemia)

      e. Decreased calcium levels can also be seen in conjunction with decreased potassium and magnesium levels

   3. Trending of results

      a. ECG tracings demonstrate characteristic changes with hypokalemia (described earlier in chapter)

      b. Trending ECG changes can help to monitor client's status and response to therapeutic treatment

E. Priority nursing diagnoses

   1. Risk for injury related to muscle weakness and hyporeflexia

   2. Risk for ineffective breathing pattern related to neuromuscular impairment

   3. Decreased cardiac output related to dysrhythmias

   4. Constipation related to smooth muscle atony

   5. Altered nutrition related to poor dietary levels

   6. Fatigue related to neuromuscular weakness

F. Therapeutic management: treatment focuses on restoring normal levels, preventing complications, and treating underlying problems

   1. Replacement therapies

      a. For clients at risk, provide a diet containing adequate potassium, about 50–100 mEq daily

      b. If the diet is insufficient to meet needs, administer potassium supplements as ordered

      c. Initiate a referral to a dietitian for assistance with meal planning to ensure adequate sources of potassium in the diet (refer to Box 3-1 for dietary sources of potassium)

   2. Continued monitoring of client (lab values and physical manifestations) to assess efficacy of treatment

   3. Restoration of balance (normal serum K^+ level) to maintain homeostasis and prevent development of further complications

      a. It is important to monitor serum calcium and magnesium levels in clients who are hypokalemic as sometimes even with appropriate potassium replacement, serum levels do not rise

NCLEX**!**

NCLEX**!**

Box 3-1
Good Food Sources of Potassium

The following foods are considered adequate sources of potassium:

- Vegetables such as spinach, broccoli, carrots, green beans, tomato juice, acorn squash, and potatoes
- Fruits such as bananas, cantaloupe, watermelon, grapefruit, and strawberries
- Milk, milk products, yogurt, and meat
- Legumes, nuts, and seeds
- Whole grains

    b. If client is also found to have hypocalcemia and/or hypomagnesemia, then correction must be aimed at restoring all three electrolyte levels in order to correct serum potassium

G. Planning and implementation

    1. Monitor pertinent client assessment data for potential effects related to hypokalemia, and for response to therapeutic treatment

        a. Vital signs, especially blood pressure (hypokalemia can cause the client to develop orthostatic hypotension) and respiratory rate, depth, and pattern

        b. Serum electrolyte levels

        c. ECG changes and heart rate and rhythm pattern

        d. Intake and output and possibly daily weight

    2. Monitor therapeutic serum drug levels for clients taking cardiac glycosides (Digoxin) and serum potassium levels for clients taking loop and thiazide diuretics

    3. Protect the client from injury and maintain a safe environment as client may experience weakness due to hypokalemia

    4. Dietary interventions to promote normal potassium levels

        a. Encourage use of high fiber diets and increased fluid intake, if not on fluid restriction, to prevent constipation

        b. Provide adequate dietary sources of potassium in the diet

        c. Maintain accurate intake and output

    5. Check for signs of metabolic alkalosis (including irritability and paresthesias) because hypokalemia is present in alkalotic states

    6. Provide replacement therapy as ordered by physician paying attention to baseline labs, client's response, and therapeutic benefit

    7. Always use an infusion pump when administering parenteral potassium

        a. Observe IV site frequently for signs of infiltration, phlebitis, and tissue necrosis as potassium-containing solutions are irritating to veins

        b. Verify additive K^+ in solution prior to hanging infusion

        c. Do not exceed maximum safe infusion rate (see section that follows)

    8. Observe client's mental status and cognition during course of therapy

H. Medication therapy (note: potassium supplements should never be given unless the client has a urine output of at least 0.5 mL/kg/hour)

    1. Oral replacement therapy

        a. Clients should be started on oral supplements if they take potassium-wasting diuretics, have poor nutritional intake, and/or have disease processes that cause further potassium losses

        b. The usual oral preparation is KCl, which is available in many preparations (K-Dur, K-Lyte, K-Lyte/Cl, K-Tab, Klotrix, Micro-K, and Slow- K)

        c. The daily prophylactic dose is 20 mEq

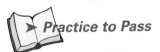

Practice to Pass

What nursing interventions should be used with clients receiving intravenous solutions containing KCl?

Prior to discharge, teach client and family to:

- Take potassium supplements with at least 4 ounces fluid or with food.
- Never crush or break potassium tablets or capsules.
- Dissolve powder form of potassium in at least 4 ounces of water or other fluids (no carbonated beverages).
- Take potassium after meals to prevent GI upset.
- Do not use salt substitutes when taking potassium supplements.
- Know the signs and symptoms of hyperkalemia and report any of these to the healthcare provider.
- Get regular serum potassium levels drawn as per healthcare provider recommendations.
- Teach client about side effects of K^+ supplements and to report them to healthcare provider if they occur.

    d. Therapeutic treatment can be given at higher doses (up to 100 mEq in divided doses), depending on the client's baseline

    d. The medication can be given in either liquid or pill form

    e. Refer to Box 3-2 for client teaching points regarding oral potassium therapy

  2. Parenteral replacement therapy

    a. Dilute potassium in a solution that provides no more than 1 mEq/10 mL

    b. Most potassium infusions are run at a rate not exceeding 5–10 mEq/hr unless there is moderate hypokalemia; peripheral IV potassium should not be infused more quickly than 20 mEq/hr or in concentrations greater than 40 mEq/L unless severe hypokalemia exists; higher concentration potassium solutions should be administered through a central line and the client should be hemodynamically monitored throughout the course of therapy

    c. The solution should be dextrose free, if possible, to prevent the release of insulin

    d. If more than 20 mEq/hour is given, the client should have continuous ECG monitoring and the serum levels should be checked every 4–6 hours until a normal level achieved

    e. Monitor IV site closely as KCl is irritating to vessels and can lead to infiltration, phlebitis, and tissue necrosis

    f. Use an infusion pump to control the infusion, paying attention to rate, intake, and output

    g. Potassium should never be administered by the IV push or intramuscular routes because this can lead to development of fatal arrhythmias

  3. Diet therapy

    a. Foods high in potassium include raisins, bananas, apricots, oranges, avocados, beans, beef, potatoes, tomatoes, cantaloupe, and spinach

    b. Avoid foods such as black licorice that, when eaten in large quantities, can cause hypokalemia

I. Client education

  1. Teach awareness of predisposing factors

a. Elderly clients are at risk for hypokalemia due to multiple medication profile

b. Clients taking diuretics (loop and thiazide) and/or digoxin (Lanoxin) are at risk to develop K^+ depletion

  2. Teach clients signs and symptoms of hypokalemia and have them report potential problems to their healthcare provider

  3. Teach clients about potassium supplement medication

a. Take with at least 4 ounces of fluid or food to prevent GI upset

b. Don't crush slow-release tablets, as this can trigger a quick release of potassium

  4. Dietary education

a. If client takes a potassium-sparing diuretic, do not encourage the use of foods high in potassium

b. Provide list of foods that are high in potassium during client education (refer to Box 3-1 for a listing of adequate food sources of potassium)

c. Collaborate with dietitian as needed

J. Evaluation

  1. Client returns to and maintains a normal serum potassium level

  2. Client complies with drug and diet therapies as ordered

  3. Client states the early signs and symptoms of hypokalemia

  4. Client has normal bowel pattern

  5. Client maintains adequate gas exchange

  6. Client maintains regular cardiac rate and rhythm

III. *Hyperkalemia:* serum level of potassium above 5.0 mEq/L; rare in those individuals with normally functioning kidneys; Table 3-3 provides a condensed overview of this electrolyte imbalance

A. Etiology and pathophysiology

  1. Cellular level transport

a. Potassium moves from the ECF to the ICF and increases cell excitability, so that cells respond to stimuli of less intensity and may actually discharge independently without a stimulus

b. The myocardium is the most excitable tissue and is most sensitive to increases in potassium levels

c. Manifestations seen with hyperkalemia depend on how rapidly the increase occurs

1) Sudden increases show profound functional changes at 6–7 mEq/L

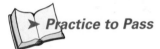

Practice to Pass

What foods would you suggest to a client who is hypokalemic?

Table 3-3	Etiology	Manifestations	Nursing Interventions
Overview of Hyperkalemia	Excessive potassium intake from foods, salt substitutes, IV infusions of KCl Decreased excretion due to adrenal insufficiency, renal failure, potassium-sparing diuretics; decreased secretion of aldosterone Massive tissue trauma Metabolic acidosis Gastrointestinal bleeds Digoxin use Overdose Insulin deficiency	Irregular, slow heart rate Decreased blood pressure ECG changes—tall, peaked T waves, widened QRS, frequent ectopy, ventricular fibrillation, standstill If levels are extremely high, can lead to muscle weakness, paralysis, and respiratory failure Muscle twitching, paralysis GI hypermotility Hyperactive bowel sounds Abdominal cramping Diarrhea Muscle cramps Irritability Anxiety Flaccid paralysis	Encourage decreased potassium intake Monitor serum potassium levels Assess for signs and symptoms Monitor cardiac status Monitor for metabolic acidosis and implement treatment for same Monitor ECG changes If blood transfusions necessary, give fresh packed red blood cells Encourage compliance with therapeutic regimen Discontinue use of IV KCl Implement safety precautions

2) Slower increases may not lead to changes until levels of 8 mEq/L are reached

2. Predisposing clinical conditions

   a. **Actual hyperkalemia** (potassium level in the ECF is elevated)

      1) Excessive potassium intake due to overingestion of potassium-rich food or medications, use of salt substitutes, or rapid infusion of K^+-containing IV solutions

      2) Decreased excretion of potassium due to adrenal insufficiency (Addison's disease), renal failure, K^+-sparing diuretics, or use of ACE inhibitors

   b. **Relative hyperkalemia** (movement of potassium from the ICF to the ECF leading to elevated serum potassium levels without a true body increase of potassium)

      1) Conditions that affect cellular release

         a) Massive cell damage

         b) Burns

         c) Hyperuricemia as a result of tumor lysis syndrome

         d) Gastrointestinal bleeds

         e) Major surgeries and hypercatabolism

      2) Conditions that are considered to cause pseudohyperkalemia

         a) Hemolysis of blood sample due to prolonged tourniquet use

         b) Clenched fist during blood draws may cause RBC hemolysis

3) Conditions that affect transcellular shifting

    a) Metabolic acidosis

    b) Insulin deficiency

    c) Rapid increase in blood osmolality

4) Conditions that result from medication therapy

    a) Digoxin use

    b) Overdose of replacement therapy

    c) Administration of stored blood, which causes hemolysis of RBCs in solution and increases serum levels

    d) Use of potassium-sparing diuretics

5) Addison's disease due to decreased aldosterone that leads to sodium depletion and potassium retention

B. Clinical manifestations

  1. Common signs

    a. Cardiovascular

      1) Irregular, slow heart rate

      2) Decreased blood pressure

      3) ECG changes (refer again to Figure 3-1): narrow, peaked T waves, widened QRS complexes, prolonged PR intervals, flattened P waves, frequent ectopy, ventricular fibrillation, and ventricular standstill

    b. Respiratory: unaffected until levels are very high, leading to muscle weakness and paralysis and causing respiratory failure

    c. Neuromuscular

      1) Early: muscle twitching

      2) Late: ascending flaccid paralysis involving arms and legs

    d. Gastrointestinal

      1) Hypermotility with hyperactive bowel sounds

      2) Diarrhea due to bowel hyperactivity

  2. Common symptoms

    a. Neuromuscular

      1) Muscle cramps

      2) Irritability

      3) Anxiety

      4) Flaccid paralysis

    b. Gastrointestinal

      1) Abdominal cramping

      2) Nausea

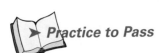

Practice to Pass

Why does a client who has massive tissue destruction get hyperkalemia?

C. Assessment

1. Monitoring expectations

    a. Serum potassium levels

    b. ECG changes

    c. Intake and output (adequate renal function is important for the excretion of potassium; intake and output must be measured accurately and frequently)

2. Identification of risk factors

    a. Assess for factors that increase the risk of hyperkalemia, such as

        1) Age: aging leads to a decrease in renal functioning

        2) Medications that can increase serum potassium levels (such as K^+-sparing diuretics or K^+ supplements, blood products, ACE inhibitors, beta adrenergic blockers, nonsteroidal anti-inflammatory drugs [NSAIDs], heparin, and sulfamethoxazole/trimethoprim [Bactrim])

    b. Dietary

        1) Clients with a high intake of potassium-rich foods

        2) Clients who use salt substitutes

        3) Clients who take potassium supplements

    c. Clients with disease states, both acute and chronic

        1) Diabetes and renal failure can lead to hyperkalemia

        2) Acute disease such as massive trauma or burns can lead to hyperkalemia

    d. Clients undergoing therapeutic treatment

        1) Recent medical or surgical intervention

        2) Blood transfusions

D. Diagnostic and laboratory findings

1. Plasma levels: a value greater than 5.0 mEq/L confirms the diagnosis of hyperkalemia

2. Associated electrolyte levels

    a. If dehydration is causing hyperkalemia, then hematocrit, hemoglobin, sodium, and chloride levels should be drawn

    b. If associated with renal failure, creatinine and BUN levels should also be drawn

    c. An arterial blood gas (ABG) is needed to monitor for metabolic acidosis

3. Trending of results

    a. ECG monitoring to determine cardiac changes

    b. ABGs to determine acid-base balance

E. **Priority nursing diagnoses**

   1. Risk for injury related to muscle weakness and seizures

   2. Risk for decreased cardiac output related to dysrhythmias

   3. Altered nutrition related to decreased renal function or increased intake

   4. Diarrhea related to neuromuscular changes and irritability

F. **Therapeutic interventions**

   1. Decrease potassium intake

      a. Stress importance of adherence to prescribed potassium restrictions

      b. Do not administer potassium supplements either orally or in parenteral fluids

      c. Refer client to a dietitian to evaluate dietary intake for hidden potassium sources

   2. Promote potassium excretion

      a. Increase urinary output

      b. Ensure adequate renal function

   3. Continued monitoring of client

      a. Serum potassium levels; report abnormals

      b. Signs and symptoms of hyperkalemia

      c. Cardiac status

      d. Metabolic acidosis

   4. Restoration of balance

      a. Since small elevations can lead to profound myocardial changes, the normal level of potassium should be restored as soon as possible to prevent lethal dysrhythmias

      b. Treatment is based on serum levels and client presentation; aggressive therapeutic management may be required to return serum levels to baseline in a timely manner

      c. Whenever possible, determine and treat the underlying cause of the client's hyperkalemia because this will help to restore balance

   5. Dialysis may be performed for intractable conditions if hyperkalemia cannot be controlled in a timely manner to prevent development of potentially lethal problems or if the client's clinical condition warrants immediate intervention

G. **Planning and implementation**

   1. Monitor pertinent client assessment data for potential effects related to hyperkalemia and for response to therapeutic treatment

      a. Notify healthcare provider of levels exceeding 5.0 mEq/L as elevations can cause serious cardiac consequences

      b. Serum electrolyte levels

      c. ECG changes and heart rate and rhythm pattern

2. Monitor client for potential serum elevations due to concomitant drug therapy (as noted in Table 3-2)

3. Check for signs of metabolic acidosis because relative hyperkalemia frequently accompanies acidotic states (and often self-corrects when the pH is corrected)

4. Do not provide any additional potassium in the form of medications (IV, supplements, and/or stored blood)

5. Dietary interventions to promote normal potassium levels

    a. Decrease catabolism by encouraging the client to consume prescribed amounts of dietary protein and carbohydrates

    b. Limit or stop additional potassium sources in the diet (such as use of salt substitutes)

    c. Refer client to a dietitian for individualized instruction as needed

6. Encourage compliance with therapeutic regimen, treat infections promptly, and decrease hypermetabolic responses

H. Medication therapy

    1. Exchange resins

        a. Sodium polystyrene sulfonate (Kayexalate) can be given either orally with an osmotic agent to decrease possible constipation or as an enema

        b. Medication works to exchange sodium with potassium in the GI tract and excrete the resin formed with potassium in the stool

        c. Sorbitol 70% can also be used as a cation exchange resin and is available in both oral and rectal forms

    2. Intravenous medications

        a. Calcium gluconate

            1) This is given to antagonize the effect of potassium on the myocardium and decrease myocardial irritability

            2) Calcium administration does not promote K^+ loss

            3) Carefully monitor clients who are taking digoxin (Lanoxin) because calcium administration can promote digitalis toxicity

        b. Regular insulin and dextrose (usually 50%) solution

            1) Combination therapy is used to shift the potassium from ECF to ICF

            2) This is not a long-term treatment method but rather a short-term treatment to reduce potassium levels

        c. Sodium bicarbonate

            1) This is used to make the cells more alkaline (elevating pH); should only be used with documented acidosis unresponsive to other treatment such as proper ventilation

            2) This shifts the potassium back into the cells (causes transcellular shifting)

3. Diuretic therapy with potassium-wasting diuretics (loop diuretics and thiazide and thiazide-like diuretics) will promote the excretion of potassium from the renal tubules

I. Client education

1. Awareness of predisposing factors

   a. Elderly clients are at risk for hyperkalemia due to multiple medication profile as are clients with multiple disease profiles (such as diabetes and renal failure)

   b. Clients taking medications that promote potassium retention should have periodic lab testing to determine serum levels

   c. Teach clients potential signs and symptoms of hyperkalemia and have them report problems to their healthcare provider

2. Dietary education

   a. Diet education includes knowledge of foods to avoid and permissible foods that contain very little potassium

   b. Teach clients to examine food labels and medication packages to determine potassium content

   c. Teach clients to avoid salt substitutes

J. Evaluation

1. The client returns to and maintains normal serum potassium level

2. The client complies with drug and diet therapies as ordered

3. The client states the early signs and symptoms of hyperkalemia

4. The client maintains adequate gas exchange

5. The client maintains regular cardiac rate and rhythm

Case Study

A 68-year-old male client is admitted to the hospital with complaints of diarrhea for three days. The client reports being weak and feels like his heart is racing.

❶ What questions will the nurse ask when assessing the client's medical history?

❷ What other manifestations might be present?

❸ What laboratory and diagnostic tests might be ordered for this client?

❹ What type of medical interventions would the nurse expect this client to receive?

❺ What information will be provided for this client by the nurse before being discharged and what are the most effective teaching methods for this client?

For suggested responses, see page 231.

Posttest

1 Which of the following serum potassium levels would most likely be seen in a client in the Emergency Department with a three-day history of diarrhea?

(1) 3.6 mEq/L
(2) 4.1 mEq/L
(3) 3.0 mEq/L
(4) 6.2 mEq/L

2 The nurse is instructing a client diagnosed with hyperkalemia about foods to avoid. Which of the following statements by the client indicates a need for further instruction?

(1) "I should avoid eating a lot of bananas."
(2) "I guess I can't eat all the tomatoes I want this summer."
(3) "I can still use my salt substitute instead of real salt."
(4) "No more avocado salads for me."

3 A client is admitted to the hospital with severe hypokalemia. Which of the following data would confirm the diagnosis?

(1) Potassium level 3.3 mEq/L, good skin turgor, and vomiting a small amount of bile-stained emesis
(2) Potassium level 3.8 mEq/L, pink nail beds, and ECG showing a normal sinus rhythm with a rate of 76
(3) Potassium level 3.3 mEq/L, respiratory rate 16 with equal bilateral breath sounds, and two loose stools this morning
(4) Potassium level 3.3 mEq/L, irregular pulse rate, and shallow respirations

4 A client receiving hydrochlorothiazide (HCTZ) should be instructed to report which of the following symptoms to the healthcare provider?

(1) Leg cramps and muscle weakness
(2) Muscle weakness and diarrhea
(3) Fatigue and irritability
(4) Nausea and irritability

5 Which of the following foods should the client who is taking spironolactone (Aldactone) be advised to avoid?

(1) Bread
(2) Cantaloupe
(3) Green beans
(4) Squash

6 A postoperative client with a serum potassium (K^+) level of 3.6 mEq/L is ordered to receive an IV with a potassium supplement (KCl). To maintain safety for this client, the nurse checks to see that the amount ordered does not exceed which of the following standard hourly amounts of KCl infusion?

(1) 10 mEq
(2) 20 mEq
(3) 30 mEq
(4) 40 mEq

7 Which of the following statements indicates the client has an understanding of the side effects of furosemide (Lasix) and its relationship to potassium levels?

(1) "I don't need to take my pulse anymore when I take my Digoxin."
(2) "I should call the doctor if I develop diarrhea."
(3) "I should call my doctor if I feel myself becoming dizzy when I stand up."
(4) "I don't need to eat bananas for breakfast anymore since I am taking this medication."

8 Which of the following is a correct statement by the nurse performing discharge teaching for a client going home with a prescription for spironolactone (Aldactone)?

(1) "Make sure you eat foods such as bananas and oranges."
(2) "Take this pill just before you go to bed."
(3) "Cut back on your intake on those foods on your list that are high in potassium."
(4) "You don't have to watch your intake of fluid while you are taking this medicine."

9 Which of the following clients admitted to the hospital would be at risk for developing hypokalemia?

(1) A client whose blood gases indicate metabolic acidosis
(2) A client who had developed metabolic alkalosis
(3) A client with acute renal failure
(4) A client with adult respiratory distress syndrome (ARDS)

10 Which of the following statements correctly describes intravenous treatment of hyperkalemia associated with severe acidosis carried out by the nurse with an appropriate order?

(1) Calcium gluconate to make the potassium shift from the intracellular fluid (ICF) to the extracellular fluid (ECF)
(2) Insulin and dextrose to make the client hypoglycemic
(3) Sodium bicarbonate to make the client alkalotic so the potassium will shift into the ECF
(4) Normal saline (NS) to provide extra sodium so the potassium will move out of the ICF into the ECF

See pages 82–83 for Answers and Rationales.

Answers and Rationales

Pretest

1 **Answer: 4** *Rationale:* Clients who take furosemide (Lasix) lose potassium and are in danger of developing hypokalemia. The other choices reflect either a normal potassium level (option 3) or elevated levels (options 1 and 2), which would not be consistent with the action of this loop diuretic.
Cognitive Level: Analysis
Nursing Process: Assessment; *Test Plan:* PHYS

2 **Answer: 3** *Rationale:* To prevent gastric irritation, oral potassium supplements should be taken with at least 4 ounces of fluid or with food. Oral potassium medication should not be crushed. The use of a salt substitute is not recommended when taking potassium as a medication because it may also contain potassium, leading to hyperkalemia. It is important for the client to have an understanding of potassium medications, potential side effects, and food/drug interactions.
Cognitive Level: Application
Nursing Process: Implementation; *Test Plan:* HPM

3 **Answer: 1** *Rationale:* Clients in chronic renal failure have diminished or no excretion of potassium from the kidneys, causing hyperkalemia. Clients with intestinal or nasogastric suction, diarrhea, and/or cirrhosis are more likely to be hypokalemic due to potassium losses.
Cognitive Level: Analysis
Nursing Process: Analysis; *Test Plan:* PHYS

4 **Answer: 1** *Rationale:* Clients with renal failure have impaired excretion of potassium resulting in hyperkalemia. Hyperkalemia leads to cardiac conduction problems and possible fatal dysrhythmias. ECG monitoring is indicated for this type of client. LOC, urinary output, and ABGs are important monitoring aspects for a client in renal failure, but hyperkalemia is potentially life-threatening and should be addressed first as the primary intervention.
Cognitive Level: Analysis
Nursing Process: Planning; *Test Plan:* PHYS

5 **Answer: 1** *Rationale:* HCTZ is a diuretic that increases the excretion of potassium, so clients should be taught to increase their intake of potassium in their diet. All of the other medications are considered K-sparing or combination diuretics and, as such, dietary supplementation would not be indicated.
Cognitive Level: Analysis
Nursing Process: Planning; *Test Plan:* PHYS

6 **Answer: 2** *Rationale:* Kayexalate (cation exchange resin) is usually administered rectally and binds potassium in exchange for sodium in the gastrointestinal tract and is then excreted through the stool. Although Kayexalate can be administered orally, it requires administration with an osmotic agent to prevent constipation and may not be tolerated as well. This drug is not given by the IV or the SC route.
Cognitive Level: Application
Nursing Process: Planning; *Test Plan:* PHYS

7 **Answer: 2** *Rationale:* Hypokalemia can lead to alterations in smooth muscle functioning. Smooth muscle alterations in the gastrointestinal tract can lead to development of a paralytic ileus. Complications of

hypokalemia are usually not associated with renal failure, diabetes, or a perforated bowel because these conditions are more likely to lead to increased potassium levels.
Cognitive Level: Analysis
Nursing Process: Assessment; *Test Plan:* PHYS

8 **Answer: 3** *Rationale:* Calcium gluconate is given to antagonize the effects of the potassium on the conduction system of the heart. It is not given to promote potassium excretion (either in urine or stool), and it has no effect on transcellular shifting. The medication acts to blunt the effects of elevated potassium on the myocardium.
Cognitive Level: Analysis
Nursing Process: Planning; *Test Plan:* PHYS

9 **Answer: 2** *Rationale:* Bran flakes are not a source of potassium in the diet. It is important for the client to communicate to the physician if symptoms develop during the course of therapy. Bananas and cantaloupe are excellent sources of dietary potassium. Taking potassium supplements on a full stomach will help to minimize gastric irritation, which is commonly associated with this medication.
Cognitive Level: Analysis
Nursing Process: Evaluation; *Test Plan:* HPM

10 **Answer: 3** *Rationale:* Potassium works to maintain cardiac contractility and normal heart rate. Hypokalemia leads to the development of potential arrhythmias that can result in ischemia and death. While the length of bed rest and actual potassium level could be associated with a complaint of dizziness, it is more likely that the dizziness is associated with orthostatic hypotension and inefficient heart pumping action due to hypokalemia. It is important for the client (and family) to understand that electrolyte imbalances may have significant complications that can affect the entire body.
Cognitive Level: Application
Nursing Process: Implementation; *Test Plan:* PHYS

Posttest

1 **Answer: 3** *Rationale:* A client who has diarrhea or nasogastric suctioning will be more likely to develop hypokalemia. A serum potassium of 3.0 mEq/L is considered to be hypokalemic. A level of 3.6 mEq/L is just within the normal range but one would expect a greater K$^+$ loss given the client's history of three days of diarrhea. A level of 4.1 mEq/L is within the normal range and does not reflect K+ loss. A level of 6.2 mEq/L is suggestive of hyperkalemia.
Cognitive Level: Analysis
Nursing Process: Assessment; *Test Plan:* PHYS

2 **Answer: 3** *Rationale:* Salt substitutes have potassium chloride as their main compound and individuals with high potassium levels should not use salt substitutes. Bananas, tomatoes, and avocados are all foods that are high in potassium and should be limited in a client with hyperkalemia. Clients should be aware of foods to avoid that are high in potassium if teaching has been successful.
Cognitive Level: Analysis
Nursing Process: Evaluation; *Test Plan:* HPM

3 **Answer: 4** *Rationale:* A client with hypokalemia manifests cardiac and respiratory problems related to the ineffective smooth muscle contractions. Option 2 reflects normal findings. The symptoms listed in options 1 and 3 do not indicate severe hypokalemia (even though the serum K$^+$ level is slightly decreased) because the associated symptoms are mild. However, a K$^+$ level of 3.3 mEq/L in conjunction with irregular pulse and shallow respirations is a symptomatic presentation in this client and suggests a severe hypokalemia. It is important to look at the whole clinical picture and not just the serum level to determine the severity of an electrolyte imbalance.
Cognitive Level: Analysis
Nursing Process: Assessment; *Test Plan:* PHYS

4 **Answer: 1** *Rationale:* HCTZ is a potassium-wasting diuretic and its use can lead to hypokalemia. Leg cramps and muscle weakness are two of the symptoms seen in a client with hypokalemia. Diarrhea, fatigue, nausea, and irritability are not usually seen with the use of this class of diuretics.
Cognitive Level: Analysis
Nursing Process: Assessment; *Test Plan:* PHYS

5 **Answer: 2** *Rationale:* Spironolactone is a potassium-sparing diuretic and clients need to be aware of their intake of foods high in potassium. Cantaloupes are very high in potassium and should be avoided. Bread, green beans, and squash are not considered to be good sources of potassium. These foods do not need to be restricted in the diet.
Cognitive Level: Analysis
Nursing Process: Planning; *Test Plan:* HPM

6 **Answer: 1** *Rationale:* The maximum routine rate of infusion for KCl is 5 to 10 mEq/h. Clients who are moderately hypokalemic may have potassium admin-

istered at a rate between 10 to 20mEq/h, but there is nothing to suggest that this client is moderately hypokalemic. Concentrations of potassium in solution can range from 10 to 40 mEq/L and are administered via a peripheral vein with an infusion pump. Higher concentrations of potassium can be administered via a central line in critically ill clients that are hemodynamically monitored.
Cognitive Level: Application
Nursing Process: Implementation; *Test Plan:* SECE

7   **Answer: 3** *Rationale:* Lasix is a potassium-wasting diuretic that can cause the client to become hypokalemic. This can manifest as a weak, thready pulse and onset of orthostatic hypotension. Diarrhea is not usually seen as a side effect of this medication. Monitoring of one's pulse is not required for clients taking diuretic therapy but is necessary for clients taking Digoxin or who have a pacemaker. Bananas are a good source of dietary potassium and may be warranted for this client in order to maintain normal serum potassium levels.
Cognitive Level: Analysis
Nursing Process: Evaluation; *Test Plan:* HPM

8   **Answer: 3** *Rationale:* Aldactone is a potassium-sparing diuretic and the intake of potassium-rich foods should be discouraged. It is important that the client be aware of potassium retaining diuretics as most clients associate diuretics with potassium loss. Diuretics should not be taken before going to bed because their primary effect is diuresis. This time frame could cause the client to experience altered sleep patterns due to nocturia. Clients taking diuretics should be aware of their fluid intake and monitor accordingly.
Cognitive Level: Analysis
Nursing Process: Implementation; *Test Plan:* HPM

9   **Answer: 2** *Rationale:* A client with metabolic alkalosis is at risk for developing hypokalemia due to the shift of potassium to the ICF from the ECF. Clients with acute renal failure are usually hyperkalemic due to a decreased ability to excrete potassium. Clients with ARDS are usually hyperkalemic due to compromised ventilation, resulting in metabolic acidosis. Metabolic acidosis is associated with hyperkalemia because potassium shifts from the ECF to the ICF as a result of increase in hydrogen ion concentration.
Cognitive Level: Analysis
Nursing Process: Analysis; *Test Plan:* PHYS

10   **Answer: 3** *Rationale:* Sodium bicarbonate will temporarily alkalinize the plasma, causing the potassium to move into the cells. NS is an isotonic solution and therefore will not cause fluid or electrolyte shifting. Calcium gluconate is given to blunt the effects on the myocardium; it does not decrease the serum K^+ level. Insulin and dextrose are given to decrease K^+ levels by increasing K^+ uptake at the cellular level.
Cognitive Level: Application
Nursing Process: Analysis; *Test Plan:* PHYS

References

Ball, J. & Bindler, R. (1999). *Pediatric nursing: Caring for children* (2nd ed.). Stamford, CT: Appleton & Lange, pp. 310–316.

Horne, M. M. & Bond, E. F. (2000). Fluid, electrolyte and acid-base imbalances. In S. M. Lewis, M. M. Heitkemper, & S. R. Dirksen (Eds.). *Medical-surgical nursing: Assessment and management of clinical problems* (5th ed.). St. Louis: Mosby, pp. 335–338.

Kozier, B., Erb, G., Berman, A., & Burke, K. (2000). *Fundamentals of nursing: Concepts, process, and practice* (6th ed.). Upper Saddle River, NJ: Prentice-Hall, Inc., pp. 1315–1317.

LeMone, P. & Burke, K. (2000). *Medical-surgical nursing: Critical thinking in client care* (2nd ed.). Upper Saddle River, NJ: Prentice-Hall, Inc., pp. 126–133.

Pagana, K. D. & Pagana, T. J. (2001). *Mosby's diagnostic and laboratory test reference* (5th ed.) St. Louis: Mosby, pp. 676–678.

Patton, K. T. & Thibodeau, G. A. (2000). *Mosby's handbook of anatomy and physiology.* St. Louis: Mosby, pp. 22, 497.

Schmidt, T. C. & Williams-Evans, S. A. (2000). How to recognize hypokalemia, *Nursing 30*(2), p. 22.

Skidmore-Roth, L. (1999). *Mosby's drug reference.* St. Louis: Mosby, pp. 825–827.

Smeltzer, S. C. & Bare, B. G. (2000). *Brunner and Suddarth's medical-surgical nursing* (9th ed.). Philadelphia: Lippincott, pp. 203–221.

Understanding hypokalemia. (2000). *Nursing 30*(11), pp. 74–76.

Williams, B. R. & Baer, C. L. (1998). *Essentials of clinical pharmacology in nursing* (3rd ed.). Springhouse, PA: Springhouse, pp. 624–628.

Workman, M. (1999). Interventions for clients with electrolyte imbalances. In D. Ignatavicius, M. Workman, & M. Mishler (Eds.), *Medical-surgical nursing across the health care continuum* (3rd ed.). Philadelphia: W. B. Saunders, pp. 243–250.

CHAPTER 4

Calcium Balance and Imbalances

Kristy A. Nielson, BSN, CCRN, BS

CHAPTER OUTLINE

OBJECTIVES

▋ Review basic functions of calcium in the body.

▋ Discuss the pathophysiology and etiology of calcium imbalances.

▋ Discuss specific assessment findings in calcium imbalances.

▋ Identify priority nursing diagnoses for a client experiencing a calcium imbalance.

▋ Discuss therapeutic management of calcium imbalances.

▋ Discuss nursing management of a client who is experiencing a calcium imbalance.

[Media Link]

Use the CD-ROM enclosed with this text, or log onto the address given to access the free, interactive Companion Website created for this series. The CD-ROM and Companion Website accompanying this book offer additional practice opportunities and information—NCLEX Review, Case Studies, Glossary, In Depth with NCLEX, and more.

www.prenhall.com/hogan

REVIEW AT A GLANCE

calcitonin *also called thyrocalcitonin; a calcium-lowering hormone produced by the thyroid gland that lowers calcium by inhibition of bone-resorbing osteoclasts and the promotion of osteoblasts that lead to bone formation*

calcitriol *the active hormone form of vitamin D; promotes absorption of calcium in intestines, decreases calcium excretion via the kidneys, and acts with PTH to maintain homeostasis*

calcium pump *a "pump" driven by ATP that takes calcium into and out of cells and is initiated by some type of mechanical or electrical stimulus during relaxation and contraction of skeletal (involves a change in membrane potential) and smooth muscle (intracellular calcium causes contraction)*

Chvostek's sign *tapping over the facial nerve just anterior to the ear and observing for ipsilateral facial muscle contraction or twitching that indicates a positive response and is a sign of hypocalcemia; a form of latent tetany*

hypercalcemia *increased total serum calcium concentration to > 10.5 mg/dL*

hyperparathyroidism *a condition caused by excess levels of parathyroid hormone in the body, demonstrated by a PTH > 55 pg/dL*

hypocalcemia *decreased total serum calcium concentration to < 8.5 mg/dL; any condition that causes a decrease in the production of PTH may result in development of hypocalcemia*

hypoparathyroidism *a condition caused by insufficient or absent secretion of the parathyroid glands, demonstrated by a PTH level < 11 pg/dL*

ionized calcium *represents approximately 40 to 50% of the calcium that is free or not bound to albumin; the calcium level that is physiologically useful and elicits the signs and symptoms of hypocalcemia*

osteoblasts *bone-forming cells that lay down new bone; responsive to PTH and are stimulated by activated vitamin D; adapt to stress on the bone by strengthening the bone mass; a form of osteocyte*

osteoclasts *cells that resorb (remove calcium from the bone) during the processes of bone growth and repair; derived from monocytes that are produced in the bone marrow; monocytes travel through the bloodstream and collect at sites of bone resorption, where they fuse together to become osteocytes (cells that erode old bone)*

osteoporosis *reduction of bone mass (or density) or the presence of a fragility fracture*

parathyroid hormone *hormone produced by the parathyroid glands; regulates serum calcium by way of a negative feedback system; main role is to increase serum calcium by stimulating bone resorption, increasing renal calcium absorption, and promoting renal conversion of vitamin D to its active metabolite, calcitriol; under normal conditions, when calcium is low, PTH increases; conversely, when calcium is high, PTH decreases; normal PTH level is 11 to 55 pg/dL*

tetany *neurologic disorder marked by intermittent spasms that are usually paroxysmal and involve the extremities; calls for immediate intervention*

Trousseau's sign *inflation of a blood pressure cuff on the upper arm to 20 mm Hg above the client's systolic pressure for about 3 minutes leads to carpal spasm; a form of latent tetany*

Vitamin D *a fat-soluble vitamin absorbed from food and synthesized in skin exposed to sunlight*

Pretest

1 A client with hypocalcemia asks the nurse why calcium is so important. The nurse would base a response on which of the following functions that is unique to calcium?

(1) Regulation of acid-base balance
(2) Activation of enzymes to stimulate chemical reactions
(3) Stimulation of cardiac muscle to produce contraction
(4) Promotion of total body water balance

2 The results of a client's laboratory tests show an elevated ionized calcium and parathyroid hormone (PTH). The nurse suspects that the cause is:

(1) Hypoparathyroidism.
(2) A malignancy.
(3) Hyperparathyroidism.
(4) Vitamin D deficiency.

3 A client becomes hypocalcemic as a result of prolonged nasogastric (NG) tube suctioning. The nurse concludes that the primary cause for hypocalcemia at this time is:

(1) Metabolic alkalosis.
(2) Fluid shifts from hypoalbuminemia.
(3) Hypermagnesemia.
(4) Metabolic acidosis.

4 A client has a diagnosis of ovarian cancer and is undergoing chemotherapy. The client's calcium level is now elevated. The nurse suspects that:

(1) Antineoplastic medications are the cause for this elevation in calcium.
(2) The ovarian cancer has metastasized, causing the increase in calcium.
(3) The client is not eating enough dairy products as a result of decreased appetite.
(4) The client is developing pancreatitis.

5 A client with a calcium imbalance has been prescribed large doses of corticosteroids for another condition. Which of the following would be a high priority nursing diagnosis for this client?

(1) Potential complication: electrolyte imbalance, hypocalcemia
(2) Altered nutrition: more than body requirements for calcium
(3) Fluid volume deficit
(4) Risk for electrolyte excess: hypercalcemia

6 The nurse is assessing a client with hypercalcemia. The nurse expects neuromuscular examination to show:

(1) Tetany.
(2) A positive Trousseau's sign.
(3) Muscle weakness.
(4) Hyperactive deep tendon reflexes.

7 A nurse is caring for a client with a diagnosis of hypercalcemia. Which of the following cardiac signs should the nurse monitor on the electrocardiogram (ECG)?

(1) Development of atrial fibrillation
(2) Shortening of the QT interval
(3) Hypotension
(4) Prolonged QT interval

8 A nurse prepares to administer calcium gluconate to a client post-thyroidectomy. The nurse explains to the licensed practical nurse (LPN) that the rationale for this replacement therapy is:

(1) Because of accidental removal of the parathyroid gland.
(2) Related to increased parathyroid hormone (PTH) release during surgery.
(3) To prevent complications from immobility postoperatively.
(4) Due to hypophosphatemia after this type of surgery.

9 A client presents with complaints of fatigue, headache, and increasing muscle weakness. The nurse anticipates medical management to include:

(1) Thiazide diuretics.
(2) Vitamin D supplements.
(3) Fluid restriction.
(4) Increased hydration.

10 The nurse evaluates that discharge teaching has been effective when the client with hypocalcemia states:

(1) "I shouldn't take antacids such as TUMS."
(2) "I should notify my healthcare provider if I start to feel tingling or numbness around my mouth."
(3) "I'll need to cut down on the protein in my diet."
(4) "I will watch my urine for signs of kidney stones."

See pages 109–110 for Answers and Rationales.

I. Overview of Calcium Regulation

    A. Calcium balance and function: major extracellular cation; mainly found in the hard part of the bones where it is stored; concentration of calcium is kept constant by a **calcium pump** that constantly moves calcium in and out of cells

        1. Serum levels

            a. Normal total serum concentration is approximately 8.5 to 10.5 mg/dL

            b. Ionized calcium level 4.0 to 5.0 mg/dL

    c. Slightly different laboratory reference ranges may appear due to differences in laboratory calibration; always check reference ranges with regard to established laboratory criteria

    d. Three forms of calcium exist in the body

        1) 45% is bound to protein, mostly albumin; part of the total serum calcium concentration

        2) 40% is **ionized calcium** (calcium that is free or unbound from proteins, specifically albumin); it is the calcium that is physiologically active and clinically important for neuromuscular transmission; many symptoms of low calcium are often not apparent until the ionized calcium is < 4.0 mg/dL; though many laboratories perform total serum calcium levels most often, ionized calcium levels are recommended for the critically ill client

        3) 15% is bound to other substances such as phosphate, citrate, or carbonate

    e. The concentration of serum proteins, specifically albumin, is an important determinant of calcium concentration; remember to evaluate the calcium in relation to the serum albumin as changes in the serum protein level can cause changes in the serum calcium level

    f. Certain formulas can be used to obtain a calcium level corrected for an albumin level; for example, the total serum calcium will decrease or increase 0.8 g/dL for every 1 g/dL decrease or increase in albumin above or below 4 mg/dL

2. Functions in the body

    a. Important in enzyme activation to stimulate many essential chemical reactions required for hormone secretion and the function of cell receptors

    b. Significant role in skeletal and heart muscle relaxation, activation, excitation, and contraction

    c. Exerts a sedating, or calming, effect on nerve cells

    d. Plays a major role in nerve impulse transmission as it determines the speed of ionic influxes through nerve membranes

    e. Plays a role in blood clotting by activating specific steps as an enzymatic cofactor in blood coagulation, the most important being the conversion of prothrombin to thrombin

    f. Assists in regulation of acid-base balance

    g. Gives firmness and rigidity to bones and teeth

    h. Maintains membrane permeability by holding body cells together

    i. Essential for lactation

3. System interactions

    a. Parathyroid hormone (PTH) raises the plasma calcium level by promoting the transfer of calcium from the bone to plasma

        1) PTH responds to the ionized calcium level, regulates the concentration of calcium in the ECF, and has bone-resorbing (removal of calcium from the bone) effects

2) PTH helps with intestinal absorption of calcium by activating **vitamin D** (a fat-soluble vitamin)

3) PTH also aids in calcium reabsorption (where calcium is taken up) in the kidneys

4) The overall effect of PTH is to increase calcium and decrease phosphorus

5) Under normal conditions, PTH responds to changes in the ionized calcium via a negative feedback system; if the ionized calcium level is low, the PTH will be elevated; conversely, if the ionized calcium level is high, the PTH will be low

6) Normal PTH level is 11–54 pg/mL

b. Calcium is dependent upon **calcitriol,** the most active form of vitamin D

1) Calcitriol makes calcium and phosphate available for new bone formation

2) It plays a major role in the prevention of symptomatic **hypocalcemia** (abnormally low serum calcium level) and hypomagnesemia (decreased serum, clinically noted by increased neuromuscular irritability)

3) Calcitriol also promotes calcium absorption from the intestine (duodenum), helps PTH mobilize calcium from the bone, and limits calcium excretion if the client has **hypercalcemia** (elevated serum calcium concentration)

c. **Calcitonin,** a calcium-lowering hormone produced by the thyroid gland, acts against PTH by transferring calcium from the plasma to the skeletal system

1) Calcitonin is directly secreted when serum calcium is high, thus lowering the plasma calcium level

2) Calcitonin inhibits osteoclastic activity and promotes osteoblasts that result in bone formation; **osteoclasts** resorb (remove) bone during the process of growth and repair, while **osteoblasts** are bone-forming cells that respond to PTH, which in turn is stimulated by the activated form of vitamin D

d. Calcium interferes with the absorption of iron, so those with high levels of calcium may be prone to iron deficiency

e. Calcium has inverse or reciprocal relationship with phosphorus; when calcium goes up, phosphorus levels go down; conversely, when calcium levels decrease, phosphorus levels increase

B. Sources of calcium

1. Cellular level

a. Over 99% of the body's calcium is deposited in the bones, but can be mobilized from bones to keep blood level constant when dietary intake is inadequate

b. The < 1% outside the bone is located in the extracellular fluid and soft tissues

c. A total of 1 to 2 kg of calcium is present in the average adult

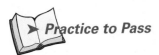

Practice to Pass

Can you identify the system interactions that control calcium concentrations in the body?

d. Calcium pump in the body helps to regulate the flow of calcium at the cellular level

e. 30% is absorbed in GI tract

NCLEX!

f. In the kidney, 98% of the filtered calcium is reabsorbed in the proximal renal tubules and then excreted by the kidneys; rates of reabsorption of filtered calcium are high

2. Dietary level

NCLEX!

a. Calcium is obtained from ingested foods; about 40% of calcium consumed is absorbed

b. Adults should consume at least 1,000–1,200 mg (1–1.2 gm) of calcium daily

c. Infants require 270 mg, children ages 1 to 3 need 500 mg, children ages 4 to 8 should have 800 mg, and the requirement of children ages 9 to 18 is 1,300 mg daily

d. Pregnant, lactating, and postmenopausal women should consume 1.2 to 1.5 grams of calcium daily

e. Upper limit for calcium intake is 2.5 grams daily

f. Foods high in dietary calcium include milk, yogurt, cheese, calcium-fortified orange juice, ice cream, canned salmon, sardines, broccoli, tofu, rhubarb, spinach, almonds, figs, and turnip greens

g. Dietary factors affecting calcium absorption include oxalic acids found in beets, spinach and peanuts, phytic acids found in grains, excess phosphorus consumption, and polyphenols (tannins) found in teas (see Box 4-1 for a listing of factors affecting calcium absorption)

NCLEX!

II. Hypocalcemia: abnormally low calcium level (< 8.5 mg/dL) or decreased availability of ionized calcium

A. Etiology and pathophysiology

NCLEX!

1. Cellular level transport

a. Moves in and out of cells via a calcium pump

Box 4-1
Factors That Affect Calcium Absorption in the Body

The following factors promote calcium absorption:

- Vitamin D
- Milk products
- Adequate stomach acid
- Growth hormones

The following factors decrease calcium absorption:

- Vitamin D deficiency
- High intake of phosphorous, protein, and/or fiber in the diet
- Phytates, oxalates, and polyphenols (tannins)
- Decreased absorption with aging

    b. Adds to bone by osteoblasts—bone-forming cells that lay down new bone

    c. Calcium is responsive to PTH and is stimulated by activated vitamin D

2. Predisposing clinical conditions result from decreased physiologic availability of calcium, decreased calcium intake or absorption, or increased calcium excretion (see Box 4-2 for a listing of clinical conditions that can lead to hypocalcemia)

    a. Hypoparathyroidism: a condition caused by insufficient or lack of secretion of PTH by the parathyroid glands

        1) Primary (or idiopathic) hypoparathyroidism is due to tumor or depressed function or a hereditary disorder and secondary hypoparathyroidism is related to surgical removal of the parathyroid glands

        2) Postsurgical symptoms of hypocalcemia may be due to impaired blood supply to the remaining parathyroid tissue or possibly the release of calcitonin from the thyroid gland

    b. Hypomagnesemia: abnormally low magnesium levels (< 1 mg/dL)

        1) Magnesium helps regulate the mechanisms that keep serum calcium within normal

        2) If magnesium is low, PTH release is impaired, lowering the serum calcium

        3) Hypomagnesemia lowers the threshold for **tetany,** the neurologic disorder marked by intermittent spasms that are usually paroxysmal and involve the extremities

---

Box 4-2	
Clinical Conditions That Lead to the Development of Hypocalcemia	• Hypoparathyroidism • Hypomagnesemia • Alkalotic states • Multiple blood transfusions • Medications (loop diuretics, anticonvulsants, citrate-buffered blood products, phosphates, antineoplastic agents, radiographic contrast media, corticosteroids, biphosphonates, antacids, and heparin) • Hypoalbuminemia • Acute pancreatitis • Hyperphosphatemia • Vitamin D deficiency • Malabsorptive states • Renal disease • Alcoholism • Neonatal hypocalcemia • Gram-negative sepsis • Medullary thyroid carcinoma • Burns

4) Hypomagnesemia is also seen with hypokalemia and hypocalcemia

5) Many medications that decrease magnesium also cause hypocalcemia

c. Alkalosis: an actual or relative increase in the alkalinity of the blood due to accumulation of bases or reduction in acid (pH > 7.45)

1) In alkalosis, more ionized calcium binds to albumin

2) Though serum calcium may be normal, symptoms such as tetany occur due to the decrease in physiologically active ionized calcium

3) Tetany may result if the pH rises above 7.6; prolonged nasogastric tube (NGT) suctioning or diarrhea lead to metabolic alkalosis

NCLEX!

d. Massive blood transfusion: citrate is a preservative added to units of red blood cells that acts as an anticoagulant; in massive rapid transfusions, citrate can combine with ionized calcium and render this inactive, leading to a transient hypocalcemia (due to citrate toxicity)

NCLEX!

e. Medications that can lead to the development of hypocalcemia include:

1) Loop diuretics such as furosemide (Lasix) and ethacrynic acid (Edecrin): promote renal excretion of calcium

2) Phenytoin (Dilantin) and phenobarbital: may alter the hepatic metabolism of vitamin D

3) Citrate-buffered blood and blood products: citrate prevents calcium from becoming ionized and causes transient hypocalcemia

4) Phosphates: oral, IV, or enema; increase phosphorus levels thus decreasing calcium level

5) Plicamycin (Mithracin), calcitonin, and etidronate disodium (Didrone): inhibit bone resorption of calcium

6) Antineoplastic drugs such as cisplatin (Platinol) and antibiotics such as gentamicin (Garamycin) and tetracycline (Achromycin): lower the magnesium level, thus lowering calcium

7) Some radiographic contrast media, such as gallium nitrate: inhibit bone resorption

8) Corticosteroids: large doses can reduce calcium absorption in intestine and increase calcium excretion

9) Biphosphonate drugs, such as pamidronate (Aredia): inhibit bone resorption in excess doses

10) Antacids containing magnesium: compete with calcium in the intestines

11) Heparin, protamine, and glucagon: promote bone resorption and lead to **osteoporosis,** a condition resulting from a reduction in bone mass or density or the presence of a fragility fracture

NCLEX!

f. Hypoalbuminemia (low serum albumin levels < 3.5 g/dL): can result in low total serum calcium concentration although the ionized calcium may be normal; signs of hypocalcemia occur when the ionized calcium level falls below normal; among the causes are malnutrition, malabsorption syndromes, burns, and chronic renal failure

g. Acute pancreatitis

   1) PTH secretion is inadequate with this disorder, thereby preventing the uptake of calcium from the bones to correct the hypocalcemia

   2) There is also a lack of pancreatic lipase from impaired fat digestion

   3) Dietary calcium and calcium secreted into the intestine from the ECF bind to undigested fat in the intestine and are excreted, which results in decreased calcium absorption and increased calcium excretion

   4) May also be the result of secretion of calcitonin when the inflamed pancreas secretes excessive glucagon

h. Hyperphosphatemia—excessive phosphorus levels (> 4.5 mg/dL): phosphorus has a reciprocal relationship with calcium; is commonly seen in clients with renal failure; may also occur with excess treatment of hypercalcemia resulting in the lowering of calcium; excessive phosphorus in total parenteral nutrition (TPN) may also contribute to hypocalcemia

i. Inadequate vitamin D: due to inadequate dietary consumption, insufficient exposure to sunlight, or malabsorption states; recall that calcium absorption occurs in the duodenum only in the presence of activated vitamin D

j. Malabsorption syndromes: may occur in conditions when effective intestinal surfaces are lost, making fewer available sites for calcium absorption

   1) It is important to remember that calcium absorption occurs primarily in the small intestine

   2) Conditions such as Crohn's disease, small bowel resection, partial gastrectomy with gastrojejunostomy, and jejunoileal bypass or excessive laxative use may interfere with calcium absorption

k. Renal disease: kidneys cannot produce activated form of vitamin D (calcitriol), which leads to reduced use of calcium, thus hypocalcemia; this also associated with renal disease, which decreases calcium levels

l. Alcoholism: may lead to intestinal malabsorption, dietary deficiencies, hypoalbuminemia, pancreatitis, and hypomagnesemia, all of which contribute to deceased calcium levels

m. Neonatal hypocalcemia: due to functional immaturity of the parathyroid glands during the first three days of life; after the first three days, hypocalcemia may be caused by milk with a high phosphate content; those at high risk are those with asphyxia at birth and infants born to Type 1 diabetic mothers

n. Gram-negative sepsis: leads to a decrease in ionized calcium and as such is a true hypocalcemia; possible causes are parathyroid gland insufficiency, inadequate dietary Vitamin D, or renal hydroxylase insufficiency

o. Medullary thyroid carcinoma: may produce hypocalcemia if excess calcitonin is secreted by the tumor

p. Burns: fluid shifts outside the cell with burn or wound injuries cause hypoalbuminemia

> **➤ Practice to Pass**
>
> What are the predisposing conditions that lead to calcium imbalance in the body?

B. Assessment

1. Clinical manifestations: due to increased neuromuscular irritability (see Table 4-1)

   a. Common signs

      1) Cardiovascular: decreased blood pressure and myocardial contractility leading to pulse rate and rhythm changes; ECG changes include prolonged QT interval and lengthened ST segment; cardiac arrest can occur

      2) Respiratory: laryngospasm can occur leading to respiratory compromise and airway failure; respiratory arrest can occur

      3) Renal: low serum calcium levels are associated with renal failure; other electrolyte disturbances are seen in conjunction with clinical manifestations of renal failure

NCLEX!

Table 4-1	System	Manifestations of Hypocalcemia	Manifestations of Hypercalcemia
Comparison of Clinical Manifestations of Hypocalcemia and Hypercalcemia	Neuromuscular	Tetany Positive Chvostek's sign Positive Trousseau's sign Hyperactive deep tendon reflexes (DTRs) Laryngospasm Seizures	Muscle weakness Increased fatigue Depressed DTRs
	Gastrointestinal	Hyperactive bowel sounds Abdominal cramps	Hypotonic bowel sounds Nausea/vomiting Constipation Anorexia
	Central nervous system	Irritability Depression Apprehension Confusion Delusions Hallucinations Memory impairment Convulsions Anxiety	Headache Personality changes Acute psychosis Confusion Bizarre behavior Lethargy Memory impairment Coma
	Cardiac	Hypotension Decreased myocardial contractility Prolonged QT interval Lengthened ST segment Cardiac arrest	Hypertension Heart block Shortened QT interval Shortened ST segment Cardiac arrest
	Respiratory	Respiratory arrest	No major manifestations
	Renal	Oliguria Anuria	Polyuria Polydipsia Renal colic Kidney stones
	Hematologic	Increased bleeding and bruising	No major manifestations
	Integumentary	Dry, brittle nails and hair	No major manifestations

4) Neuromuscular

    a) Positive **Trousseau's sign:** inflation of blood pressure cuff on upper arm to 20 mm above the systolic BP for about 3 minutes results in carpopedal spasm

    b) Positive **Chvostek's sign:** tapping over the facial nerve just anterior to the ear results in ipsilateral facial muscle contracting or twitching

    c) Above signs are clinical indicators of tetany; characterized by hyperactive deep tendon reflexes; seizures can occur

NCLEX!

5) Gastrointestinal: possible hyperactive bowel sounds and diarrhea

6) Musculoskeletal: possible bone fractures due to demineralization; in children, chronic hypocalcemia may retard growth and cause rickets; can lead to osteomalacia and osteoporosis in adults

7) Other systems: increased bleeding from abnormal clotting mechanisms; development of cataracts and calcification of basal ganglia

NCLEX!

b. Common symptoms

1) Neuromuscular: paresthesias and tingling in the hands and feet; muscle spasms of the extremities and face; hyperactive reflexes and increased irritability and apprehension; mental status changes ranging from depression, memory impairment, delusion, and hallucinations to convulsions

2) Other system complaints: intestinal cramps; dry, brittle nails and dry hair; complaints of bone pain; increased bleeding or bruising may occur

2. Diagnostic and laboratory findings

  a. Plasma levels, urinary levels, and radiology measurements

1) Total serum calcium < 8.5 mg/dL

2) Ionized calcium level < 4.0 mg/dL or < 40%

3) 24-hour urinary calcium level (reference levels): low calcium diet < 150 mg/24 hours; average calcium diet 100–250 mg/24 hours; high calcium diet 250–300 mg/24 hours; useful for determining parathyroid gland disorders

4) X-rays to detect bone fractures and thinning

5) Bone mass density tests for signs of osteoporosis

6) CT scan to detect tumors of the parathyroid gland

  b. Associated electrolyte levels

1) Hypomagnesemia (< 1 mg/dL)

2) Hypokalemia (< 3.5 mg/dL)

3) Hyperphosphatemia (> 2.6 mg/dL)

4) Albumin < 3.5 g/dL

5) PTH < 11 mg/dL if caused by hypoparathyroidism

6) Elevated creatinine from renal insufficiency

7) Elevated alkaline phosphatase

    c. Trending of results

        1) ECG tracings demonstrate characteristic changes with hypocalcemia; trending ECG changes can help to monitor client's status and response to therapeutic treatment

        2) Monitor appropriate electrolyte levels (calcium, phosphorus, magnesium, potassium) and serum chemistry findings (albumin, BUN, and creatinine levels)

        3) Monitor albumin and PTH levels

        4) Review results of x-rays and bone density tests

  3. Identification of risk factors

    a. Assess for factors that increase the risk of hypocalcemia

NCLEX!

        1) Postmenopausal women not taking estrogen

        2) Post-thyroidectomy or parathyroidectomy

        3) Family history of hereditary hypoparathyroidism

        4) Clients with history of Crohn's or small bowel dysfunction

        5) Clients with an increased incidence of fractures

NCLEX!

        6) Clients who are immobile (or bedfast), due to inadequate calcium stores present in the body as a consequence of immobility

        7) Clients who have osteoporosis and/or osteopenia

    b. Medications

        1) Obtain pertinent client history of medications that can alter calcium levels

        2) Examine both prescription and over-the-counter (OTC) medications and supplements that the client is taking for possible interactions

    c. Dietary

NCLEX!

        1) Dietary patterns that lack adequate calcium and vitamin D sources

        2) Excessive use of dietary phosphorous supplements

        3) Clients with eating disorders who use laxatives as part of their dietary pattern

        4) Lactose-intolerant clients who may be at risk for not meeting adequate calcium intake needs unless alternative form products are used

        5) Dietary factors that limit absorption of calcium (oxalates, phytates, and tannins)

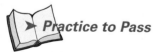

Practice to Pass

Explain how the neurologic system is affected by hypocalcemia.

C. Priority nursing diagnoses: Potential complication: hypocalcemia; Decreased cardiac output; Risk for injury related to tetany and seizures; Risk for impaired gas exchange; Potential complication: fracture; Potential complication: respiratory arrest; Potential complication: osteoporosis; Altered nutrition: less than body requirement of calcium; Knowledge deficit; Risk for noncompliance

D. Therapeutic management: treatment focuses on restoring normal levels, preventing complications, and treating underlying problems

1. Replacement therapies

   NCLEX!

   a. Calcium gluconate 10% solution, 500 mg to 2 g at a rate of < 0.5 mL/min (10–20 mL) by slow IV push or calcium chloride 10% solution, 500 mg to 1 g (5–10 mL) at a rate < 1 mL/min by slow IV push in an emergency

   b. All calcium preparations can cause venous irritation, but calcium chloride causes more venous irritation and may cause sloughing of tissue, so calcium gluconate is the most commonly used preparation

   c. Administer with D_5W or normal saline (NS) and do not add to solutions containing bicarbonate because rapid precipitation may occur

   d. May give slow IV infusion of calcium gluconate until tetany has been controlled or until calcium reaches 8–9 mg/dL

   NCLEX!

   e. Daily oral doses of elemental calcium, usually 1.0–3.0 grams/day

   f. Postoperative clients may require an additional supplement with calcitriol 0.5–1.0 mcg/dL; dosage range based upon cause or complication of hypocalcemia

   g. Vitamin D supplements may be ordered: 1–3 mg/dL with supplemental calcitriol 0.25–1.0 mcg/dL if hypocalcemia from vitamin D dietary deficiency

   h. Phosphorus binding antacids may be ordered to increase calcium

   i. If hypomagnesemia present, must be corrected with 50% magnesium sulfate 2–4 mL over 15 minutes, followed by infusion of 48 mEq in one liter or more over 24 hours

   j. Thiazide diuretics may be used to decrease urinary excretion of calcium

2. Continued monitoring of client (laboratory values and physical manifestations) to watch for efficacy of treatment

   NCLEX!

   a. Continuous ECG monitoring, especially during calcium gluconate or calcium chloride administration

   b. Continually reassess neurologic, respiratory, and cardiac status

   c. Monitor clients receiving calcium replacement who are also on digitalis for enhanced digitalis effect—check pulse

   d. Monitor clients who may experience hypocalcemia as a result of surgical intervention and/or possible endocrine dysfunction

3. Restoration of balance (normal serum Ca^{++} level) to maintain homeostasis and prevent development of further complications

   a. Monitor serum magnesium and potassium levels in clients who are hypocalcemic because sometimes there can be concurrent electrolyte abnormalities that may require correction

   b. Monitor endocrine function and evaluate PTH status

E. Planning and implementation

1. Obtain thorough nursing history and physical examination

   NCLEX!

   a. Subjective: such as symptoms, family history, previous thyroid, or parathyroid surgeries

   b. Objective: such as signs of hypocalcemia, predisposing clinical conditions, risk factors

   NCLEX!

   c. Medication history: medications that may cause hypocalcemia, hypomagnesemia, or hyperphosphatemia; OTC and herbal therapies that may interfere with calcium function

2. Monitor pertinent client assessment data for potential effects related to hypocalcemia and for response to therapeutic treatment

   a. Monitor serum calcium, phosphate, magnesium, albumin, creatinine, PTH, and potassium levels and report abnormal findings to healthcare provider

   b. ECG changes and heart rate and rhythm pattern

   NCLEX!

   c. Observe for signs of tetany and document findings relative to Chvostek's and Trousseau's signs; check reflexes

3. Monitor therapeutic serum drug levels for clients taking cardiac glycosides because calcium replacement therapy can enhance effects of digitalis

4. Assess for signs of dehydration that may result from diarrhea or renal insufficiency

   NCLEX!

5. Assess intake and output: maintain intake of 2,000–3,000 mL/day and an output of 1,000–1,500 mL/day; monitor daily weight

   NCLEX!

6. Protect the client from injury and maintain a safe environment, as the client is likely to present with neuromuscular changes

   a. Be knowledgeable and prepared for emergencies as a result of hypocalcemia, such as tetany, seizures, laryngospasm, and respiratory and cardiac arrest

   b. Initiate seizure precautions and maintain a quiet environment

   c. Closely observe respiratory and airway status; have emergency tracheostomy kit available and IV calcium gluconate at bedside for postoperative thyroidectomy clients (may have inadvertent removal of parathyroid gland)

   d. Observe for signs of tetany for clients receiving multiple blood transfusions

   e. Observe for signs of bleeding or increased bruising

7. Monitor for the possibility of hypercalcemia as a result of replacement therapy

F. Medication therapy

   NCLEX!

1. Oral replacement therapy

   a. Approximately 1.5–3.0 grams/day of oral calcium gluconate is needed to raise total calcium by 1 mg/dL

   b. Calcium citrate and calcium lactates are other oral calcium salts that are more soluble and may be better absorbed in the elderly; calcium is best absorbed when taken in divided doses vs. all at once

    c. Calcitonin may by be prescribed instead of calcium salts for post-menopausal women who cannot take estrogen; subcutaneous or IM salmon calcitonin doses are 100 IU/d or intranasally: 1 spray (200 IU) daily, alternating nostrils

    d. Vitamin D supplements may be ordered, initially 400–1,000 IU/day if dietary deficiency is present or calcitriol (Rocatrol) 0.25–0.5 mg/capsule, then maintenance

2. Parenteral replacement therapy

    a. For severe hypocalcemia, 10% calcium gluconate solution, 500 mg–2 g at a rate of < 0.5 mL/min (10–20 mL) by slow IV push or 10% calcium chloride solution, 500 mg–1 g (5–10mL) at a rate < 1 mL/min by slow IV push in emergency; too-rapid administration can cause bradycardia and cardiac arrest; may give slow IV infusion of calcium gluconate in D_5W or NS until signs of tetany are controlled or calcium is 8–9 mg/dL; may cause precipitation with bicarbonate

    b. Calcium chloride produces a higher ionized calcium level and is more irritating to the vein, so it is used less frequently than calcium gluconate

    c. For post operative hypocalcemia from thyroidectomy, radical neck dissection, or parathyroidectomy, an infusion of calcium gluconate may be needed in the first 24 to 48 hours; titrate to clinical signs and calcium levels; this hypocalcemia is usually transient

3. Dietary therapy

    a. Recommendation for older clients is 1,000–1,500 mg daily

    b. Encourage adequate calcium intake from the various food groups daily; encourage foods high in calcium, such as dairy products

    c. Be aware of foods that decrease the absorption of calcium and possibly limit them in the diet pattern

G. Client education

1. Awareness of predisposing factors associated with developing hypocalcemia

    a. Teach clients that paresthesias and tingling and numbness in extremities are early warning signs of tetany

    b. Instruct clients to report the onset of signs of tetany or seizures immediately to healthcare provider

    c. Instruct clients to take oral replacements as prescribed

    d. Instruct clients to avoid overuse of antacids containing phosphorus

    e. Instruct clients to avoid overuse of laxatives

    f. Teach clients importance of regular exercise

2. Dietary education

    a. Educate clients about foods rich in calcium and protein

    b. Teach clients that sources of vitamin D and protein are important to keep calcium within normal

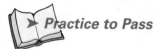

> **Practice to Pass**
>
> A client has received calcium gluconate IV push for severe hypo-calcemia. How will you evaluate the therapeutic response to calcium gluconate and what nursing interventions are appropriate for this therapy?

    c. Provide information on appropriate substitutes for milk and dairy products if client is lactose intolerant

    d. Teach clients to avoid foods or antacids high in phosphorus

    e. Teach clients about foods that decrease absorption of calcium and limit them in the diet pattern

    f. Collaborate with dietitian to meet dietary goals

H. Evaluation

    1. Total serum calcium is between 8.5–10.5 mg/dL; ionized calcium level is between 4.0 and 5.0 mg/dL; urine calcium within normal reference range

    2. Resolution of signs and symptoms of hypocalcemia

    3. Levels of magnesium, potassium, and phosphorus are within normal limits

    4. PTH levels are within normal limits if caused by hypoparathyroidism

    5. Intake and output are within normal limits; daily weight is stabilized

    6. Priority nursing diagnosis goals are met

    7. Client demonstrates compliance with interventions

III. Hypercalcemia: an abnormally elevated serum calcium level (> 10.5 mg/dL); symptoms may not appear until the serum calcium > 12 mg/dL

    A. Etiology and pathophysiology

        1. Cellular level transport

        a. Movement occurs via a calcium pump

        b. Removed from bone by osteoclasts that are derived from monocytes that are produced in the bone marrow

        c. Monocytes travel through the bloodstream and collect at sites of bone resorption, where they fuse together to become osteocytes (cells that erode old bone)

        2. Predisposing clinical conditions

        a. Can result from increased calcium intake or absorption, a shift from calcium from the bone to the ECF, or decreased calcium excretion (see Box 4-3 for a listing of clinical conditions that can lead to hypercalcemia)

        b. Hyperparathyroidism: increased PTH causes calcium release from bone, adds to absorption of calcium in the intestines, and increases renal absorption of calcium; adenoma of the parathyroid gland is most common cause

        c. Metastatic cancer: most common cause of hypercalcemia; multiple myeloma, pulmonary, breast, and ovarian cancers most commonly associated with hypercalcemia; related to increased release of calcium from bone that is destroyed; occurs locally when tumor cell products stimulate osteoclastic bone resorption or systemically stimulate bone resorption and increased calcium excretion

        d. Thiazide-diuretic use: potentiates the action of PTH on the kidneys and decreases calcium excretion; results in small to moderate increases in calcium

Box 4-3	
Clinical Conditions That Lead to the Development of Hypercalcemia	• Hyperparathyroidism • Metastatic cancer • Use of thiazide diuretics • Sarcoidosis • Immobility • Hypophosphatemia • Hyperthyroidism (thyrotoxicosis) • Renal tubular acidosis • Milk-alkali syndrome • Familial hypocalciuric hypercalcemia • Lithium therapy • Vitamin D intoxication

NCLEX!

NCLEX!

NCLEX!

e. Sarcoidosis: from increased active metabolite of vitamin D made in the cells with this and other granulomatous diseases

f. Immobility: related to an imbalance between the rates of bone formation and bone resorption; seen in clients with Paget's disease or adolescents during growth spurts

g. Hypophosphatemia (< 3.0 mg/dL): phosphorus is inversely related to calcium

h. Thyrotoxicosis (hyperthyroidism): associated with high bone turnover; excessive bone resorption

i. Renal tubular acidosis: increases ionized portion of the calcium

j. Milk-alkali syndrome: can occur in clients with peptic ulcer disease who use milk or antacids, especially calcium carbonate (TUMS or Oscal), for prolonged periods of time

k. Familial hypocalciuric hypercalcemia: a rare autosomal dominant disorder

l. Lithium therapy: competes with calcium and other important cations affecting neurotransmitters, cell membranes, and body water

m. Vitamin D intoxication: increases absorption of calcium

B. Assessment

1. Clinical manifestations: due to decreased neuromuscular irritability (refer again to Table 4-1)

   a. Common signs

   1) Cardiovascular: hypertension, decreased ST segments, and shortened QT interval on ECG, cardiac dysrhythmias such as heart block and cardiac arrest

   2) Neuromuscular: depressed neuromuscular excitability as evidenced by decreased deep tendon reflexes; impairment of memory and bizarre behavior, lethargy, or coma (seizures are rare)

NCLEX!

3) Gastrointestinal: hypotonic bowel sounds, constipation, history of peptic ulcer disease

4) Renal: polyuria and polydipsia due to altered renal function; decreased ability of the kidneys to concentrate urine; renal colic can occur from development of kidney stones due to excess calcium levels; renal failure may occur

5) Musculoskeletal: pathologic bone fractures; bone thinning

b. Common symptoms

1) Neuromuscular: headache and confusion, subtle changes in personality to acute psychosis, impairment of memory, fatigue

2) Gastrointestinal: anorexia, nausea and vomiting; abdominal pain; constipation

3) Renal: altered voiding patterns due to polyuria and polydipsia; pain from renal colic or kidney stones

4) Musculoskeletal: deep bone pain; altered mobility and transfer due to presence of bone pain and increased risk of pathologic fractures

2. Diagnostic and laboratory findings

a. Plasma, urinary levels, and radiology measurements

1) Plasma level of > 11 mg/dL; in malignancies, total serum calcium may be > 14 mg/dL

2) Ionized plasma level of > 5.0 mg/dL or > 40%

3) 24-hour urinary level of > 400 mg/24 hours

4) PTH level > 55 pg/dL if due to hyperparathyroidism

5) Radiology findings that confirm the presence of pathologic fractures, presence of kidney stones, and bone mineral density evaluations

b. Associated electrolyte levels: hypophosphatemia (< 3.0 mg/dL)

c. Trending of results

1) Monitor calcium and phosphorus levels

2) Assess for signs and symptoms of resolving hypercalcemia

3) Monitor creatinine and BUN

4) Monitor daily weight in response to therapeutic regimens

5) Monitor strict intake and output

6) Monitor ECG for shortening of the ST segment and QT interval

7) Results of x-rays for bone changes and fractures; results of bone density tests

8) Monitor for renal calculi and calcium deposits in renal parenchyma on x-ray

9) If parathyroid tumor, surgical removal should bring PTH to normal; control of tumor from malignancy should aid in restoration of balance

NCLEX!

NCLEX!

NCLEX!

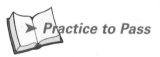
Practice to Pass

How would you compare the differences and similarities that occur in the central nervous system between hypocalcemia and hypercalcemia?

3. Identification of risk factors: assess for factors that increase the risk of hypercalcemia

    a. Clients with cancer or known metastasis

    b. Clients who are post-parathyroidectomy

    c. Clients who are immobile due to clinical conditions or sedentary lifestyle

    d. Excessive dietary intake of calcium rich foods

    e. Excessive intake of antacids for gastric distress

C. Priority nursing diagnoses: Potential complication: hypercalcemia; Potential complication: renal insufficiency; Decreased cardiac output; Risk for constipation; Risk for injury related to neuromuscular and sensorium changes; Fluid volume excess; Fluid volume deficit; Potential complication: dysrrhythmias; Altered nutrition: more than body requirements for calcium; Knowledge deficit; Risk for noncompliance

D. Therapeutic management

1. Decrease calcium intake

    a. Limit milk and dairy products

    b. Eliminate use of calcium carbonate antacids until calcium levels return to within normal limits

2. Promote calcium excretion

    a. Use loop diuretics, such as furosemide (Lasix) or ethacrynic acid (Edecrin), to promote increased urine output, thus more calcium will be excreted

    b. Maintain hydration of 3,000–4,000 mL (3–4 L) of fluid/day; oral fluids should be high in acid-ash, such a cranberry or prune juice

    c. Give 0.9% saline (NS) infusion of 300–500 mL/hour up to 6 liters as ordered until volume status restored, then 0.45% NaCl may be used; watch for fluid overload as a consequence of therapy, especially if the client has preexisting cardiac or respiratory disease

    d. Corticosteroids to decrease GI absorption of calcium: prednisone 20–50 mg po BID is usual dose or 40–100 mg daily in four divided doses; may take 5–10 days for calcium levels to fall

    e. Chronic management of hypercalcemia is effective only with parathroidectomy for primary hyperparathyroidism

3. Continued monitoring of client

    a. Monitor serum calcium and phosphorus levels

    b. Continuous ECG monitoring to detect cardiac arrhythmias

    c. Strict intake and output

    d. Daily weight

    e. If plicamycin (Mithracin) is used, client must be monitored for tissue sloughing in the area of the intravenous site as plicamycin (Mithracin) has vesicant properties; it is also nephrotoxic therefore renal function must be closely monitored

NCLEX!

    f. Monitor client for side effects of corticosteroids such as hyperglycemia, weight gain, mood changes, bearing in mind the long-term side effects

4. Restoration of balance

    a. Monitor calcium and phosphorus levels

    b. Monitor neurologic and cardiac status

    c. Monitor for therapeutic effect of medications to reduce calcium

    d. Monitor PTH post-parathyroidectomy

    e. Monitor for balanced intake and output

    f. Monitor for stable daily weight

    g. Monitor for absence of signs of heart failure from treatment

    h. Monitor for absence of signs of hypocalcemia from treatment

5. Treatment of hypercalcemic crisis

    a. Isotonic saline (0.9% NaCl) at 300–500 mL/hr initially and up to 6 liters until intravascular volume restored or calcium 8–9 mg/dL; promotes calcium excretion; loop diuretics should be used if heart failure develops

    b. Biphosphonates, such as pamidronate (Aredia) intravenously to inhibit bone resorption—90 mg in 1 liter NS or D_5W over 4 hours for severe hypercalcemia (> 13.5 mg/dL), returns calcium to normal within 24–48 hours with effects lasting for weeks in most clients

    c. Plicamycin (Mithracin) intravenously to inhibit bone resorption specifically if hypercalcemia induced by metastasis; doses of 24 mcg/kg in 500 mL D_5W over 4–6 hours gradually reduce calcium

    d. Salmon calcitonin may temporarily lower level by 1–3 mg/dL in clients with severe hypercalcemia; starting dose is 2–8 units/kg intramuscularly, subcutaneously every 6–12 hours; effective within 2 hours after initial dose, peaks in 24–48 hours, and duration is 4–7 days

    e. Intravenous phosphorus to decrease calcium by increasing phosphorus: dose greater than or equal to 1,500 mg over 6–8 hours in emergency situations only

6. Dialysis: during oliguric/anuric stage, severe renal dysfunction can lead to life-threatening fluid and electrolyte imbalances

E. Planning and implementation

1. Monitor pertinent client assessment data for potential effects of hypercalcemia and for response to therapeutic treatment

    a. Obtain a thorough nursing history

        1) Subjective (family history, history of previous cancer, history of kidney stones, postoperative parathyroidectomy)

        2) Objective (signs of hypercalcemia, predisposing conditions, risk factors)

        3) Medication history (medications that may cause hypercalcemia or excess of medications to treat hypocalcemia)

        4) OTC or herbal therapies that may lead to hypercalcemia

    b. Inspection of particular systems for specific findings

        1) Neurologic system for changes in level of consciousness or subtle personality changes

        2) Cardiovascular system to determine if client is on digitalis preparations (because hypercalcemia can enhance digitalis effects) and to detect presence of arrhythmias

        3) Genitourinary system for flank and thigh pain from renal calculi and for polyuria

        4) Gastrointestinal system for nausea, vomiting, constipation, and decreased bowel sounds

        5) Musculoskeletal system for weakness of muscles, diminished deep tendon reflexes, and observable fractures

    c. Hypercalcemic crisis is considered a medical emergency; report laboratory results immediately to healthcare provider for therapeutic treatment

    d. Monitor PTH if hypercalcemia is from primary hyperparathyroidism

    e. Frequently assess for heart failure in clients receiving hydration therapy

    f. Identify symptoms of digitalis toxicity when client has hypercalcemia and is also receiving digitalis

    g. Monitor client for signs of hypocalcemia as a result of treatment

2. Prevent injuries and maintain safe environment

    a. Monitor for pathologic fractures in clients with long-term hypercalcemia

    b. Assist client with mobility and transfer attempts in order to prevent injury and maintain safety

3. Administer medications as ordered checking for therapeutic response and evaluating client condition during the course of drug therapy

4. Assess intake and output

    a. Encourage clients to drink 3–4 liters of fluid per day, especially fluids such as cranberry juice or prune juice so that calcium salts will not deposit in the urine

    b. Monitor color and characteristics of urine

    c. Observe urine for presence of kidney stones

    d. Obtain daily weight

5. Assess for signs of fluid volume excess from treatment or dehydration from polyuria

6. Dietary interventions to decrease calcium levels

    a. Limiting calcium sources in the diet

    b. Limiting medications that provide hidden sources of calcium in the diet

    c. Referral to a dietician

7. If client's hypercalcemic state is due to malignancy, long-term treatment may be indicated to correct this problem

8. Encourage compliance with therapeutic regimen

F. Medication therapy

NCLEX!

1. Hydration therapy

   a. Isotonic saline (0.9%) at a rate of 300–500 mL/hr, up to 6 liters, in emergency or 0.45 % NaCl until serum calcium level is diluted

   b. Titrate to prevent signs of heart failure

NCLEX!

2. Specific drug therapies

   a. Loop diuretics: such as furosemide (Lasix) 20–40 mg every 2 hours; enhance calcium excretion and prevent volume overloading during hydration

   b. Plicamycin (Mithracin): inhibits osteoclastic bone resorption and decreases bone turnover; intended use is in malignant hypercalcemia due to its nephrotoxicity; use cautiously in clients with impaired renal function; dosage is single dose of 25 mcg/kg in 500 mL D_5W intravenously over 4–6 hours

   c. Corticosteroids (glucocorticoids): inhibit calcium absorption in the intestine, inhibit osteoclastic bone resorption and increase urinary excretion of calcium; prednisone 20–50 mg po BID initially, then change to maintenance dose; may not reduce calcium significantly for 5–10 days so use in conjunction with other measures to decrease calcium

   d. Phosphate salts: Phospho-Soda or Neutra-Phos orally 1.0–1.5 grams for several days or rectally by Fleet retention enema 100 mL BID; phosphate therapy should be limited to clients with phosphate levels < 3.0 mg/dL and whose renal function is not impaired; a dose of 0.5–1.0 g elemental phosphorus po TID modestly lowers serum calcium; controversy exists about use of IV phosphates

   e. Biphosphonate drugs: retard bone turnover by inhibiting activity of osteoclasts; pamidronate disodium (Aredia) 60–90 mg/L in 0.9% NaCl or D_5W infused over 24 hours

   f. Calcitonin, salmon: 4 to 8 U/kg IM or subcutaneously every 6–12 hours to temporarily lower serum calcium

   g. Gallium nitrate: inhibits bone resorption; 200 mg in 1 liter D_5W or NS IV over 24 hours for 5 days along with saline diuresis; do not use if creatinine > 2.5 mg/dL

G. Client education

1. Awareness of predisposing factors associated with hypercalcemia

   a. Teach client causes of hypercalcemia

   b. Instruct client to take phosphorus agents as prescribed

   c. Teach client correct method of taking prescribed medications

   d. Instruct client to notify healthcare provider if flank pain develops

Practice to Pass

A client has hypercalcemia due to milk-alkali syndrome. Which foods and antacids will you teach this client to avoid?

    e. Demonstrate to client how to check for kidney stones (straining of urine) if indicated

    f. Instruct client to notify healthcare professional if symptoms worsen

  2. Dietary education

    a. Instruct client as to which over-the-counter antacids contain high amounts of calcium and to avoid these

    b. Discuss with client foods highest in calcium and offer alternative options; a low calcium diet (< 400 mg/day) is recommended if hypercalcemia is because of vitamin D toxicity

    c. Instruct client to increase fluid intake to 2,000–3,000 mL in 24 hours, especially fluids high in acid-ash such as prune or cranberry juice

    d. Teach client to increase dietary fiber and fluid to prevent constipation

    e. Caution client not to take large doses of vitamin D supplements

    f. Refer client to a dietician to meet dietary goals

H. Evaluation

  1. Total serum calcium is between 8.5 and 10.5 mg/dL

  2. Serum ionized calcium is between 4.0 and 5.0 mg/dL

  3. Phosphorus level is between 2.5 and 4.5 mg/dL

  4. 24-hour urine calcium is within normal limits

  5. PTH is within normal limits if cause was primary hyperparathyroidism or surgery

  6. Signs of heart failure from hydration therapy are absent

  7. Serum creatinine and BUN are within normal limits

  8. There is resolution of signs and symptoms of hypercalcemia

  9. There is an absence of clinical manifestations of hypocalcemia as result of treatment

  10. There are no signs of complications of hyper- or hypocalcemia

  11. The client demonstrates compliance with therapeutic management regime

Case Study

A 54-year-old male with a diagnosis of multiple myeloma has been admitted to your unit. The client has chief complaints of increasing fatigue, muscle weakness, and bone pain. Lab work indicates pancytopenia, hyperuricemia, hypercalcemia, and elevated creatinine. Bone scans and x-rays have been ordered.

❶ What do you suspect is the cause of these signs and symptoms?

❷ What is the pathophysiologic mechanism for the calcium imbalance?

❸ What immediate medical treatment do you anticipate and why?

❹ What are your priority nursing interventions?

❺ How will you determine if therapy has been effective?

For suggested responses, see pages 231–232.

Posttest

1   The nurse notes a decreased total serum calcium level on the client's lab work. The client has no symptoms of hypocalcemia at this time. The nurse interprets that:

(1) This level reflects only the ionized calcium.
(2) The client's magnesium is high resulting in false levels of calcium.
(3) Phosphorus is low resulting in low serum calcium levels.
(4) This does not reflect the ionized calcium that results in symptomatology.

2   A client is admitted with chronic renal failure. The nurse concludes that this client may also be hypocalcemic because:

(1) There is decreased renal excretion of calcium.
(2) The serum creatinine will be low.
(3) Renal colic is present.
(4) Diseased kidneys are unable to produce calcitriol.

3   A client presents with a mildly elevated calcium level. During a nursing history, the client states that current medications include hydrochlorothiazide (HydroDiuril), a thiazide diuretic. The nurse explains to the client that thiazide diuretics can cause hypercalcemia by:

(1) Increasing urinary output.
(2) Excreting calcitriol.
(3) Inhibiting calcium excretion.
(4) Stimulating calcitonin secretion.

4   A client with hypercalcemia is receiving digoxin (Lanoxin). The nurse plans to incorporate which of the following in client assessments?

(1) Checking for Trousseau's sign
(2) Frequent pulse checks to determine any change in heart rhythm
(3) Auscultation of bowel sounds
(4) Inspection of skin for signs of bleeding

5   A client returns to the unit following a thyroidectomy. The nurse plans to frequently assess which of the following?

(1) Respiratory sign of laryngospasm
(2) Renal sign of polyuria
(3) Cardiac sign of hypertension
(4) Neurologic sign of hypoactive deep tendon reflexes

6 When determining a plan of care for a client with hypocalcemia, the nurse chooses which of the following as a high priority nursing diagnosis?

(1) Potential complication: electrolyte excess
(2) Risk for injury related to sensorium changes
(3) Risk for injury related to tetany and seizures
(4) Fluid volume deficit

7 The client presents with signs of severe hypocalcemia. The nurse anticipates administration of:

(1) Isotonic normal saline as a rapid infusion.
(2) 10% calcium gluconate by slow IV push.
(3) Intravenous phosphorus over 6 to 8 hours.
(4) 10% calcium chloride by rapid IV push.

8 A client is receiving a 0.9% (normal) saline infusion for hypercalcemia. The nurse determines that hydration has been effective when:

(1) Chvostek's sign is positive.
(2) Volume status has been restored.
(3) Calcium level is 11 to 12 mg/dL.
(4) Serum creatinine is elevated.

9 The nurse caring for a client with a calcium imbalance places highest priority on nursing interventions that help to manage:

(1) Renal signs and symptoms.
(2) Cardiac changes.
(3) Hematologic disorders.
(4) Neuromuscular clinical manifestations.

10 The nurse determines that a client with hypercalcemia understands client teaching when the client states:

(1) "If my stomach becomes upset, I can just take more TUMS."
(2) "I'll need to take my phosphorus supplements once a day."
(3) "I'll need to be on strict bedrest to help with this problem."
(4) "I'll need to drink many more fluids than I have been, even up to 2 to 3 liters each day."

See pages 110–111 for Answers and Rationales.

Answers and Rationales

Pretest

1 **Answer: 2** *Rationale:* Calcium plays a unique role in the regulation of many enzymes and intracellular signaling. Although calcium does play an important role in acid-base balance, other electrolytes do this as well. Sodium and potassium are also needed for heart muscle contraction. Sodium is primarily responsible for shifts in body water.
Cognitive Level: Application
Nursing Process: Analysis; *Test Plan:* PHYS

2 **Answer: 3** *Rationale:* In hyperparathyroidism, the ionized calcium is almost always elevated. In hyperparathyroidism, the level of intact PTH is elevated and is best interpreted in conjunction with ionized calcium. PTH is suppressed in clients with most other causes of hypercalcemia, which makes the other options incorrect.
Cognitive Level: Application
Nursing Process: Analysis; *Test Plan:* PHYS

3 **Answer: 1** *Rationale:* Prolonged NGT suctioning leads to metabolic alkalosis. Changes in pH will alter the level of ionized calcium. Alkalosis increases calcium binding to albumin, leading to a decrease in ionized calcium. There may be fluid shifts from hypoalbuminemia, but this would not be from NG tube suctioning. Hypomagnesemia can be a cause of hypocalcemia. Metabolic acidosis decreases calcium binding to albumin, leading to more ionized calcium.
Cognitive Level: Application
Nursing Process: Analysis; *Test Plan:* PHYS

4 **Answer: 2** *Rationale:* Many malignant tumors produce chemicals that are carried in the blood to cause release of calcium from the bones; most commonly in association with ovarian cancer, renal cell carcinoma, breast cancer, among others. Several antineoplastic medications cause hypocalcemia and lack of dairy products and pancreatitis cause hypocalcemia.
Cognitive Level: Application
Nursing Process: Analysis; *Test Plan:* PHYS

5　**Answer: 1** *Rationale:* Large doses of glucocorticoids decrease calcium absorption in the intestines. Glucocorticoids (corticosteroids) cause increased output of calcium and phosphorus, which may lead to conditions such as osteoporosis. All of the other options would indicate hypercalcemia, not hypocalcemia.
Cognitive Level: Application
Nursing Process: Analysis; *Test Plan:* PHYS

6　**Answer: 3** *Rationale:* Hypercalcemia causes decreased neuromuscular irritability, while hypocalcemia has clinical manifestations that indicate increased neuromuscular irritability. Options 1, 2, and 4 are all signs of increased neuromuscular irritability—signs of hypocalcemia.
Cognitive Level: Application
Nursing Process: Assessment; *Test Plan:* PHYS

7　**Answer: 2** *Rationale:* The cardiac effects of hypercalcemia include shortened plateau phase of the action potential, which causes shortening of the QT interval. Atrial fibrillation may develop, but heart block is more of a concern with hypercalcemia due to delayed atrioventricular conduction. Hypotension is not observed on ECG. Prolonged QT interval is a finding with hypocalcemia.
Cognitive Level: Application
Nursing Process: Assessment; *Test Plan:* PHYS

8　**Answer: 1** *Rationale:* Hypoparathyroidism is characterized by hypocalcemia and hyperphosphatemia and is often associated with tetany. Hypoparathyroidism usually results from accidental removal of or damage to parathyroid glands during thyroidectomy. Because hypocalcemia may be severe, prolonged parenteral administration of calcium may be necessary to avoid serious postoperative complications. Hypoparathyroidism results from a deficiency or absence of PTH so therefore option 2 is incorrect. Immobility results in hypercalcemia, making option 3 incorrect.
Cognitive Level: Application
Nursing Process: Implementation; *Test Plan:* PHYS

9　**Answer: 4** *Rationale:* Symptoms of fatigue, headache, and increasing muscle weakness are clinical manifestations of hypercalcemia. Increased hydration is needed to reduce the serum concentration and aid in elimination. All of the other options will worsen client's symptoms and increase hypercalcemia. Thiazide diuretics inhibit calcium excretion; Vitamin D supplements will increase absorption of vitamin D in the intestine; and fluid restriction will cause hemoconcentration leading to increased serum calcium.
Cognitive Level: Analysis
Nursing Process: Planning; *Test Plan:* PHYS

10　**Answer: 2** *Rationale:* Tingling or numbness around the mouth is called circumoral paresthesia and is a sign of impending tetany. A healthcare provider should be notified immediately. TUMS is a brand name for calcium carbonate that can be used as a calcium supplement when calcium intake is inadequate. To prevent hypocalcemia, the client should increase the protein in the diet. Kidney stones are a sign of hypercalcemia.
Cognitive Level: Application
Nursing Process: Evaluation; *Test Plan:* HPM

Posttest

1　**Answer: 4** *Rationale:* Ionized calcium is approximately 40 to 50% of the total serum calcium. Ionized calcium is the portion of the serum calcium that is not bound to protein and is physiologically active and clinically important. Hypocalcemia that is due to reduced protein binding is asymptomatic. The question states that the total serum calcium is low; therefore option 1 is not correct. Ionized calcium levels may remain normal even when total calcium levels are low. Option 2 is incorrect, as hypocalcemia may be a result of hypomagnesemia, not hypermagnesemia. Option 3 is incorrect, as phosphorus and calcium are inversely proportional, so phosphorus would be high.
Cognitive Level: Analysis
Nursing Process: Analysis; *Test Plan:* PHYS

2　**Answer: 4** *Rationale:* Renal failure can result in hypocalcemia from diminished formation of calcitriol from renal cell damage as well as from hyperphosphatemia. In renal disease, severe hypocalcemia can occur from abnormal renal losses of calcium. Serum creatinine would be high due to nephron destruction in renal failure. Renal colic occurs from hypercalcemia.
Cognitive Level: Application
Nursing Process: Analysis; *Test Plan:* PHYS

3　**Answer: 3** *Rationale:* Thiazide diuretics can cause mild hypercalcemia because they have calcium-retaining effects on the kidney. Increasing urinary output would lead to hypocalcemia. Calcitriol excretion would lead to hypocalcemia as well as an increase in calcitonin secretion.
Cognitive Level: Application
Nursing Process: Analysis; *Test Plan:* PHYS

4 **Answer: 2** *Rationale:* The hypercalcemic client is more sensitive to the toxic effects of digitalis. Frequent apical and radial pulse checks by the nurse will aid in detecting potential complications. Options 1 and 4 are assessment priorities in hypocalcemia. Auscultation of bowel sounds is appropriate, but not of high priority with digitalis therapy.
Cognitive Level: Application
Nursing Process: Assessment; *Test Plan:* PHYS

5 **Answer: 1** *Rationale:* Hypocalcemia frequently results from accidental removal or destruction of parathyroid tissue or its blood supply during surgery. Clinical manifestations of tetany include laryngospasm postoperatively. The other options are assessment criteria representative of hypercalcemia.
Cognitive Level: Application
Nursing Process: Assessment; *Test Plan:* PHYS

6 **Answer: 3** *Rationale:* Tetany and seizures are clinical manifestations of hypocalcemia. The nurse must be aware of all potential risks to the client based on physiological factors of the presenting illness and must plan for the client's safety. The other nursing diagnoses are appropriate for hypercalcemia.
Cognitive Level: Analysis
Nursing Process: Planning; *Test Plan:* SECE

7 **Answer: 2** *Rationale:* 10% calcium gluconate is the treatment option for symptomatic severe hypocalcemia. All IV calcium preparations are administered slowly to prevent arrhythmias and damage to veins. Normal saline and IV phosphorus are used to treat hypercalcemia.
Cognitive Level: Application
Nursing Process: Planning; *Test Plan:* SECE

8 **Answer: 2** *Rationale:* The mainstay of treatment of hypercalcemia is to increase renal calcium excretion with extracellular volume expansion. Chvostek's sign indicates hypocalcemia, which would not be an overcorrection of treatment. Calcium levels of 11 to 12 mg/dL indicate hypercalcemia. Serum creatinine elevation indicates that renal function is diminished and is therefore not an effective response to therapy.
Cognitive Level: Application
Nursing Process: Evaluation; *Test Plan:* PHYS

9 **Answer: 4** *Rationale:* Although all systems are impacted by calcium imbalance, the major clinical manifestations of calcium imbalance are due to either increased or decreased neuromuscular irritability.
Cognitive Level: Analysis
Nursing Process: Implementation; *Test Plan:* PHYS

10 **Answer: 4** *Rationale:* The client should increase fluid intake to 2 to 3 liters a day. Hydration leads to increased calcium excretion and prevents the development of kidney stones. TUMS is a calcium carbonate supplement that can be used to increase calcium; the client in the question already has hypercalcemia. Phosphorus supplements can decrease calcium, but need to be taken more than once a day. Strict bedrest leads to increased calcium from osteoclastic activity.
Cognitive Level: Application
Nursing Process: Evaluation; *Test Plan:* HPM

References

American Association of Critical-Care Nurses (1998). *Core curriculum for critical care nurses.* (5th ed.). Philadelphia: W. B. Saunders, pp. 474, 543–548.

Beers, J. H. & Berkow, R. (Eds.) (1999). *Merck manual of diagnosis and therapy* (17th ed.). Whitehouse Station, NJ: Merck Research Laboratories, pp. 137–151.

Braunwald, E., Fauci, A. S., Kasper, D. L., Hauser, S. L., Longo, D. L., & Jameson, J. L. (2001). *Harrison's principles of internal medicine* (15th ed.). New York: McGraw-Hill, pp. 2194–2195, 2209–2226.

Copstead, L. E. & Banasik, J. L. (2000). *Pathophysiology: Biological and behavioral perspectives* (2nd ed.). Philadelphia: W. B. Saunders, pp. 603–604, 1127–1128.

Horne, M. & Bond, E. (2000). Fluid, electrolyte, and acid-base imbalances. In S. Lewis, M. Heitkemper, & M. Dirksen (Eds.), *Medical–surgical nursing: Assessment and management of clinical problems* (5th ed.). St. Louis: Mosby, pp. 338–346.

Huether, S. E. & McCance, K. L. (2001). *Understanding pathophysiology.* (2nd ed.). St. Louis: Mosby, pp. 118–123, 468, 1007–1008.

Kee, J. L. (2001). *Handbook of laboratory and diagnostic tests with nursing implications* (4th ed.). Upper Saddle River, NJ: Prentice Hall, Inc., pp. 16–17, 22–23, 61–65, 92–93, 233–239, 244–257, 333, 454, 477.

Kidd, P. S. & Wagner, K. D. (2001). *High acuity nursing.* (3rd ed.). Upper Saddle River, NJ: Prentice-Hall, Inc., pp. 67–69, 660, 663, 757.

Kozier, B., Erb, G., Berman, A., & Burke, K. (2000). *Fundamentals of nursing: Concepts, process, and practice* (6th ed.). Upper Saddle River, NJ: Prentice Hall, Inc., pp. 1318–1319.

LeMone, P. & Burke, K. (2000). *Medical-surgical nursing: Critical thinking in client care* (2nd ed.). Upper Saddle River, NJ: Prentice Hall, Inc., pp. 99–162.

Nettina, S. (2001). *Lippincott manual of nursing practice* (7th ed.). Philadelphia: Lippincott Williams & Wilkins, pp. 678–679, 815, 827–830.

Venes, D. & Thomas, C. *Taber's cyclopedic medical dictionary* (2001). (19th ed.). Philadelphia: F. A. Davis.

Twin Cities Dietetic Association. (1999). *Patient education handout,* pp. 666–672.

Webster's third world medical dictionary. (2000). Foster City, CA: IDG Books Worldwide, pp. 58–59.

Wilson, B. A., Shannon, M. T., & Stang, C. L. (2001). *Nursing drug guide 2001.* Upper Saddle River, NJ: Prentice Hall, Inc., pp. 195, 197–199, 202–205.

Magnesium Balance and Imbalances

Julie A. Adkins, RN, MSN, FNP

CHAPTER OUTLINE

Overview of Magnesium Regulation   *Hypomagnesemia*   *Hypermagnesemia*

OBJECTIVES

▮ Review basic functions of magnesium in the body.

▮ Discuss the pathophysiology and etiology of magnesium imbalances.

▮ Discuss specific assessment findings in magnesium imbalances.

▮ Identify priority nursing diagnoses for a client experiencing a magnesium imbalance.

▮ Discuss therapeutic management of magnesium imbalances.

▮ Discuss nursing management of a client who is experiencing a magnesium imbalance.

 [Media Link]

Use the CD-ROM enclosed with this text, or log onto the address given to access the free, interactive Companion Website created for this series. The CD-ROM and Companion Website accompanying this book offer additional practice opportunities and information—NCLEX Review, Case Studies, Glossary, In Depth with NCLEX, and more.

www.prenhall.com/hogan

Review at a Glance

hypermagnesemia *an excess of magnesium in the blood, with a serum level of greater than 2.1 mEq/L*

hypomagnesemia *a deficit of magnesium in the blood, with a serum level of less than 1.4 mEq/L*

magnesium *the second most abundant cation in the body, found mainly in bone and within the cells*

Pretest

1 The nurse would expect a client to have a high serum level of magnesium after seeing which of the following health problems listed in the medical history?

(1) Malabsorption
(2) Anemia
(3) Overuse of laxatives
(4) Alcoholism

2 The nurse would assess for which of the following classic manifestations in a client suspected of having hypermagnesemia?

(1) Diarrhea
(2) Hyperreflexia
(3) Hypertension
(4) Diminished deep tendon reflexes

3 The nurse is educating the client who has a decreased magnesium level. What information is most important for the nurse to include in discussions with the client?

(1) Avoid hazardous activities
(2) Weekly laboratory evaluation
(3) Diet counseling
(4) Moderate alcohol consumption

4 The client complains of leg cramps. The nurse is aware that this client takes a mild diuretic on a daily basis. Besides potassium, the nurse suspects that which of the following could cause this client's symptom?

(1) Elevated calcium level
(2) Elevated sodium level
(3) Elevated magnesium level
(4) Decreased magnesium level

5 The nurse would conclude that a client's serum magnesium level is normal if it falls within which of the following ranges?

(1) 1.4 to 2.1 mEq/L
(2) 0.8 to 1.6 mEq/L
(3) 2.0 to 4.0 mEq/L
(4) Less than 5 mEq/L

6 The nurse would interpret that a magnesium level of 3.2 indicates which of the following?

(1) Hypomagnesemia
(2) Concurrent hypokalemia
(3) Hypermagnesemia
(4) Concurrent hypocalcemia

7 The nurse who is teaching nutrition is discussing the effects of various electrolytes and minerals in the body. In describing the action of magnesium, the nurse would explain that it diminishes acetylcholine and thus acts as a:

(1) Muscle stimulant.
(2) Muscle relaxant.
(3) Vitamin metabolizer.
(4) Stimulant for blood glucose.

8 The nurse is aware that most of the magnesium in the body is found in which of the following areas?

(1) Small intestine
(2) Kidney
(3) Blood
(4) Bone

9 The nurse doing health promotion recommends that a client take in how many milligrams of magnesium to be within the recommended dietary allowance (RDA) for magnesium?

(1) 75 mg
(2) 200 mg
(3) 350 mg
(4) 500 mg

10 | The nurse recalls that magnesium is absorbed where in the body?

(1) Ascending colon
(2) Descending colon
(3) Stomach
(4) Small intestine

See pages 124–125 for Answers and Rationales.

I. Overview of Magnesium Regulation

A. *Magnesium* **balance and function:** the second most abundant cation in the human body; absorbed in the small intestine; conserved by the kidney during times of inadequate dietary intake and excreted by the kidneys during times of excessive intake

1. Serum levels

NCLEX!

   a. Normal plasma levels of magnesium range from 1.4 to 2.1 mEq/L

   b. The maintenance of magnesium levels in the body is mostly a function of dietary intake

   c. Serum concentration of magnesium does not parallel tissue concentration; body stores may be more adequately measured by urinary magnesium excretion

2. Functions in the body

   a. Plays a major role in at least 300 fundamental enzymatic reactions

NCLEX!

   b. Powers the sodium-potassium pump in the body

   c. Aids in converting adenosine triphosphate (ATP) to adenosine diphosphate (ADP) for energy release

   d. Transmits electrical impulses across nerves and muscles; is important for skeletal muscle relaxation following contraction

NCLEX!

   e. Maintains normal heart rhythm

   f. Is involved in nucleic acid metabolism

   g. Is needed for thiamine activity and for calcium and vitamin B_{12} absorption and utilization

   h. May be involved in stabilization of DNA and RNA

   i. Relaxes lung muscles that open airways

NCLEX!

   j. Fights tooth decay by binding calcium to tooth enamel

   k. Decreased magnesium levels may contribute to secondary decreases in potassium, calcium, and phosphate levels

   l. Is involved in fatty acid oxidation and is a cofactor in carbohydrate metabolism and protein synthesis

NCLEX!

   m. Decreases or blocks the release of acetylcholine thereby acting as a smooth muscle relaxant

3. System interactions

   a. Plays a central role in secretion and action of insulin thereby controlling blood glucose

   b. Is necessary for the release of parathyroid hormone (PTH) and plays a role in pre-eclampsia

   c. PTH and aldosterone indirectly affect magnesium reabsorption or excretion in the kidney

   d. High amounts of calcium and poorly digested fats and phosphates interfere with magnesium absorption due to the binding mechanism in the small intestine

B. Sources of magnesium

1. Cellular level

   a. More than 50% of magnesium is found in the bone

   NCLEX!

   b. Much of the remaining magnesium in the body is intracellular (approximately 45%), and the remaining small amount is present in extracellular spaces

   c. Most of the magnesium within the cells is found in the mitochondria and only 5 to 10% is free in cytosol

   NCLEX!

   d. Potassium, magnesium, and calcium are tied together intracellularly to maintain a neutral electrical charge; therefore, an altered level of any of these would ultimately affect the others

2. Dietary level

   a. The average diet contains between 168 and 720 mg of magnesium per day

   NCLEX!

   b. The recommended allowance for magnesium is 300 to 350 mg for young men and women with an extra 150 mg per day during pregnancy and lactation; another way to calculate magnesium need is to base it on 4.5 mg per kilogram of body weight

   NCLEX!

   c. Sources of magnesium in the diet include green leafy vegetables, nuts, legumes, seafood, whole grains, bananas, oranges, cocoa, and chocolate

II. *Hypomagnesemia:* a serum magnesium level that falls below 1.4 mEq/L

A. Etiology and pathophysiology

1. Cellular level

   a. Hypomagnesemia usually occurs with nutritional or metabolic abnormalities; can occur because of altered absorption, increased renal loss, or redistribution of body magnesium

   b. Approximately 50% of dietary magnesium is usually absorbed; absorption is inhibited by phytates, oxalates, and fat

2. Predisposing clinical conditions

   a. Chronic alcoholism is the most common cause

   b. Decreased magnesium intake may be due to dietary factors or prolonged intravenous therapy without magnesium supplementation; in parenteral nu-

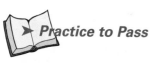

Practice to Pass

What foods would you recommend to a client who needs to increase magnesium intake?

trition therapy, magnesium moves into the cells from the bloodstream, leading to low serum magnesium levels

c. Decreased absorption may be caused by inflammatory bowel disease, small bowel resection (less surface available to absorb), GI cancer, chronic pancreatitis, or medications such as gentamicin (Garamycin)—an aminoglycoside antibiotic, or cisplatin (Platinol)—an antineoplastic agent

d. Increased intestinal (lower GI) losses may occur because of prolonged diarrhea, draining intestinal fistulas, and ileostomy

e. Increased renal excretion may result from diuretic use (furosemide [Lasix] or ethacrynic acid [Edecrin]), hyperaldosteronism that leads to volume expansion, diabetes that leads to osmotic diuresis

f. Losses can also occur because of burns and debridement therapy

B. Assessment

1. Clinical manifestations

   a. Do not usually occur until the serum level drops below 1 mEq/L

   b. Muscle twitching, tremors, hyperreactive reflexes occur due to the effect of magnesium on neuromuscular function and hypocalcemic effect

   c. Laryngeal stridor can occur

   d. Cardiovascular manifestations include supraventricular tachycardia and ventricular dysrhythmias (premature ventricular contractions and ventricular fibrillation) and increased susceptibility to digitalis toxicity (possibly enhanced by concurrent hypokalemia)

   e. Electrocardiogram (ECG) changes include diminished voltage of P wave, T waves that are broad, flat, or inverted; ST segments that are depressed; and QT intervals that are prolonged; a prominent U wave may be present

   f. Central nervous system manifestations include mood changes, such as apathy, depression, and confusion

   g. GI manifestations include nausea and vomiting, diarrhea, and anorexia, which occur because of concurrent hypokalemia

   h. Growth failure in children can occur

   i. Severe deficiency can lead to convulsions, hallucinations, or tetany

   j. Signs and symptoms are somewhat similar to those of hypokalemia or hypocalcemia because they are all cations; positive Chvostek's sign can occur

2. Diagnostic and laboratory findings

   a. Plasma magnesium levels < 1.4 mEq/L

   b. Associated electrolyte levels: concurrent decreases in calcium, potassium, and phosphate levels

    c. Trending of results

        1) Since most magnesium is stored in the cells, serum plasma levels may be normal despite an overall body depletion of magnesium

        2) Hypomagnesemia should be considered with reference to presenting clinical manifestations or in the presence of other electrolyte imbalances, such as hypocalcemia or hypokalemia

   3. Identification of risk factors: dietary insufficiency or previously identified co-existing medical conditions that lead to or exacerbate hypomagnesemia

C. Priority nursing diagnoses

   1. Altered nutrition: less than body requirements related to decreased magnesium intake

   2. Knowledge deficit related to magnesium content in food and alternative food choices

   3. Risk for injury related to neuromuscular manifestations

   4. Risk for decreased cardiac output related to increased risk of cardiac arrhythmias

D. Therapeutic management

   1. Replacement therapies

     a. Vary depending on presenting signs and symptoms and severity of condition

     b. Include any of the following:

       1) Intravenous infusion of magnesium sulfate

       2) Intramuscular magnesium sulfate

       3) Oral magnesium salts

       4) Dietary interventions

   2. Continued monitoring of client

     a. Monitor serum magnesium levels

     b. Assess the client for neuromuscular manifestations

     c. Assess the client for altered GI function

     d. Monitor the client for cardiovascular changes/arrhythmias

     e. Monitor for other electrolyte imbalances

     f. Monitor for unresolved signs and symptoms after therapy

     g. Monitor ECG for T waves that are broad, flat or inverted; ST segments that are depressed; and QT intervals that are prolonged

   3. Restoration of balance

     a. Promote dietary changes to increase magnesium intake

     b. Administer magnesium supplements as ordered

     c. Continue to assess those clients at risk

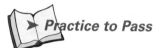

Practice to Pass

By what mechanism does hypokalemia occur with hypomagnesemia?

    d. Provide parenteral administration if warranted

    e. Monitor the client taking digitalis, as there is increased susceptibility to digitalis toxicity with hypomagnesemia

E. Planning and implementation

  1. Identify risk factors: malabsorption and/or GI dysfunction, renal disease, diabetes, alcohol intake, and medications such as diuretics

  2. Monitor the diabetic client for hyperglycemia leading to osmotic diuresis resulting in decreased magnesium

  3. Monitor the client with continuous IV fluid therapy; this client may need addition of magnesium in fluid solution

  4. Monitor the client with hyperaldosteronism because volume expansion may result in decreased magnesium

  5. Monitor the client taking a diuretic for increased renal excretion of magnesium

  6. Institute ECG monitoring and seizure precautions

  7. Monitor for stridor and/or difficulty swallowing

  8. Keep bed rails raised if client is confused; take other safety precautions as needed

  9. Maintain accurate intake and output records

  10. Monitor DTRs in clients receiving IV magnesium solutions; depressed deep tendon reflexes indicate an elevated magnesium level

F. Medication therapy

  1. Oral replacement therapy

    a. Magnesium-containing antacids

    b. Magnesium oxide 300 mg/day in divided doses

    c. Use caution because oral administration may cause diarrhea, leading to decreased absorption

  2. Parenteral replacement therapy

    a. Magnesium sulfate 2 gm (16 mEq) in 50% solution every 8 hours IM

    b. Magnesium chloride 48 mEq/day by continuous IV infusion; give slowly as per manufacturer's recommendations; giving too rapidly could cause respiratory or cardiac arrest

    c. Ensure that client maintains a urine output of at least 30 mL/hr or 120 mL every 4 hours during therapy to avoid rebound hypermagnesemia if renal insufficiency is present

    d. Monitor deep tendon reflexes (such as patellar reflex) before each dose of parenteral magnesium; if reflex is present, hypermagnesemia from previous doses has not occurred

    e. Watch for signs of rebound hypermagnesemia

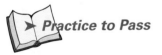

Practice to Pass

What commonly used antacids are high in magnesium?

3. Dietary therapy: for mild hypomagnesemia, encourage foods high in magnesium, such as legumes, whole grain cereals, nuts, dark green vegetables, and cocoa

G. Client education

1. Teach awareness of predisposing factors, including the following:

   a. Diabetes mellitus

   b. Anorexia, nausea, and vomiting

   c. Chronic diarrhea or chronic aluminum-based laxative abuse

   d. Alcoholism

   e. Hyperaldosteronism

   f. Renal tubular disorders

   g. Chronic diuretic therapy

2. Dietary education

   a. Review foods high in magnesium

   b. Increase intake of hard water or mineral water as these are high in magnesium

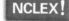

   c. Recommend 300 to 350 mg magnesium intake daily with an extra 150 mg for pregnant or lactating women

   d. Collaborate with dietician as necessary

H. Evaluation

1. Serum magnesium, calcium, and other electrolyte levels are within normal limits

2. Client remains is safe and free from injury

3. Manifestations of hypomagnesemia resolve

III. *Hypermagnesemia:* a serum magnesium level greater than 2.1 mEq/L

A. Etiology and pathophysiology

1. Cellular level: is usually due to iatrogenic causes

   a. Decreased renal excretion of magnesium, such as with decreased urine output or renal failure

   b. Increased magnesium intake, such as with overuse of magnesium-containing antacids, cathartics, or enemas; total parenteral nutrition; or hemodialysis using hard water dialysate

2. Predisposing clinical conditions

   a. Untreated diabetic ketoacidosis (glucose carries cations across cell membranes)

   b. Adrenal insufficiency (Addison's disease): causes fluid and electrolyte shifts

   c. Magnesium treatment in pre-eclampsia of pregnancy

        d. Lithium ingestion

        e. Volume depletion

B. Assessment

  1. Clinical manifestations

        a. Neuromuscular symptoms are the most common, including decreased deep tendon reflexes and depressed neuromuscular activity; these are similar to those seen in hyperkalemia

        b. Cardiovascular manifestations include hypotension, bradycardia, bradyarrhythmias, flushing and sensation of warmth, possible cardiac arrest

        c. ECG may show prolonged PR interval, widened QRS complex, and elevated T wave

        d. CNS depression may include somnolence, weakness and lethargy, respiratory depression, and coma

  2. Diagnostic and laboratory findings

        a. Plasma magnesium levels are > 2.1 mEq/L

        b. Associated electrolyte levels: none

        c. Trending of results: the degree of elevation of magnesium is proportionate to the severity of the symptoms

C. Priority nursing diagnoses

  1. Risk for alteration in cardiac function

  2. Risk for injury

  3. Risk for altered respiratory status

  4. Knowledge deficit related to causes of elevated magnesium levels

D. Therapeutic management

  1. Decrease magnesium intake; withdraw all magnesium-containing agents including antacids and enemas

  2. Promote magnesium excretion using diuretics (in stable renal function)

  3. Continued monitoring of client

        a. Continue to monitor the client for overhydration, magnesium toxicity

        b. Monitor cardiac status and ECG changes

        c. Monitor for symptoms of CNS depression

        d. Monitor respiratory status and changes

  4. Restoration of balance

        a. Correct diabetic ketoacidosis by administration of insulin and IV dextrose to halt cellular catabolism

        b. Provide rehydration to promote increased urinary output and magnesium excretion

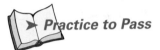

NCLEX!

Practice to Pass

What cardiovascular symptoms may occur with hypermagnesemia?

NCLEX!

NCLEX!

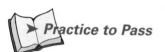

NCLEX!

    c. Emergency treatment includes IV calcium gluconate to antagonize the effect of magnesium and counteract cardiac and respiratory symptoms

    d. Dialysis: in clients with renal failure, dialysis may be necessary for magnesium removal; if hemodialysis is not feasible, peritoneal dialysis is an option

E. Planning and implementation

1. Monitor intake and output

2. Identify risk factors such as antacid use, laxative use, diabetic instability, and renal failure

3. Monitor for potential complications

4. Promote client safety

F. Medication therapy

1. Parenteral administration

    a. IV calcium gluconate 10% for emergency situations

    b. IV diuretics to promote urinary excretion and output

    c. Rehydration to increase urinary output

2. Specific drug therapies: as above

G. Client education

1. Awareness of predisposing factors

    a. Educate the client to avoid medications and supplements high in magnesium

    b. Educate the client about risks of chronic antacid and enema use

    c. Review diabetic control measures

    d. Educate the client about signs and symptoms of high or low magnesium levels

2. Dietary education: avoid high magnesium foods such as legumes, whole grain cereals, nuts, dark green vegetables, and cocoa

H. Evaluation

1. Manifestations of hypermagnesemia resolve and serum levels return to normal

2. Client verbalizes an understanding of importance of diet and followup visits and laboratory testing

Practice to Pass

What role does calcium gluconate have in the treatment of hypermagnesemia?

Case Study

A 32-year-old female tells the nurse she feels her heart is racing and she has been getting frequent cramps in her legs and hands for the past week or so. She has had no recent illness or injury. She has no known allergies and denies any medication or drug use. Her review of systems is negative except for constipation. Intake information for this visit is as follows: height 5'8", weight 120 lbs, B/P 110/72, pulse 98, respirations 18.

❶ What data from the above may indicate a risk factor for hypomagnesemia?

❷ What other subjective data is necessary to gather?

❸ What diagnostic evaluation measures would be helpful?

❹ What collaborative measures should be considered?

❺ What instructions would you give this client to avoid fluctuating magnesium levels?

For suggested responses, see page 232.

Posttest

1   The nurse who is working with a client with a magnesium deficiency understands that magnesium is bound to ATP, which is responsible for what body activity?

(1) Sugar absorption
(2) Energy
(3) Bone absorption
(4) Vitamin conservation

2   The nurse doing health promotion with a group of clients explains that magnesium has which of the following important functions to maintain the health of teeth?

(1) Binds calcium to tooth enamel
(2) Decreases risk of gum disease
(3) Protects teeth from bacteria
(4) Raises serum calcium levels

3   The nurse would recommend to a client with hypomagnesemia to increase intake of which of the following foods that contains high amounts of magnesium?

(1) Rice
(2) Bread
(3) Legumes
(4) Fresh fruit

4   The nurse anticipates that which of the following treatments would be used for a client just diagnosed with hypermagnesemia?

(1) Laxative
(2) Diuretic
(3) Antacid
(4) Fluid restriction

5   The nurse anticipates that which of the following clients is at risk for hypermagnesemia?

(1) An anorexic teen
(2) An alcoholic
(3) A client with a history of partial gastrectomy
(4) A client with renal failure

6   The nurse explains to a new nurse orientee that a hyperglycemic diabetic client may experience low magnesium levels due to which of the following?

(1) Liver toxicity
(2) Osmotic diuresis
(3) Kidney failure
(4) Low serum osmolarity

7   The nurse would assess for which of the following common side effects when administering oral magnesium?

(1) Decreased appetite
(2) Anuria
(3) Polydipsia
(4) Diarrhea

8   The nurse would assess for signs of hypomagnesemia in which of the following clients?

(1) A client with laxative abuse
(2) A client who is noncompliant with diuretic therapy
(3) A client who takes magnesium-containing antacids
(4) A client who is taking gentamicin (Garamycin)

9   A client is admitted with new onset renal failure. The nurse would observe for which of the following most common clinical manifestations of hypermagnesemia?

(1) Cardiac arrest
(2) Neuromuscular symptoms
(3) Respiratory depression
(4) Hypertension

10   After treating hypomagnesemia with IV fluids, a repeat serum magnesium level is 4.0 mEq/L. The nurse anticipates receiving an order for which of the following medications?

(1) Dextrose
(2) Calcium gluconate
(3) Potassium chloride
(4) Sodium chloride

See page 125 for Answers and Rationales.

Answers and Rationales

Pretest

1   **Answer: 3** *Rationale:* Many laxatives are magnesium-based compounds. Overuse could result in increased absorption of magnesium and decreased kidney excretion. The other problems listed do not elevate magnesium levels.
Cognitive Level: Application
Nursing Process: Assessment; *Test Plan:* PHYS

2   **Answer: 4** *Rationale:* Deep tendon reflexes (DTRs) may be diminished or absent when magnesium levels are high. This is because magnesium diminishes acetylcholine activity at the myoneural junction, thus impairing impulse transmission.
Cognitive Level: Application
Nursing Process: Assessment; *Test Plan:* PHYS

3   **Answer: 3** *Rationale:* Clients should be instructed to eat foods that are high in magnesium in order to raise blood levels to within the normal range.
Cognitive Level: Application
Nursing Process: Planning; *Test Plan:* HPM

4   **Answer: 4** *Rationale:* Magnesium deficiency often coexists with other electrolyte imbalances, especially decreased calcium and potassium. Leg cramps are a manifestation of hypomagnesemia.
Cognitive Level: Application
Nursing Process: Assessment; *Test Plan:* PHYS

5   **Answer: 1** *Rationale:* Normal blood levels of magnesium range from 1.4 to 2.1 mEq/L. The other ranges listed are incorrect.
Cognitive Level: Analysis
Nursing Process: Assessment; *Test Plan:* PHYS

6   **Answer: 3** *Rationale:* Normal levels of magnesium in the blood are between 1.4 and 2.1 mEq/L. A level of 3.2 mEq/L indicates hypermagnesemia. Symptoms of hypermagnesemia may be similar to those of hyperkalemia, because it is responsible for neuromuscular transmission.
Cognitive Level: Analysis
Nursing Process: Analysis; *Test Plan:* PHYS

7   **Answer: 2** *Rationale:* Magnesium decreases the amount of acetylcholine activity, thereby causing muscle relaxation. The other responses are incorrect.
Cognitive Level: Application
Nursing Process: Implementation; *Test Plan:* PHYS

8   **Answer: 4** *Rationale:* Most magnesium exists within the cells of the body, with more than 50% being located in the bone. The other responses are incorrect.
Cognitive Level: Comprehension
Nursing Process: Analysis; *Test Plan:* PHYS

9   **Answer: 3** *Rationale:* The RDA for magnesium is 300 to 350 mg for young men and women. Extra re-

quirements beyond this amount are needed during pregnancy and lactation.
Cognitive Level: Application
Nursing Process: Implementation; *Test Plan:* HPM

10 **Answer: 4** *Rationale:* Magnesium is absorbed in the small intestine and is excreted mostly by the kidney.
Cognitive Level: Knowledge
Nursing Process: Analysis; *Test Plan:* PHYS

Posttest

1 **Answer: 2** *Rationale:* ATP (adenosine triphosphate) is responsible for producing energy for the body and accomplishes this by splitting ATP into adenosine diphosphate (ADP). Magnesium is bound to the ATP molecule and is thus needed for this reaction.
Cognitive Level: Knowledge
Nursing Process: Analysis; *Test Plan:* PHYS

2 **Answer: 1** *Rationale:* Magnesium binds calcium to tooth enamel and thus helps to maintain the health of teeth. The other responses are incorrect statements.
Cognitive Level: Application
Nursing Process: Implementation; *Test Plan:* HPM

3 **Answer: 3** *Rationale:* Legumes are high in magnesium. The other options listed contain either low or trace amounts of magnesium.
Cognitive Level: Application
Nursing Process: Implementation; *Test Plan:* HPM

4 **Answer: 2** *Rationale:* Treatment for hypermagnesemia is to promote urinary excretion of magnesium to decrease serum levels, so a diuretic may be indicated. Laxatives and antacids often contain magnesium, which could worsen the imbalance. Fluid restriction would be contraindicated, because it would prevent flushing of excess magnesium from the body.
Cognitive Level: Analysis
Nursing Process: Planning; *Test Plan:* PHYS

5 **Answer: 4** *Rationale:* Renal failure interferes with excretion of electrolytes, including magnesium. All of the conditions listed in the incorrect options increase

risk of hypomagnesemia by interfering with the magnesium absorption in the small intestine.
Cognitive Level: Analysis
Nursing Process: Analysis; *Test Plan:* PHYS

6 **Answer: 2** *Rationale:* The hyperglycemic diabetic client experiences osmotic diuresis and polyuria, which then increases risk of excess urinary excretion of magnesium, leading to lowered magnesium levels. The other options are incorrect.
Cognitive Level: Application
Nursing Process: Implementation; *Test Plan:* PHYS

7 **Answer: 4** *Rationale:* Oral administration of magnesium may cause diarrhea, which would then further decrease magnesium absorption. The other options are incorrect items.
Cognitive Level: Application
Nursing Process: Assessment; *Test Plan:* PHYS

8 **Answer: 4** *Rationale:* Gentamicin is one medication that may lead to hypomagnesemia. All the conditions or circumstances listed in the other options increase serum magnesium levels by enhancing the absorption of magnesium by the small intestine or interfering with its excretion by the kidney.
Cognitive Level: Analysis
Nursing Process: Assessment; *Test Plan:* PHYS

9 **Answer: 2** *Rationale:* Neuromuscular symptoms are the most common clinical manifestations of hypermagnesemia and may include decreased deep tendon reflexes. Decreased respirations, cardiac arrhythmias, and hypotension may also occur in some clients, but are not the most common signs.
Cognitive Level: Application
Nursing Process: Assessment; *Test Plan:* PHYS

10 **Answer: 2** *Rationale:* The repeat serum magnesium level is high. Calcium gluconate is an antagonist of magnesium and is used intravenously to counteract toxicity.
Cognitive Level: Analysis
Nursing Process: Planning; *Test Plan:* PHYS

References

Beers, J. H. & Berkow, R. (Eds.) (1999). *Merck manual of diagnosis and therapy* (17th ed.). Whitehouse Station, NJ: Merck Research Laboratories, pp. 137–151.

Dudek, S. (2001). *Nutrition essentials for nursing practice* (4th ed.). Philadelphia: Lippincott, Williams & Wilkins, pp. 142–144, 639.

Horne, M. & Bond, E. (2002). Fluid, electrolyte, and acid-base imbalances. In S. Lewis, M. Heitkemper, & M. Dirksen. *Medical–surgical nursing: Assessment and management of clinical problems* (5th ed.). St. Louis: Mosby, pp. 341–342.

Kee, J. L. (2001). *Handbook of laboratory and diagnostic tests with nursing implications* (4th ed.). Upper Saddle River, NJ: Prentice-Hall, Inc., pp. 300–302.

Kozier, B., Erb, G., Berman, A. J., & Burke, K. (2000). *Fundamentals of nursing: Concepts, process, and practice* (6th ed.). Upper Saddle River, NJ: Prentice-Hall, Inc., pp. 1302–1334.

LeMone, P. & Burke, K. (2000). *Medical-surgical nursing: Critical thinking in client care* (2nd ed.). Upper Saddle River: NJ: Prentice-Hall, Inc., pp. 146–149.

McCance, K. & Huether, S. (1998). *Pathophysiology: The biological basis for disease in adults and children* (4th ed.). St. Louis: Mosby.

Pagana, K. & Pagana, T. (1999). *Mosby's diagnostic and laboratory test reference* (4th ed.). St. Louis: Mosby.

CHAPTER 6

Chloride Balance and Imbalances

Linda Wilson Covington, PhD, RN

CHAPTER OUTLINE

OBJECTIVES

- Review basic functions of chloride in the body.
- Discuss the pathophysiology and etiology of chloride imbalances.
- Discuss specific assessment findings in chloride imbalances.
- Identify priority nursing diagnoses for a client experiencing a chloride imbalance.
- Discuss therapeutic management of chloride imbalances.
- Discuss nursing management of a client who is experiencing a chloride imbalance.

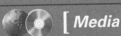

[Media Link]

Use the CD-ROM enclosed with this text, or log onto the address given to access the free, interactive Companion Website created for this series. The CD-ROM and Companion Website accompanying this book offer additional practice opportunities and information—NCLEX Review, Case Studies, Glossary, In Depth with NCLEX, and more.

www.prenhall.com/hogan

REVIEW AT A GLANCE

halogen *a nonionized form of a halide that combines with alkali metals in the body to form salts such as sodium chloride or potassium chloride*

hyperchloremia *a serum chloride level greater than 108 mEq/L*

hypochloremia *a serum chloride level less than 95 mEq/L*

Pretest

1 A client is being discharged with a prescription for glucocorticoid steroids. Which statement would indicate the client's understanding of the side effects of this type of drug?

(1) "I should limit my salt intake."
(2) "I should stop taking my diuretics."
(3) "I should increase salt in my diet."
(4) "I should eat more spinach and celery."

2 Which of the following should be included in the plan of care for a client who received multiple ampules of sodium bicarbonate over several days time?

(1) Administer dextrose 5% in water infusion at 125 mL/hour for 5 days.
(2) Draw a serum chloride level periodically.
(3) Draw a stat serum magnesium level.
(4) Administer diuretics to prevent metabolic acidosis.

3 Which of the following laboratory test results would you expect to see in a client admitted with Cushing's syndrome who has a serum osmolality of 298 mOsm/kg?

(1) Serum chloride level of 111 mEq/L
(2) Serum sodium level of 130 mEq/L
(3) Serum potassium level of 5 mEq/L
(4) Urine chloride level of 90 mEq/L

4 Which one of the following interventions should be implemented when the nurse is preparing to draw a serum chloride level?

(1) Draw the blood from an implanted port used for chemotherapy, if possible.
(2) Have the client clench and unclench the hand prior to drawing the blood.
(3) Draw a 3 to 5 mL blood sample without a tourniquet if possible.
(4) Send hemolyzed blood to the laboratory if no other specimen is available.

5 Which one of the following clients would be the least likely to benefit from the administration of 3% saline solution for hypochloremia?

(1) A client diagnosed with Addison's disease
(2) A client who has been NPO for several days
(3) A client diagnosed with congestive heart failure (CHF)
(4) A client diagnosed with alkalosis

6 A client has developed weakness, lethargy, and fatigue due to a chloride imbalance. Which of the following statements to the client by the nurse is most accurate?

(1) "Your symptoms are permanent but you can learn to live with them."
(2) "If you increase your exercise routine, your chloride level will return to normal."
(3) "You will have to increase your salt intake in order to eliminate your symptoms."
(4) "Your symptoms will be disappear after your chloride level decreases to normal."

7 The nurse should place highest priority on which of the following interventions in the care of a client admitted with symptoms related to a chloride level of 70 mEq/L and extracellular fluid (ECF) loss?

(1) Monitoring blood pressure for decrease in value
(2) Assisting client to the restroom to prevent injury
(3) Starting an IV with dextrose in water
(4) Monitoring pulse for pounding slow rate

8 Which of the following nursing diagnoses would be a priority for a client experiencing neuromuscular abnormalities related to a chloride imbalance?

(1) Fluid volume excess
(2) Fluid volume deficit
(3) Risk for injury
(4) Ineffective individual coping

9 An alert client is admitted with a diagnosis of hyperchloremia. The nurse should place highest priority on doing which of the following interventions first?

(1) Place the client on isolation precautions.
(2) Document the client's history.
(3) Allow the client to ambulate ad lib unassisted to maintain independence.
(4) Start an IV of 3% saline infusion stat.

10 Which of the following activities would be least acceptable for a client diagnosed with hypochloremia?

(1) Decrease salt in the diet.
(2) Use soy sauce sparingly in the diet.
(3) Decrease canned soups.
(4) Decrease bananas and dates.

See pages 141–142 for Answers and Rationales.

I. Overview of Chloride Regulation

A. Chloride balance and function: major extracellular anion (average level 104 mEq/L) that also exists in a lesser concentration in the cell (average 4 mEq/L); it is closely associated with serum sodium levels and affects acid-base balance in the body

1. Chloride levels

   a. Adult norm 95 to 108 mEq/L

   b. Newborn norm 96 to 106 mEq/L

   c. Normal urinary chloride level ranges from 110 to 254 mEq/24 hours in adults and varies significantly in children depending on age (see Table 6-1)

   d. Chloride sweat levels: adults 10 to 70 mEq/L and 5 to 45mEq/L in children

2. Functions in the body

   a. Chloride is a **halogen** (nonionized form of a halide) that combines with alkali metals to form salts in the body, such as sodium chloride or potassium chloride

   b. Chloride circulates primarily with sodium and water and helps to maintain cellular integrity by maintaining a balance between intracellular and extracellular fluids in the body; it also helps to control osmotic pressure

Table 6-1	Age	Normal Range
Normal Urine Chloride Levels	**24-Hour Urine**	
	Adult Age 18–59	110–254 mEq/24h
	Age 60 and older	95–195 mEq/24h
	Child	2–10 mEq/24h
	Infant	15–40 mEq/24h

c. In addition to its function as a passive transport companion for sodium and potassium in the body, active transport mechanisms may also be involved

d. Chloride is essential for maintaining acid-base and electrolyte balance and is an enzyme activator; it serves as a buffer in the exchange of oxygen and carbon dioxide in red blood cells

e. When joined with hydrogen (a cation), the chloride anion plays an important role in digestion by forming hydrochloric acid (HCl) in the stomach; chloride regulates the pH of the stomach and helps in digestion of protein

f. In conjunction with calcium and magnesium, chloride helps to maintain nerve transmission and normal muscle contraction and relaxation

g. The kidneys eliminate or retain chloride mainly as sodium chloride to regulate acid-base levels

h. Chloride may also assist the liver in clearing waste products

i. Chloride is also found in significant amounts in sweat

j. Refer to Table 6-2 for a listing of chloride concentration in body fluids

3. System interactions

a. There is a correlation between chloride levels and serum osmolality and sodium levels

1) When serum osmolality is increased to > 295 mOsm/kg, there are a greater number of sodium and chloride ions in proportion to body water, leading to elevated serum chloride levels

2) When serum osmolality is decreased to < 280 mOsm/kg, there are relatively fewer sodium and chloride ions in proportion to body water, leading to decreased serum chloride levels

3) When sodium is retained, chloride is frequently retained, causing water retention

b. The kidneys excrete the chloride anion or bicarbonate, and sodium reabsorbs either chloride or bicarbonate to maintain acid-base balance

c. Chloride combines with hydrogen ion in the stomach to form hydrochloric acid

Table 6-2	Fluid	Chloride (mEq/L)
Concentration of Chloride in Body Fluids	Saliva	34
	Cecal fluid	48
	Sweat	< 60 adults; < 50 children
	Pancreatic juice	77
	Gastric juice	84
	Bile	101
	Ileal fluid	116
	Cerebrospinal fluid	127

Table 6-3	Food Group	Examples
Foods High in Chloride	Fruits	Dates and bananas only
	Dairy products	Cheese, milk
	Vegetables	Canned vegetables and soup, spinach, celery, olives, and rye
	Meat, fish, and poultry	Eggs, crabs, fish, turkey

B. Sources of chloride

    1. Cellular level

        a. Chloride passively diffuses from the tubule to the capillary; reabsorption depends on active reabsorption of sodium into the cell

        b. Chloride is absorbed from the small intestine and is primarily found in the extracellular fluid

        c. It is secreted in the gastric juice as hydrochloric acid

        d. The kidneys play a role in chloride regulation that affects acid-base balance in the body

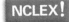

    2. Dietary level

        a. Chloride is obtained primarily from salt, such as standard table salt or sea salt

        b. Foods with high chloride levels include canned vegetables, dates, bananas, cheese, spinach, milk, eggs, celery, crabs, fish, olives, and rye (refer to Table 6-3 for a list of foods high in chloride)

        c. Processed foods are high in chloride content

        d. Chloride is a constituent part of sodium chloride as well as other dietary salts

        e. There is no RDA for this micronutrient but there is an adult estimated minimum requirement of 750 mg/day

II. *Hypochloremia:* a serum chloride level that falls below 95 mEq/L

    A. Etiology and pathophysiology

        1. Cellular level

            a. Decreases in chloride usually are accompanied by decreases in sodium and potassium

            b. A reduction in hydrochloric acid decreases chloride

            c. Chloride is excreted with cations during massive diuresis and when the bicarbonate level is elevated

            d. When the serum level falls, the urinary excretion of chloride is decreased in an attempt to retain more of the electrolyte

Table 6-4		Hypochloremia (serum level < 95 mEq/L adults)	Hyperchloremia (serum level > 108 mEq/L adults)
Chloride Imbalances with Abnormal Values and Etiologies	**Etiology**		
	Metabolic imbalance Gastrointestinal disorders and dietary changes	Metabolic alkalosis GI suctioning, vomiting, diarrhea, GI surgery, hypokalemia, excessive ingestion of alkaline substances	Metabolic acidosis Increased retention or intake, hyperkalemia, hypernatremia, severe vomiting, salicylate intoxication
	Renal disorders	Advanced renal disorders, diuretics	Reduced glomerular filtration
	Hormonal influences	SIADH, Addison's disease	Excess adrenocortical hormone production, IV or oral cortisone therapy
	Altered cellular function	Hypervolemic CHF and cirrhosis	
	Skin/environmental changes Head injury	Burns, fever, large skin wounds	Profuse perspiration Head trauma

NCLEX!

2. Predisposing clinical conditions (see Table 6-4)

   a. Fluid and electrolyte imbalances

      1) Hyponatremia

      2) Metabolic alkalosis (due to ingestion of alkaline substances or as a consequence of elevated bicarbonate concentration due to disease processes—can be chloride responsive or chloride resistant depending on urinary chloride levels)

      3) Hypokalemia

      4) Prolonged administration of D_5W IV therapy

   b. Chronic respiratory acidosis

   c. Clients with chronic lung disease have high pCO_2 levels with chronic elevation of bicarbonate levels that results in a decreased serum chloride

   d. Diabetic acidosis because of increased anion gap

   e. Acute infections, although the mechanism by which they lower serum chloride level is unclear

NCLEX!

   f. Vomiting (loss of HCl), GI suctioning, perspiration, diarrhea, and presence of fistulas

   g. Metabolic stress conditions, such as severe burns, fever, heat and exhaustion states

   h. Disease states such as Addison's disease, anorexia, salt-wasting renal nephropathy, syndrome of inappropriate antidiuretic hormone (SIADH), and hypervolemic states such as congestive heart failure (CHF) and cirrhosis

Table 6-5	Increase Serum Chloride Levels	Decrease Serum Chloride Levels
Pharmacologic Agents Affecting Chloride Balance	Acetazolamide (Diamox) Ammonium chloride Boric acid Chlorothiazide (Diuril) Cyclosporine (Neoral) Glucocorticoids Guanethidine sulfate (Ismelin) Phenylbutazone Sodium bromide 0.9% Sodium chloride solution 3% Sodium chloride solution	Aldosterone Amiloride (Midamor) Bumetanide (Bumex) Corticotropin (ACTH) Dextrose infusion (prolonged) Ethacrynic acid (Edecrin) Furosemide (Lasix) Mercurial diuretics Prednisolone (Delta-Cortef) Sodium bicarbonate (Citrocarbonate) Triamterene (Dyrenium) Thiazide diuretics

     i. Various medications that promote electrolyte loss, have diuretic activity, or promote alkalosis (see Table 6-5 for a listing of medications that contribute to hypochloremia)

B. Assessment

  1. Clinical manifestations (refer to Table 6-6)

    a. Hyperexcitability of nerves and muscles leads to tremors and twitching

    b. Respiratory abnormalities include slow and shallow breathing

    c. Cardiac abnormalities include hypotension when there are severe chloride and extracellular fluid (ECF) losses

NCLEX!

    d. Alterations in serum chloride levels are seldom a primary problem; there are usually associated electrolyte imbalances (such as hyponatremia or hypokalemia) and acid-base disturbances such as metabolic alkalosis and hypokalemic alkalosis

    e. Decreased levels are associated with diarrhea, emphysema, gastric suction, fluid volume excess states (such as CHF, hyponatremia, and SIADH), pyloric obstruction, malabsorption syndrome, diabetes with ketoacidosis, excess of mineralcorticoids, and salt-wasting renal disease

Table 6-6	System Alteration	Hypochloremia	Hyperchloremia
Clinical Manifestations of Chloride Imbalances	Respiratory	Slow and shallow respirations (signs of metabolic alkalosis due to bicarbonate retention)	Deep rapid respirations (signs of metabolic acidosis due to loss of bicarbonate)
	Cardiac	Hypotension with severe chloride and extracellular fluid loss	
	Neurological	Muscle tremors and twitching	Weakness, lethargy, stupor, unconsciousness
	Serum laboratory value	< 95 mEq/L	> 108 mEq/L

f. Decreased chloride sweat levels are seen in hypoaldosteronism, sodium depletion, and the administration of mineralocorticoids

2. Diagnostic and laboratory findings

a. Serum chloride level is < 95 mEq/L

b. Panic value for serum chloride level is < 80 mEq/L (see Box 6-1)

c. Urinary chloride concentration varies with salt intake and urine volume and is helpful when discriminating between chloride responsive (< 10 mEq/L) and chloride resistant (> 10 mEq/L) metabolic alkalosis disturbances

d. Obtaining ABG results and serum sodium and potassium levels may provide information necessary for the management of clients with chloride deficit

e. Trending of results

1) Helpful in differentiating between types of metabolic alkalosis

2) Hypochloremia should be considered with reference to presenting clinical manifestations or the presence of other electrolyte imbalances, such as hyponatremia or hypokalemia

3. Identification of risk factors: dietary insufficiency or previously identified co-existing medical conditions that lead to or exacerbate hypochloremia

C. Priority nursing diagnoses

1. Altered nutrition: less than body requirements related to decreased chloride intake or increased loss

2. Fluid volume excess related to disease process

3. Risk for sensory/perceptual alterations related to neurological changes

4. Fatigue related to muscle weakness

5. Risk for injury related to weakness and lethargy

6. Self-care deficit related to altered respiratory status

7. Anxiety related to increased muscle irritability

D. Therapeutic management

1. Replacement therapies

a. If chloride levels are slightly low and client is able to tolerate PO feedings, then administer oral salt tablets or increase chloride dietary sources

---

NCLEX!

NCLEX!

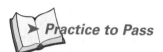
Practice to Pass

A client is being treated for metabolic alkalosis and is at risk for altered serum chloride level because of this condition. Would you expect the serum chloride level to be increased or decreased? Why?

Box 6-1

Severe Serum Chloride Imbalance (Panic Level)

Laboratory Values: < 80 or > 115 mEq/L

Manifestations
• Impaired mentation
• Hypotension or hypertension
• Cardiac dysrhythmias

Treatment: correct the underlying disorder

      b. Provide IV infusion of chloride if levels are critical or if client is unable to tolerate PO administration

  2. Continued monitoring of client

      a. Monitor serum and urinary chloride levels

      b. Monitor intake and output because excess water administration can cause dilutional hypochloremia and hyponatremia

      c. Monitor blood pressure because a drop in blood pressure can occur if hypochloremia is due to ECF volume loss

      d. Monitor ABG results if client's clinical presentation or underlying medical history suggests accompanying acid-base imbalance

      e. When drawing a serum chloride specimen:

         1) Client should be NPO (8 to 12 hours) prior to test to obtain most accurate result

         2) Do not draw specimen from hemodialysis access because this can lead to unreliable results due to coagulation factors

         3) Draw specimen from an extremity that does not have saline infusing into it because this can affect results

         4) When possible, do not use a tourniquet and prevent the client from pumping the fist, because this can lead to hemolysis of blood specimen and yield inaccurate results

  3. Restoration of balance

      a. Promote dietary changes to increase chloride intake

      b. Administer chloride supplements as ordered

      c. Continue to assess those clients at risk

      d. Provide parenteral administration if warranted

      e. Monitor the client with underlying or contributory disease processes and/or medication therapy that would lead to chloride deficiencies

E. Planning and implementation

  1. Identify risk factors specific to development of chloride loss, such as dietary factors, GI losses, renal losses, altered hormone secretion, altered cellular states, and metabolic alkalosis

  2. Monitor the client during the course of therapy, looking at pertinent lab values and clinical manifestations

  3. Monitor vital signs (VS) and intake and output (I & O) parameters

  4. Maintain safety precautions by keeping bedrails up and assisting client with ambulation if client presents with muscle tremors and/or decreased blood pressure

F. Medication therapy

  1. Oral replacement therapy

      a. Utilize salt tablets or potassium chloride salts to raise serum chloride levels

b. Chloride is usually not administered as a separate medication but rather is found in combination with other elements in salt formation products or as an additive/buffer

2. Parenteral replacement therapy

a. Chloride can be given parenterally as a constituent part of a medication such as potassium chloride or sodium chloride in the clinical setting

b. Monitoring of IV solutions containing chloride depends on concentration of overall solution and may require the use of IV administration pumps

3. Dietary therapy: include foods that are high in chloride, such as salt, processed foods, canned vegetables, dates, bananas, cheese, spinach, milk, eggs, celery, crabs, fish, olives, and rye (refer back to Table 6-3)

G. Client education

1. Teach awareness of predisposing factors, including contributory conditions

a. Endocrine states that result in adrenocortical insufficiency or primary aldosteronism

b. Acid-base imbalances that result in metabolic acidosis (high anion gap), such as diabetic ketoacidosis, Addison's disease, and nephritis

c. Acid-base imbalances that result in metabolic alkalosis, such as pyloric obstruction

d. Acid-base imbalances that result in chronic respiratory acidosis

e. Use of medications that would likely increase chloride loss (refer back to Table 6-5)

f. Recognition of fluid volume states that would cause fluid shifting and electrolyte deficit

2. Dietary education

a. Review foods that are high in chloride

b. Advise client to include in the diet sodium and processed foods that are also high in chloride

c. Advise client that electrolyte replacement as well as fluid replacement is important if activity level is increased and client has excessive perspiration

d. Collaborate with dietician as needed

H. Evaluation

1. Chloride serum levels and other pertinent electrolyte levels return to normal baseline

2. Acid-base balance returns to normal baseline

3. Clinical manifestations resolve

III. *Hyperchloremia:* a serum chloride level that is greater than 108 mEq/L

A. Etiology and pathophysiology

1. Cellular level

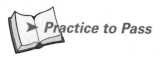

Practice to Pass

A client is diagnosed with hypochloremia. How would you explain the disorder? What strategies can be used to correct the problem?

a. Cellular chloride shifts are seen in response to acid-base changes and volume disturbances in the body

b. Increases in serum chloride are seen in conjunction with other electrolyte imbalances and are usually assessed with sodium, potassium, water, and CO_2 levels in the body

2. Predisposing clinical conditions (refer again to Table 6-4)

   a. Fluid and electrolyte imbalances

     1) Hypernatremia

     2) Metabolic acidosis (loss of sodium bicarbonate because of prolonged diarrhea), hyperchloremic metabolic acidosis (renal disease that causes decreased excretion of hydrogen ions and prevents reabsorption of bicarbonate), or respiratory alkalosis (hyperventilation)

   b. Ingestion or administration of drugs that promote chloride retention, such as IV saline, certain diuretics, salicylate intoxication, corticosteroids, guanethidine, and phenylbutazone (refer back to Table 6-5)

   c. Fluid volume disturbances that result in dehydration states

   d. Endocrine disturbances that result in diabetes insipidus (DI) and certain cases of hyperparathyroidism (seen in association with hypercalcemia)

   e. Gastrointestinal losses involving severe vomiting, diarrhea, or intestinal fistula may cause elevated serum chloride levels

   f. Renal changes that manifest as renal tubular acidosis or acute renal failure can result in elevated serum chloride levels

B. Assessment

1. Clinical manifestations (refer again to Table 6-6)

   a. Neuromuscular symptoms include weakness and lethargy and can progress to significant CNS damage

   b. Respiratory abnormalities include deep, rapid, vigorous breathing that can lead to unconsciousness as the client attempts to compensate for acidotic state due to loss of bicarbonate

   c. Cardiac abnormalities include risk of dysrhythmias due to retained chloride levels and accompanying acid-base disturbances

   d. Alterations in hormonal response as a result of increased aldosterone levels can lead to elevations of both sodium and chloride due to greater reabsorption

   e. Fluid volume disturbances can lead to increased chloride levels, including dehydration, retention of salt and water due to drug administration, and a greater sodium loss than chloride loss, leading to imbalance

   f. Presence of disease states such as DI, certain types of hyperparathyroidism, and renal tubular diseases result in hydrogen ion retention and decreased reabsorption of bicarbonate

   g. Increased chloride sweat levels are seen in DI, hypothyroidism, malnutrition, acute renal failure, and certain genetic disorders such as cystic fibrosis and glucose-6-phosphate-dehydrogenase (G6PD) deficiency

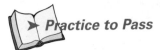

> **Practice to Pass**
>
> A client is taking both furosemide (Lasix) for treatment of hypertension and a steroid Medrol dose pack for an allergic reaction. Which of these medications would intensify hyperchloremia?

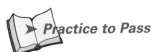

> **Practice to Pass**
>
> A client diagnosed with hyperchloremia should be monitored for respiratory abnormalities. Which symptoms should the nurse assess for?

2. Diagnostic and laboratory findings

NCLEX!

   a. Panic value for serum chloride is > 115 mEq/L (refer again to Box 6-1)

   b. Urine chloride level > 250 mEq/L in 24 hours is significant and is associated with sodium and fluid imbalances

NCLEX!

   c. In dehydration states, serum chloride levels are increased due to hemoconcentration

   d. Increased chloride sweat levels are seen in many disease states and can be used as a diagnostic tool in the work-up for cystic fibrosis

NCLEX!

   e. Associated electrolyte imbalances that usually occur with elevated chloride levels are elevated potassium and sodium levels and decreased bicarbonate levels

   f. Trending of results

      1) It is important to monitor the client with attention to acid-base values and trend results by examining anion gap

      2) Hyperchloremic acidosis is associated with a normal anion gap

      3) There can be artifact disturbances seen in acid-base imbalances resulting in falsely elevated chloride levels; it is therefore important to trend results and evaluate the client using complete assessment parameters and not merely one lab value

C. Priority nursing diagnoses

1. Altered nutrition: greater than body requirements related to increased chloride intake or decreased loss

2. Impaired skin integrity related to dehydration

3. Altered health maintenance related to weakness

4. Risk for sensory/perceptual alterations related to lethargy

5. Risk for injury related to weakness and lethargy

6. Self-care deficit related to altered respiratory status

7. Anxiety related to increased lethargy

D. Therapeutic management

1. Decrease chloride intake; withdraw all chloride-containing agents used as treatment measures

2. Promote chloride excretion by administering diuretics

NCLEX!

3. Continue monitoring client, including acid-base, respiratory, and cardiac status

4. Restoration of balance

   a. Administer appropriate IV therapy to restore fluid and electrolyte balance

NCLEX!

   b. Correct dehydration states with oral and parenteral fluids as needed to restore serum chloride levels

   c. Promote dietary changes to decrease chloride intake

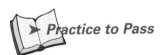

Practice to Pass

A client with a high fever and severe diarrhea and vomiting is admitted to the hospital. Which chloride imbalance is occurring and what are the most likely etiologies for the suspected imbalance?

d. Continue to assess those clients at risk due to underlying or contributory disease and implement appropriate therapies to decrease serum chloride levels

E. Planning and implementation

1. Identify risk factors specific to the development of chloride excess, such as dietary factors, specific disease states, medical therapies, and acidotic states

2. Monitor the client during the course of therapy, trending pertinent laboratory test results and response to treatment

3. Monitor VS and I & O parameters

4. Promote client safety

F. Medication therapy

1. Parenteral administration

   a. Hypotonic solutions such as 0.45% NaCl or D_5W to restore balance

   b. IV administration of diuretics may be utilized to restore acid-base disturbances

2. Additional drug therapies maybe indicated based on underlying clinical conditions and presence of contributory disease

G. Client education

1. Awareness of predisposing factors

   a. Educate the client to avoid medications and supplements containing chloride

   b. If client is experiencing other electrolyte imbalances (sodium, potassium, and water), have a high index of suspicion for possible development of hyperchloremia

2. Dietary education

   a. Avoid foods that are high in chloride levels and restrict use of processed foods because they are high in both sodium and chloride content

   b. Maintain adequate hydration status

   c. Collaborate with dietician as needed

H. Evaluation

1. Chloride serum levels and other pertinent electrolyte levels return to normal baseline

2. Client is able to identify restricted foods, medications, and therapies that would cause serum chloride elevations

3. Correction of underlying disease states and contributory clinical conditions that will assist in returning chloride levels to normal

4. Resolution of symptoms relative to hyperchloremia

Case Study

A 38-year-old male client is being admitted to the hospital with a diagnosis of vomiting related to a gastrointestinal virus. Vital signs reveal BP 100/70, pulse 88, and respirations 18. Client has been unable to keep solid food down for two days and has been drinking liquids (water, soda, and tea) during that time period.

❶ What questions will you ask the client on admission?

❷ What assessments will you make before starting interventions?

❸ What nursing diagnoses are applicable for this client?

❹ What nursing interventions would you implement?

❺ What discharge instructions will you include in your plan of care?

For suggested responses, see page 232.

Posttest

1. A client diagnosed with hyperchloremia is exhibiting neuromuscular abnormalities. The nurse should assess for which of the following manifestations?

   (1) Tremors and flaccid muscles
   (2) Twitching and spastic reflexes
   (3) Hyperreflexia and tremors
   (4) Weakness and lethargy

2. Which of the following should be included as a priority intervention for a client diagnosed with metabolic alkalosis?

   (1) Assess for muscle tremors and slow deep respirations.
   (2) Assess for rapid deep respirations and stupor.
   (3) Restrict salt in the diet.
   (4) Administer diuretics.

3. Which of the following is the most appropriate intervention for a client admitted with a chloride level of 80 mEq/L?

   (1) Administration of 5% dextrose and water
   (2) Administration of 0.9% NaCl
   (3) Administration of 0.45% saline with 20 mEq of potassium
   (4) Administration of free water

4. Which of the following statements would the nurse make during dietary teaching for a client who has been diagnosed with hypochloremia?

   (1) Avoid eating foods containing rye.
   (2) Take a diuretic daily.
   (3) Increase the amount of fruit in the diet.
   (4) Increase dates and bananas in the diet.

5. After checking the medical record of a client who was admitted with shortness of breath and lethargy, the nurse noted a chloride level of 110 mEq/L. Which of the following coexisting medical diagnoses would be the nurse suspect?

   (1) Addison's disease
   (2) Cushing's syndrome
   (3) Metabolic alkalosis
   (4) Syndrome of inappropriate antidiuretic hormone (SIADH)

6. Which of the following nursing diagnoses would the nurse most likely identify for a client with a serum chloride level of 112 mEq/L?

   (1) Altered health maintenance related to nasogastric suctioning
   (2) Altered electrolytes related to hypochloremia
   (3) Altered nutrition: more than body requirements related to excess intake of foods rich in salt
   (4) Altered renal function (chronic) related to acid base imbalance of metabolic alkalosis

7 The nurse should monitor the urine chloride level for a client diagnosed with a serum chloride level of less than 100 mEq/L because urinary excretion of chloride:

(1) Decreases to retain more of the serum chloride.
(2) Increases with a level of 100 mEq/L or less.
(3) Is not influenced by serum chloride level.
(4) Increases with levels greater than 100 mEq/L.

8 A client is admitted to the intensive care unit (ICU) with metabolic alkalosis, hypokalemia, and hyponatremia. The nurse should expect to implement which of the following appropriate actions?

(1) Place the client on a low sodium diet.
(2) Start IV administration of dextrose and water.
(3) Draw stat serum magnesium level.
(4) Draw serum chloride level.

9 Which of the following items in a client's recent history could contribute to a state of hyperchloremic acidosis?

(1) Administration of acetazolamide (Diamox)
(2) Administration of antacids
(3) Administration of thiazide diuretics
(4) Chronic laxative use

10 Which of the following changes in urine levels would be expected in a cardiac client who is experiencing pitting edema?

(1) Increased sodium
(2) Decreased chloride
(3) Increased chloride
(4) Decreased calcium

See pages 142–143 for Answers and Rationales.

Answers and Rationales

Pretest

1 Answer: 1 *Rationale:* Glucocorticoids cause retention of chloride and sodium leading to fluid retention. All of the other options, such as decreasing diuretic intake, increasing salt, and eating foods such as spinach and celery (high in chloride content), will increase the serum chloride level.
Cognitive Level: Analysis
Nursing Process: Evaluation; *Test Plan:* HPM

2 Answer: 2 *Rationale:* Increased use of sodium bicarbonate causes excretion of chloride or hypochloremia; therefore, it would be appropriate to have serum chloride levels drawn to monitor serum level for potential deficits. Option 1 is incorrect because D_5W infusion is hypotonic and will cause further fluid shifting and more potential electrolyte imbalances given the high rate. This will decrease chloride levels if administered over a prolonged time. Option 4 is incorrect, because diuretics will decrease chloride levels. Option 3 is incorrect because a stat magnesium value will not give any additional information and is, therefore, unnecessary.
Cognitive Level: Analysis
Nursing Process: Implementation; *Test Plan:* PHYS

3 Answer: 1 *Rationale:* When serum osmolality is > 295 mOsm/kg, there are more sodium and chloride ions in proportion to water. Therefore, you would expect to see a higher serum chloride level. In a client who has Cushing's syndrome, one would expect to see elevated serum chloride and sodium levels, elevated urinary chloride, and a decreased potassium level. All of the other options are inconsistent with the clinical presentation of Cushing's syndrome.
Cognitive Level: Analysis
Nursing Process: Assessment; *Test Plan:* PHYS

4 Answer: 3 *Rationale:* A tourniquet can potentially cause turbulence in blood flow and alter results by hemolyzing erythrocytes. If possible, blood should be drawn without the use of a tourniquet. Option 1 is incorrect because drawing blood from an implanted port used for chemotherapy is not recommended procedure. Option 2 is incorrect because the action of clenching and unclenching the fist can lead to hemolysis of RBCs and cause altered test results. Option 4 is incorrect because hemolyzed blood will provide altered results of serum electrolytes.
Cognitive Level: Application
Nursing Process: Implementation; *Test Plan:* SECE

5 Answer: 3 *Rationale:* In CHF, chloride is increased; in addition, the administration of hypertonic saline may cause a lethal hypervolemia. Furthermore, mechanisms for excretion of sodium, chloride, and water

are compromised in the client with CHF, causing significant fluid and electrolyte alterations if such a therapy were to be utilized. The clients in options 1 and 2 would benefit from administration of a hypertonic solution in a closely monitored situation. Option 4 is incorrect because a client diagnosed with alkalosis would benefit from administration of a hypertonic solution, since the client would most likely be experiencing chloride and sodium deficits.
Cognitive Level: Analysis
Nursing Process: Planning; *Test Plan:* PHYS

6 **Answer: 4** *Rationale:* The clinical symptoms noted above (weakness, lethargy, and fatigue) are associated with hyperchloremia. Option 1 is incorrect because the symptoms related to chloride deficiency can be reversed with clinical treatment that restores serum chloride levels to normal. Option 2 is incorrect because there is no correlation between exercise and increase in serum chloride level. It is likely that increased exercise would lead to a chloride deficiency through sweat and perspiration losses. Option 3 is incorrect because merely increasing salt intake will not automatically increase serum chloride levels.
Cognitive Level: Application
Nursing Process: Implementation; *Test Plan:* PHYS

7 **Answer: 1** *Rationale:* With severe chloride and ECF losses, the blood pressure drops, potentially leading to shock if it not corrected. The nurse should place the highest priority on monitoring the client to prevent development of potential complications and to maintain client safety. Although it may be necessary to assist the client to the bathroom, this is not the priority intervention. If there is sufficient ECF loss, then the client would more likely be too weak to ambulate and bedrest would be indicated. Option 3 is incorrect because starting IV therapy with a hypotonic solution may further exacerbate the client's clinical condition. Although it would be important to monitor the client's pulse, this again is not the priority intervention at this point in time.
Cognitive Level: Analysis
Nursing Process: Implementation; *Test Plan:* PHYS

8 **Answer: 3** *Rationale:* Neurological alteration related to chloride imbalance includes tremors and twitching of the muscles with hypochloremia or weakness and lethargy with hyperchloremia. These manifestations place the client at risk for injury. Options 1, 2, and 4 may be potential diagnoses but more data would be needed to determine the priorities.
Cognitive Level: Application
Nursing Process: Planning; *Test Plan:* PHYS

9 **Answer: 2** *Rationale:* Documenting the history can assist in determining the cause of the elevated chloride level. This should occur, if possible, prior to intervention. Option 1 is incorrect because isolation is not indicated for hyperchloremia. Option 3 is incorrect because ambulating independently without assessment is unsafe since the client will probably have weakness and lethargy. Option 4 is incorrect because infusing 3% saline is an unsafe intervention that would lead to increased chloride levels.
Cognitive Level: Analysis
Nursing Process: Implementation; *Test Plan:* PHYS

10 **Answer: 1** *Rationale:* Decreasing salt intake will further decrease serum chloride level. The client should increase salt in the diet with hypochloremia. All of the other options reflect foods that are high in chloride and therefore should not be limited in a client with hypochloremia.
Cognitive Level: Application
Nursing Process: Planning; *Test Plan:* HPM

Posttest

1 **Answer: 4** *Rationale:* Weakness and lethargy occur with hyperchloremia. All of the other options reflect manifestations that are associated with hypochloremia.
Cognitive Level: Application
Nursing Process: Assessment; *Test Plan:* PHYS

2 **Answer: 1** *Rationale:* In metabolic alkalosis, bicarbonate ions are retained and the kidneys respond by excreting chloride ions, which in turn causes reciprocal hypochloremia. Option 2 is incorrect because deep, rapid respirations and stupor are symptoms of hyperchloremia. Options 3 and 4 are incorrect because serum chloride levels are decreased and the restriction of salt and administration of diuretics will normally cause further chloride losses to occur, which could further compromise the client's status.
Cognitive Level: Analysis
Nursing Process: Planning; *Test Plan:* PHYS

3 **Answer: 3** *Rationale:* The client presents with hypochloremia and most likely is experiencing other electrolyte deficiencies as well, most notably sodium and potassium. A solution with 0.45% saline with added potassium would be an appropriate option because this would correct all fluid and electrolyte imbalances. Option 2 would not be appropriate because it does not address the issue of additional electrolyte deficiencies. Options 1 and 4 are incorrect because

these fluids can further dilute the plasma and the serum chloride level.
Cognitive Level: Analysis
Nursing Process: Planning; *Test Plan:* PHYS

4 Answer: 4 *Rationale:* Dates and bananas are high in chloride and therefore can be included in a dietary pattern to increase chloride levels. Option 1 is incorrect—foods containing rye should be included in the diet because they are high in chloride. Option 2 is incorrect because diuretics can increase the excretion of chloride and thereby reduce serum chloride levels. Although increasing the amount of fruit in the diet provides nutritional benefit, it does not increase chloride levels.
Cognitive Level: Application
Nursing Process: Implementation; *Test Plan:* HPM

5 Answer: 2 *Rationale:* A serum value of 110 mEq/L reflects an elevated serum chloride level. Cushing's syndrome causes retention of excess sodium and chloride and potassium deficit. Option 1 is incorrect because Addison's disease is associated with decreased levels of sodium and chloride and potassium excess. Option 3 is incorrect because elevated chloride levels are usually associated with metabolic acidosis. Option 4 is incorrect because SIADH is associated with chloride deficit.
Cognitive Level: Analysis
Nursing Process: Assessment; *Test Plan:* PHYS

6 Answer: 3 *Rationale:* The stated value represents an elevated chloride level. Increased use of table salt will cause increase in both sodium and chloride levels. Option 1 is incorrect because the use of NG suctioning causes HCl acid to be lost, thereby decreasing chloride level. Option 2 is incorrect because the client has hyperchloremia, not hypochloremia. Option 4 is incorrect because chloride excess is associated with metabolic acidosis and is seen in clients who have acute renal failure.
Cognitive Level: Analysis
Nursing Process: Planning; *Test Plan:* PHYS

7 Answer: 1 *Rationale:* When the serum chloride level drops below 100 mEq/L, the kidney retains chloride in order to maintain fluid and electrolyte balance. All of the other options are not accurate statements.
Cognitive Level: Comprehension
Nursing Process: Assessment; *Test Plan:* PHYS

8 Answer: 4 *Rationale:* An admitting clinical diagnosis of metabolic alkalosis, hypokalemia, and hyponatremia is usually associated with chloride deficit. It would be prudent to check serum chloride levels in order to ascertain client's baseline and acknowledge multiple electrolyte deficiencies. Option 1 is incorrect because the client's sodium level is low and sodium should not be restricted. Option 2 is incorrect because IV administration of D_5W may cause further complications and fluid shifting if other electrolyte deficiencies are not corrected. Option 3 is incorrect because there is insufficient information to warrant a stat magnesium level to be drawn.
Cognitive Level: Application
Nursing Process: Planning; *Test Plan:* PHYS

9 Answer: 1 *Rationale:* The use of acetazolamide (Diamox) can lead to the development of hyperchloremic acidosis because it increases chloride levels. All of the other options are incorrect because they would lead to chloride deficiencies that would result in an alkalotic state.
Cognitive Level: Analysis
Nursing Process: Analysis; *Test Plan:* PHYS

10 Answer: 2 *Rationale:* A low urine chloride indicates chloride retention in the body, especially with overhydration or fluid excess. Options 1 and 3 are incorrect because they indicate fluid deficit. Option 4 is incorrect, because calcium is not altered by fluid retention due to cardiac disorders.
Cognitive Level: Application
Nursing Process: Assessment; *Test Plan:* PHYS

References

Brody, T. (1999). *Nutritional biochemistry* (2nd ed.). New York: Academic Press, pp. 118–120, 694–698, 702–703, 705.

Corbett, J. (2000). *Laboratory tests and diagnostic procedures with nursing diagnoses* (5th ed.). Upper Saddle River, NJ: Prentice-Hall, Inc., pp. 129–132.

Ignatavicius, D., Workman, M., & Mischler, M. (1999). *Medical-surgical nursing: A nursing approach* (3rd ed.). Philadelphia: W. B. Saunders, pp. 243–264.

Kee, J. & Paulanka, B. (2000). *Fluids and electrolytes with clinical applications: A programmed approach* (6th ed.) Albany, NY: Delmar.

Kozier, B., Erb, G., Berman, A., & Burke, K. (2000). *Fundamentals of nursing: Concepts, process, and practice* (6th ed). Upper Saddle River, NJ: Prentice-Hall, Inc., pp. 1302–1339.

LeMone, P. & Burke, K. (2000). *Medical surgical nursing: Critical thinking in client care* (2nd ed). Upper Saddle River, NJ: Prentice-Hall, Inc., pp. 99–162.

Wallach, J. (2000). *Interpretation of diagnostic tests* (7th ed.). Philadelphia: Lippincott, Williams & Wilkins, pp. 48, 72–73, 489–500.

Whitney, E. N., Cataldo, C. B., & Rolfes, S. R. (1998). *Understanding normal and clinical nutrition* (5th ed.). New York: West Wadsworth, pp. 423–424.

CHAPTER 7

Phosphorus Balance and Imbalances

Mary Catherine Rawls, RN, MS

Mary Ann Hogan, RN, CS, MSN

CHAPTER OUTLINE

OBJECTIVES

■ Review basic functions of phosphorus in the body.

■ Discuss the pathophysiology and etiology of phosphorus imbalances.

■ Discuss specific assessment findings and diagnostic tests as they relate to phosphorus imbalances.

■ Identify priority nursing diagnoses for phosphorus imbalances.

■ Discuss therapeutic management of phosphorus imbalances.

■ Discuss nursing management of a client who is experiencing a phosphorus imbalance.

[Media Link]

Use the CD-ROM enclosed with this text, or log onto the address given to access the free, interactive Companion Website created for this series. The CD-ROM and Companion Website accompanying this book offer additional practice opportunities and information—NCLEX Review, Case Studies, Glossary, In Depth with NCLEX, and more.

www.prenhall.com/hogan

REVIEW AT A GLANCE

2,3-diphosphoglycerate (2,3-DPG) *a substance found in red blood cells that facilitates the delivery of oxygen to tissues*

adenosine triphosphate (ATP) *a compound stored in muscle containing three phosphorus groups that produces energy when split*

glycolysis *the breakdown of glucose*

hyperphosphatemia *serum phosphate level greater than 4.5 mg/dL*

hypophosphatemia *serum phosphate level less than 2.5 mg/dL*

metastatic calcification *the precipitate of calcium phosphate in the soft tissues, joints, and arteries as a complication of hyperphosphatemia*

parathyroid hormone (PTH or parathormone) *secreted by the parathyroid gland, which regulates calcium and phosphorus metabolism*

phospholipids *a lipid substance containing phosphorus and fatty acids*

phosphorus/phosphate *a nonmetallic element usually found in combination with other elements; terms are often used interchangeably*

refeeding *a process to provide nutrition by infusing high levels of calories into clients who have alcoholism, anorexia, or are otherwise malnourished*

rhabdomyolysis *destruction of skeletal (striated) muscle*

tetany *a nervous system disorder marked by intermittent tonic spasms that are usually paroxysmal and involve the extremities*

total parenteral nutrition (TPN) *the intravenous provision of total nutritional needs for a client unable to take appropriate amounts of food by the enteral route*

vitamin D *a fat-soluble vitamin essential for calcium and phosphorus absorption from the small intestine and for their metabolism*

Pretest

1 The physician orders a high phosphorus diet for the client with hypophosphatemia. You would expect to see which of the following dietary items on the meal tray?

(1) Fresh fruits
(2) Dairy products
(3) Noncarbonated soft drinks
(4) White bread

2 The nurse uses which of the following scientific principles when caring for the pediatric client with hypophosphatemia?

(1) Phosphorus is the primary cation of intracellular fluid.
(2) The least abundant mineral in the body is phosphorus.
(3) Serum phosphate levels are higher in children because of their rapid skeletal growth rate.
(4) Serum phosphate levels are consistent throughout the day.

3 The client asks the nurse to explain the role of phosphorus in the body. The nurse's best response would be which of the following?

(1) Phosphorus is essential for muscle function.
(2) Phosphorus is the end product of metabolism of 2,3-DPG.
(3) Phosphorus is essential for the metabolism of carbohydrates but not fats or proteins.
(4) Cell membranes contain large amounts of phosphorus combined with calcium.

4 The nurse would assess for signs and symptoms of hypophosphatemia in the client who had which of the following predisposing clinical conditions?

(1) First-degree burns
(2) Diabetic ketoacidosis
(3) Hypermagnesemia
(4) Oliguria

5 Discharge teaching for the client with hypophosphatemia would be to include which of the following foods in the diet as the source that is richest in phosphorus?

(1) Green leafy vegetables
(2) White breads
(3) Citrus fruits
(4) Eggs

6 Which of the following is consistent with the nurse's understanding of hypophosphatemia in the adult?

(1) Insulin promotes the movement of phosphorus out of the cell.
(2) Hypophosphatemia is a result of the movement of phosphorus out of the cell.
(3) This condition occurs as a result of increased renal re-absorption of phosphorus.
(4) This is defined as a serum level of less than 2.5 mg/dL.

7 Which of the following findings in a client's history would alert the nurse to assess for signs and symptoms of hypophosphatemia?

(1) Withdrawal from alcohol
(2) The oliguric phase of acute tubular necrosis
(3) Short-term gastric suction
(4) Occasional use of aluminum-containing antacids

8 Which of the following concurrent electrolyte imbalances should the nurse anticipate while working with a client who has hyperphosphatemia?

(1) Hyperkalemia
(2) Hyponatremia
(3) Hypocalcemia
(4) Hypermagesemia

9 A client has developed hyperphosphatemia as a result of massive cell kill during cytotoxic drug therapy. Which of the following medications would the nurse expect to be ordered to combat the concurrent rise in uric acid levels that is likely to occur?

(1) Aluminum hydroxide (Amphogel)
(2) Allopurinol (Zyloprim)
(3) Acetazolamide (Diamox)
(4) Hydralazine (Apresoline)

10 Discharge teaching for the client who requires a diet high in phosphates would include which of the following statements?

(1) "High levels of phosphates are found in food additives."
(2) "Increase your Vitamin A intake to enhance phosphorus absorption."
(3) "Aluminum-based antacids increase phosphorus absorption."
(4) "Soy and soy products are excellent sources of phosphorus."

See pages 161–162 for Answers and Rationales.

I. Overview of Phosphorus Regulation

A. Phosphorus balance

1. Serum levels

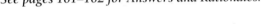

    a. Normal serum **phosphate** levels range from 2.5 to 4.5 mg/dL

    b. Levels are greater in children because of their higher rate of skeletal growth

    c. Newborns have almost twice the adult level of **phosphorus**

    d. Serum levels may vary throughout the day

    e. Most phosphorus (P^+) exists in the body as the phosphate ion (PO_4^-)

    f. Phosphorus is the second most abundant mineral in the body

        1) 85% is combined with calcium in the teeth and bones, also in skeletal muscle

2) 14% is found in intracellular fluid

3) 1% is found in extracellular fluid and viscera

   g. Phosphorus is the primary anion of intracellular fluid

   h. Ionized calcium and phosphorus exist in a reciprocal balance in the blood

2. Functions in the body

   a. Essential for muscle function, red blood cells, nervous system function and plays a part in the metabolism of carbohydrates, fats, and proteins

   b. Plays a crucial role in the formation of teeth and bones

   c. Plays a part in the cellular metabolism of DNA and **adenosine triphosphate (ATP),** a compound stored in muscle that contains three phosphorus groups and produces energy when split

   d. Assists in regulating calcium levels

   e. Aids renal regulation of acids and bases through its role in the phosphate buffer system

   f. Found in cell membranes as **phospholipids** that help maintain cell membrane integrity

   g. Required for the release of oxygen from hemoglobin in the form of **2,3-diphosphoglycerate (2,3-DPG)**

3. System interactions

   a. Serum levels vary throughout the day related to glucose intake, insulin administration, and hyperventilation, which increases cellular uptake of phosphorus

   b. Assists in maintaining acid-base balance

   c. An inverse relationship exists between phosphorus and calcium

      1) When calcium levels increase, phosphorus levels decrease; thus, calcium influences phosphorus regulation

      2) When phosphorus levels increase, calcium levels decrease; thus, calcium levels are influenced by phosphorus

   d. Phosphorus imbalances are often related to therapeutic interventions for other disorders

B. Sources of phosphorus

   1. Cellular level

      a. Major anion of intracellular fluid; also found in extracellular fluid

      b. Kidneys are responsible for 90% of phosphate excretion

      c. Normal phosphate balance requires an efficient renal conservation mechanism

      d. During times of low phosphate intake, kidneys retain more phosphorus

   2. Dietary level

      a. Adequate intake is ensured by consumption of a balanced diet

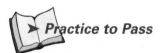

Practice to Pass

The school nurse is putting together a bulletin board that highlights foods high in various nutrients as a teaching tool for children and school visitors, including parents. What types of foods would the nurse identify on the display as being rich in phosphorus?

b. Average dietary intake ranges from 800 to 1,600 mg/dL and is consistent with the recommended daily intake

c. Found in high amounts in red and organ (brain, liver, kidney) meats, fish, poultry, eggs, milk and milk products, legumes, whole grains, and nuts

d. Absorption via active and passive transport in the duodenum and jejunum

e. Absorption influenced by **vitamin D,** a fat soluble vitamin, and **parathyroid hormone (PTH),** a hormone secreted by the parathyroid gland that regulates calcium and phosphorus levels

f. Absorption inhibited by glucocorticoids, high magnesium diet, hypothyroidism, and aluminum-containing antacids

g. Increased consumption of foods that contain food additives will result in increased ingestion of phosphates

II. *Hypophosphatemia*

A. Etiology and pathophysiology

1. Cellular level

   a. Defined as a serum phosphorus level of less than 2.5 mg/dL

   b. Can result from transient shifts of phosphorus into the cells, as in respiratory or metabolic acidosis

   c. Increased releases of PTH decrease serum phosphorus levels

   d. The mobilization of calcium from other sources may reduce phosphorus levels

   e. Renal excretion of phosphorus may be increased

   f. Administration of highly concentrated glucose solutions may cause the release of insulin, which promotes the movement of glucose and phosphorus into the cell

2. Predisposing clinical conditions

   a. A depletion of ATP, which impairs the cell's energy supply, and a decrease in the level of 2,3-DPG in the red blood cell; this in turn influences the release of oxygen from hemoglobin, keeping it bound and therefore less available to the tissues

   b. A complication of **refeeding** severely malnourished clients (infusing high levels of calories into clients who have alcoholism or are anorexic or otherwise malnourished) and has a high mortality rate

   c. Decreased intestinal absorption from vitamin D deficiency, malabsorption disorders, and starvation

   d. Increased intestinal losses from prolonged use of aluminum- and magnesium-containing antacids, which bind to phosphorus

   e. Severe vomiting and diarrhea

   f. Diabetic ketoacidosis

   g. Alcoholism and severe alcohol abuse (especially during withdrawal) related to poor nutritional intake, vomiting, diarrhea, and the use of antacids

h. Poor dietary intake, malnutrition, hypomagnesemia

i. Administering **total parenteral nutrition (TPN)**—the intravenous provision of total nutritional needs—without adequate levels of phosphorus

j. Increased renal excretion from hyperparathyroidism, hypomagnesemia, hypokalemia, thiazide diuretic therapy, the diuretic phase of acute tubular necrosis, renal tubular disorders, polyuria, and glycosuria from uncontrolled diabetic ketoacidosis

k. May be found more frequently in clients in critical care units because of nutritional deficiencies

l. A side effect of extracellular fluid volume expansion

m. Prolonged gastric suction

n. Severe burns, possibly from hyperventilation and the acceleration of **glycolysis** (breakdown of glucose)

o. Respiratory alkalosis (is thought to stimulate glycolysis, which stimulates the movement of phosphorus into the cells)

p. Hypercalcemia (may cause phosphaturia through the stimulation of parathyroid hormone release)

B. Assessment

1. Clinical manifestations

   a. Signs begin to appear when serum phosphorus levels drop below 2.0 mg/dL

   b. Hematologic effects

   1) Anemia from the increased fragility of red blood cells from low ATP levels

   2) Altered granulocyte functioning

   3) Bruising and bleeding from platelet dysfunction and destruction

   c. Central nervous system effects

   1) Slurred speech

   2) Confusion, apprehension

   3) Seizures

   4) Coma

   d. Neuromuscular effects

   1) Reports of circumoral and fingertip/extremity numbness and tingling

   2) Muscle weakness, paresthesias

   3) Tremors, spasms, tetany

   e. Cardiovascular effects

   1) Reports of chest pain

   2) Dysrhythmias related to decreased oxygenation

   3) Heart failure and shock from decreased myocardial contractility

NCLEX!

      f. Respiratory effects

        1) Alkalosis from an increased rate/depth of breathing in response to hypoxemia

        2) Respiratory muscle fatigue leading to respiratory failure

      g. Gastrointestinal effects

        1) Hypoactive bowel sounds

        2) Anorexia, dysphagia, vomiting

        3) Gastric atony and ileus related to reduced gastric motility

  2. Diagnostic and laboratory findings

    a. Plasma levels

      1) Mild hypophosphatemia: serum values of 1.0–2.5 mg/dL

      2) Severe hypophosphatemia: <1.0 mg/dL

    b. Associated electrolyte levels

      1) Serum magnesium: may be decreased because of increased renal excretion of magnesium

      2) Serum calcium: may be elevated because of the inverse relationship of calcium and phosphorus

      3) Arterial blood gases: may show respiratory or metabolic acidosis

    c. Trending of results

      1) Monitor laboratory values over time to determine effectiveness of therapy

      2) In prolonged hypophosphatemia, osteomalacia and pseudofractures may occur

    d. X-rays may show skeletal changes of osteomalacia

  3. Identification of risk factors

    a. Alcohol withdrawal

    b. Malnourished clients

    c. TPN administration

    d. Altered ability to eat normally

    e. Diabetic and uremic clients

C. Priority nursing diagnoses

  1. Impaired physical mobility related to bone pain and fractures

  2. Risk for injury (fractures) related to shifting of phosphorus out of bone tissue

  3. Impaired gas exchange related to weakened muscles of respiration

  4. Decreased cardiac output related to effects of hypophosphatemia on myocardial functioning

  5. Risk for falls related to sensory or neuromuscular dysfunction

> **Practice to Pass**
>
> What neuromuscular manifestations should be assessed for in a client at risk for developing hypophosphatemia?

D. Therapeutic management

1. Replacement therapies

    a. Administer phosphorus via oral supplements or intravenous replacement

    b. Avoid the use of phosphorus-binding antacids

    c. Adjust subsequent doses of replacement medication based on clinical presentation and serum phosphate levels

2. Continued monitoring of the client

    a. Check serum levels periodically in clients at risk

    b. Assess diabetic clients for ketoacidosis

    c. Anticipate problems in clients who have a long history of antacid use

    d. Be alert to clients who have difficulty speaking

    e. Note weakening respiratory efforts

    f. Monitor the ventilated client for increased incidence of hypophosphatemia from respiratory alkalosis

    g. Assess serial hand grasps for increasing weakness

    h. Monitor for client reports of joint stiffness and arthralgia

    i. Investigate episodes of bleeding and/or bruising

    j. Watch for hypomagnesemia with the start of anabolism after prolonged periods of catabolism

    k. Monitor for other associated fluid and electrolyte imbalances, especially in those with nausea, vomiting, and/or diarrhea

E. Restoration of balance

1. Achieved through oral, enteral, or parenteral replacement

2. Normal phosphate levels should be achieved in 7–10 days

F. Planning and implementation

1. Identify client populations at risk, especially those who are malnourished, receiving TPN, or receiving calories via enteral (tube) feedings

2. Identify and eliminate the causes of hypophosphatemia

3. Consult physician for orders to give appropriate supplementation

4. Assess and document level of consciousness

5. Assess orientation and neurologic status with each set of vital signs

6. Inform client/significant other that altered sensorium is temporary and will improve as phosphorus levels improve

7. Use reality therapy by encouraging presence of family members and use of clock and calendar at the bedside

8. Incorporate seizure precautions into care

9. Have an appropriate size airway readily available

10. Assist client in activities of daily living and ambulating

11. Monitor breath sounds for crackles, rhonchi, and shortness of breath

12. Monitor for elevated blood pressure and increased heart rate

13. Check temperature every 4 hours

14. If a wound infection is suspected, culture the wound(s) and drainage

15. Use meticulous aseptic technique when giving care

16. Promote oral hygiene and skin care

17. Monitor for paresthesias, muscle weakness, pain, and mental changes

18. Medicate for pain

19. Assess serum phosphate levels and trends; watch for concurrent development of hypercalcemia in the presence of hypophosphatemia

20. Monitor for possible hyperphosphatemia after the initiation of therapy

21. Assess dietary intake and output

    a. Carefully monitor fluid intake and output (I & O)

    b. Complete a diet history

    c. Log dietary intake

    d. Determine client's food preferences

G. Medication therapy

1. Oral replacement therapy

   a. Monobasic potassium and sodium phosphates (K-Phos Neutral); potassium and sodium phosphates (Neutra-Phos)

      1) Usual dose is 250 mg 4 times a day

      2) Well-absorbed following oral administration; vitamin D may enhance absorption

      3) Enters extracellular fluids and is then transported to sites of action

      4) Excreted mainly by the kidneys; acidifies the urine

      5) Contraindicated in hyperkalemia, hyperphosphatemia, hypocalcemia, severe renal impairment, untreated Addison's disease

      6) Diarrhea is most frequent side effect

      7) Oxalates (in spinach and rhubarb) and phytates (in bran and whole grains) may decrease the absorption of phosphates by binding them in the GI tract

      8) Monitor serum phosphate, potassium, sodium, and calcium levels prior to and periodically throughout therapy

      9) Monitor renal function studies

    b. Phosphate/biphosphate (Fleet Phospho-Soda)

       1) Osmotically active bowel preparation and oral preparation used for its laxative effect

       2) Enema contains 7 g sodium phosphate, 19 g sodium biphosphate; oral preparation contains 18 g sodium phosphate and 48 g sodium biphosphate

       3) Up to 20% of rectally administered sodium and phosphate may be absorbed

       4) Excreted by the kidneys

       5) Side effects include cramping, nausea

       6) May cause increased serum sodium and phosphorus levels, decreased serum calcium levels, and acidosis

NCLEX!

       7) Oral preparations should be thoroughly dissolved in a full glass of water and administered after meals to minimize gastric irritation and the laxative effect, and to enhance palatability

NCLEX!

       8) Do not administer simultaneously with antacids containing aluminum, magnesium, or calcium

       9) Advise clients to maintain a high fluid intake to decrease the risk of developing kidney stones

      10) Instruct the client to promptly report diarrhea, weakness, fatigue, muscle cramps, unexplained weight gain, swelling of lower extremities, shortness of breath, unusual thirst or tremors

2. Parenteral replacement therapy

    a. Usually reserved for severe hypophosphatemia (<1 mg/dL)

    b. Potassium phosphate (KPO_4) or sodium phosphate ($NaPO_4$) used

    c. May be added to TPN solutions

NCLEX!

    d. When giving potassium phosphate, do not exceed 10 mEq/hr; give slowly over 2 to 6 hours

    e. Complications of IV therapy may include:

       1) Tetany from hypocalcemia

       2) Calcium and phosphorus in the tissues may combine and form deposits

       3) Hypotension from too rapid an infusion rate

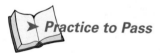
Practice to Pass

What are the important elements of care during administration of potassium phosphate in intravenous fluids for a client who has hypophosphatemia?

    f. Monitor infusion site for signs of infiltration, which may lead to tissue necrosis or sloughing

3. Dietary therapy

    a. Daily requirements are 0.15 mM/kg/day or 10 mM/day; if under stress, requirements increase to 30–45 mM/day

    b. Milk and milk products are an excellent source

    c. Phosphorus is plentiful in a normal diet and improved nutritional intake may be sufficient for replacement

NCLEX!

H. Client education

1. Teach client and family to recognize signs and symptoms of hypophosphatemia

2. Discuss the importance of avoiding phosphorus-binding antacids

3. Discuss with client the pertinent conditions that cause hypophosphatemia

4. Carry out dietary education and provide a list of foods high in phosphorus

I. Evaluation

1. The client will regain a serum phosphorus value within the normal range

2. The client can identify signs and symptoms of hypophosphatemia

3. The client exhibits no evidence of injury caused by neurosensory changes

4. The client exhibits adequate gas exchange as evidenced by a respiratory rate of 12 to 20 with normal depth and pattern and oxygen saturation (SaO_2) level of at least 92%

5. Within 24 hours of the initiation of therapy, the client exhibits purposeful movement and has full range of motion and muscle strength

6. The client has no signs or symptoms of heart failure and vital signs are within normal limits

III. *Hyperphosphatemia*

A. Etiology and pathophysiology

1. Cellular level

   a. Occurs when phosphate shifts from the cells into the extracellular fluid

   b. May be a result of respiratory or lactic acidosis or diabetic ketoacidosis because of the movement of phosphorus out of the cell

   c. Occurs with neoplastic diseases (leukemia, lymphoma) when treated with cytotoxic agents

   d. Can be a consequence of **rhabdomyolysis** (breakdown of striated muscle), which releases phosphorus from the cell because of tissue trauma, viral infections, heat stroke, increased metabolism, and catabolic states

   e. Can occur with other conditions that cause cellular destruction and release phosphorus into the extracellular fluid

2. Predisposing clinical conditions

   a. Acute and chronic renal failure, most commonly chronic glomerulonephritis and decreasing glomerular filtration rates, which prevent excretion of adequate amounts of phosphates

   b. Hypocalcemia from antacids, diuretic agents, steroids

   c. Chemotherapy for malignant tumors

   d. Hypoparathyroidism (primary or secondary), which causes a decrease in calcium and increased renal absorption of phosphorus

NCLEX!

NCLEX!

e. Prolonged or massive administration of Vitamin D, antacids, heparin, tetracycline, pituitary extract, and salicylates

f. Excess human growth hormone

NCLEX!

g. Excessive intake of phosphorus or its supplements

h. Decreased urinary losses unrelated to decreased renal function such as in hypoparathyroidism or volume depletion

i. Vitamin D excess or increased GI absorption

j. Massive transfusions because phosphorus can leak from cells during the storage of blood

k. Hyperthyroidism, hyperparathyroidism

NCLEX!

l. Infants fed cows' milk instead of human milk (940 mg of phosphorus in cows' milk compared to 150 mg in an equal amount of human milk)

m. Large milk intake for the treatment of peptic ulcers

n. Overzealous administration of oral or intravenous phosphorus supplements

B. **Assessment**

1. Clinical manifestations

    a. Common signs

        1) Most signs relate to the development of hypocalcemia or soft tissue calcification

        2) **Metastatic calcification** includes oliguria, corneal haziness, conjunctivitis, irregular heart rate

        3) ECG changes and conduction disturbance, tachycardia

        4) The deposition of calcium-phosphate in the cardiac tissues

        5) **Tetany,** which may increase in severity and spread to the limbs and face and be followed by numbness, muscle spasms, and pain

        6) The precipitation of calcium phosphate in nonosseous sites such as the kidney or heart

    b. Common symptoms

        1) Numbness and tingling around the mouth and in the fingertips, muscle spasms, and tetany from the increased phosphorus and corresponding decreased calcium

        2) Anorexia, nausea, vomiting

        3) Muscle weakness, hyperreflexia, tetany

2. Diagnostic and laboratory findings

    a. Serum phosphorus plasma levels are greater than 4.5 mg/dL

    b. In clients with chronic renal failure, phosphorus values may be kept slightly higher (4–6 mg/dL) to ensure adequate levels of 2,3-DPG and thereby minimize the effects of chronic anemia on oxygen delivery to the tissues

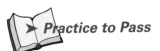

c. With increased phosphorus levels, serum calcium levels drop and hypocalcemia develops

1) Hypocalcemia is more likely to occur in sudden, severe hyperphosphatemia (such as after intravenous administration of phosphates)

2) Hypocalcemia may also occur in a client with chronic renal failure

d. Chronic hyperphosphatemia in the client with chronic renal failure may contribute to the development of renal osteodystrophy, which may be assessed by skeletal x-rays

1) A primary complication of hyperphosphatemia is metastatic calcification, the precipitation of calcium phosphate in the soft tissues, joints, and arteries

2) Calcification formation and precipitation in the soft tissues may be anticipated if the product of the serum calcium level multiplied by the serum phosphorus level is greater than 70 mg/dL (normal product is about 30–40 mg/dL)

3. Identification of clients at risk

a. Infants being fed cows' milk

b. Clients using Phospho-Soda as an enema solution or regular laxative

C. Priority nursing diagnoses

1. Knowledge deficit related to the purpose of phosphate-binding medications and the importance of reducing GI absorption of phosphorus to control hyperphosphatemia and prevent long-term complications

2. Risk for injury related to internal factors associated with calcium phosphate precipitation in the soft tissues (corneas, lungs, kidneys, gastric mucosa, heart, blood vessels) and periarticular regions of the large joints (hips, shoulders, elbows) and development of hypocalcemic tetany

D. Therapeutic management

1. Decrease phosphorus intake

a. Restrict or eliminate phosphorus intake in the diet

b. Eliminate medications containing phosphorus, particularly over-the-counter preparations

2. Promote phosphorus excretion

a. Increase gastrointestinal and renal excretion of phosphorus

b. Perform renal dialysis in clients with renal failure

c. Maintain fluid volume to ensure adequate blood pressure to enhance the excretion of phosphorus, particularly in clients receiving cytotoxic medications

3. Continue to monitor client for increasing hypocalcemia

a. Monitor for numbness and tingling of the fingers and circumoral region, hyperactive reflexes, muscle cramps

Practice to Pass

What clinical manifestations may be seen in a client diagnosed with hyperphosphatemia?

b. Consult physician promptly if symptoms of hypocalcemia develop to avoid tetany

c. Consult physician if client develops positive Trousseau's or Chvostek's sign

d. Monitor renal function carefully, particularly urine output, BUN, creatinine

e. Calcium supplements and products containing Vitamin D may be limited until phosphorus levels approach normal

f. In clients with renal failure, serum phosphate values may be kept higher to ensure adequate levels of 2,3-DPG to improve tissue oxygenation

E. Planning and implementation

1. Monitor serum phosphorus and calcium levels

2. Calculate the calcium-phosphorus product and consult physician for abnormally high results

3. Identify clients at risk; treat the underlying cause

4. Monitor intake and output; keep clients well hydrated; pay particular attention to the types of fluids being ingested (avoid carbonated beverages, which are high in phosphates); monitor urine output to be sure that it is adequate for phosphate excretion

5. Consult physician if client develops indications of soft tissue (metastatic) calcification (oliguria, corneal haziness, conjunctivitis, irregular heart rate, papular eruptions)

6. Monitor for signs and symptoms of tetany, such as positive Trousseau's and Chvostek's signs

7. Administer IV and oral phosphorus supplements cautiously in clients with normal phosphorus levels to avoid hyperphosphatemia; monitor serum phosphate levels periodically throughout administration

8. Avoid use of phosphate-containing enemas, especially in children and those with slowed bowel emptying times

9. Encourage client to avoid intake of foods that are high in phosphorus content (previously described)

F. Medication therapy

1. Specific drug therapies

   a. Avoid phosphate-containing laxatives and enemas

   b. Use phosphate binders that are available in liquid, tablet, and capsule forms

   c. Use aluminum-containing antacids to bind phosphates in the GI tract; be aware that aluminum-based products may lead to dementia if used over prolonged periods of time (such as those with renal failure) and cause constipation; examples include aluminum carbonate (Basaljel) and aluminum hydroxide (Amphojel)

   d. Calcium carbonate (Tums) is useful as a supplement for clients with renal failure because this will help to counteract hypocalcemia, the imbalance that tends to accompany hyperphosphatemia

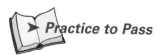

➤ Practice to Pass

What are the three main types of phosphate binders that may be used to treat hyperphosphatemia?

NCLEX!

NCLEX!

    e. In clients with hyperphosphatemia from use of cytotoxic drugs, use allopurinol (Zyloprim) as ordered to decrease uric acid production, which prevents the formation of uric acid calculi in the kidney and uric acid nephropathy

G. Client education

    1. Awareness of precipitating factors

NCLEX!

      a. Teach the client the purpose of phosphate binders and to take them as prescribed with or after meals to maximize their effectiveness

      b. Symptoms of hyperphosphatemia may be minimal; therefore, the client needs to be aware of preventing long-term complications through education

NCLEX!

      c. Teach to avoid over-the-counter phosphorus medications such as laxatives, enemas, and vitamin-mineral supplements

      d. Instruct the client to identify signs and symptoms of hyperphosphatemia

      e. Teach to read labels to identify phosphorus and phosphate inclusions

    2. Dietary education

      a. Use bulk-building supplements or stool softeners to combat the constipating effects of some phosphate-binders, especially those with an aluminum base

      b. Avoid or limit foods high in phosphorus, as previously described, and avoid carbonated beverages, which have low nutrient value and are also high in phosphates

H. Evaluation

    1. The client describes the symptoms of hyperphosphatemia and the ways in which it can be prevented

    2. The client creates a three-day meal plan using foods low in or without phosphorus

    3. The client verbalizes how to take medication therapy properly

Case Study

Mr. G. is a 56-year-old client with newly diagnosed chronic renal failure as a complication of diabetes mellitus. He will be beginning therapy with hemodialysis. He is married and lives at home with his wife; he has three grown children who do not live in the area. You have been assigned as his case manager and need to coordinate plans for his treatment and for client and family education.

❶ Do you expect Mr. G. to have hypophosphatemia or hyperphosphatemia? What is the rationale for your choice?

❷ How will you explain the etiology of this electrolyte imbalance to Mr. G?

❸ What dietary modifications need to be made in order to keep serum phosphorus levels under control?

❹ What role will dialysis play in managing phosphorus levels?

❺ What medication therapy teaching do you anticipate will be needed?

For suggested responses, see page 232.

Posttest

1 The nurse utilizes which of the following information about phosphate levels in the newborn when implementing client care?

(1) Phosphate levels are consistent throughout the day.
(2) Phosphate levels in newborns are nearly twice the adult level.
(3) Normal serum phosphate levels range from 1.5 to 2.0 mg/dL.
(4) Phosphorus is the most abundant mineral in the body.

2 Which of the following statements would the nurse make when teaching the client about phosphorus?

(1) Phosphorus levels in the body remain consistent throughout the day.
(2) Ionized calcium and serum phosphorus exist in a reciprocal balance in the blood.
(3) The primary cation in fluid within the cell is phosphorus.
(4) Adults have a high rate of skeletal growth that requires a large amount of phosphorus.

3 The nurse is aware that which of the following statements is true regarding the cellular sources of phosphorus?

(1) The lungs are responsible for 90% of the excretion of phosphorus.
(2) When serum phosphate levels are high, the kidney will retain more phosphorus.
(3) Most phosphate is excreted through the intestine.
(4) The kidneys are the main route of phosphate excretion.

4 The nurse would assess for signs and symptoms of hypophosphatemia in the client who has which of the following predisposing clinical conditions?

(1) Severe vomiting and diarrhea
(2) Occasional use of magnesium-containing antacids
(3) Infusion of balanced TPN solutions
(4) Vitamin D excess

5   The client's serum phosphorus level is 1.9 mg/dL. The nurse should be alert to which of the following signs?

(1) Hyperactive bowel sounds
(2) Dysrhythmias related to decreased oxygenation
(3) Increased muscle tone
(4) Polycythemia

6   When caring for the client with hypophosphatemia, the nurse should anticipate complaints of which of the following?

(1) Euphoria
(2) Hunger
(3) Chest pain
(4) Thirst

7   The nurse would report which of the following to the healthcare provider as an abnormal phosphorus level?

(1) 2.6 mEq/L
(2) 2.9 mEq/L
(3) 4.0 mEq/L
(4) 5.1 mEq/L

8   A history of which of the following disorders in a client would lead the nurse to suspect a problem with phosphorus excretion?

(1) Bowel obstruction
(2) Chronic renal failure
(3) Chronic obstructive pulmonary disease
(4) Coronary artery disease

9   A client with hyperphosphatemia indicates an understanding of dietary instructions by stating to limit intake of which of the following food items?

(1) Pork chops
(2) White rice
(3) Sirloin steak
(4) Green peas

10   A client chronically using which of the following types of over-the-counter products is at greatest risk for developing hyperphosphatemia?

(1) Enemas
(2) Cough preparations
(3) Cold preparations
(4) Bedtime sleeping aids

See pages 162–163 for Answers and Rationales.

Answers and Rationales

Pretest

1   **Answer: 2** *Rationale:* Dairy products are naturally high in phosphorus. Although many food sources contain phosphorus, the greatest amounts are found in red and organ meats, fish, poultry, eggs, dairy products, nuts, whole grains, and legumes. Carbonated soft drinks are also high in phosphorus, although they are low in nutrient value.
Cognitive Level: Application
Nursing Process: Analysis; *Test Plan:* PHYS

2   **Answer: 3** *Rationale:* Children have higher phosphate levels than adults because of their more rapid bone development rate. Phosphorus is an anion, not a cation (option 1). Phosphorus is the second most abundant mineral in the body (option 2). Serum phosphate levels vary throughout the day (option 4).
Cognitive Level: Comprehension
Nursing Process: Analysis; *Test Plan:* PHYS

3   **Answer: 1** *Rationale:* Phosphorus is needed for muscle cell energy. 2,3-DPG requires phosphorus for the release of oxygen from hemoglobin (option 2). Phosphorus plays a role in the metabolism of carbohydrates, fats, and proteins (option 3). Cell membranes contain phosphorus in the form of phospholipids (option 4).
Cognitive Level: Application
Nursing Process: Implementation; *Test Plan:* HPM

4   **Answer: 2** *Rationale:* Clients in diabetic ketoacidosis lose excessive amounts of phosphate in the urine. Clients with first-degree burns do not experience severe fluid shifts that affect phosphorus levels (option 1). Hypomagnesemia can result in renal excretion of phosphorus (option 3). Decreased urine output results in less renal filtration of phosphorus (option 4).
Cognitive Level: Application
Nursing Process: Assessment; *Test Plan:* PHYS

5 Answer: 4 *Rationale:* Although phosphorus is found in a large number of food items, it is found in greatest quantities in red and organ meats, fish, poultry, eggs, milk and milk products, legumes, whole grains, and nuts. The other options identify foods that have lesser amounts of phosphorus.
Cognitive Level: Application
Nursing Process: Implementation; *Test Plan:* HPM

6 Answer: 4 *Rationale:* Normal phosphorus levels in the adult are 2.5 to 4.5 mg/dL. Transporting and shifting phosphorus out of the cell and increasing the renal reabsorption of phosphorus will result in hyperphosphatemia (options 2, 3, and 4).
Cognitive Level: Comprehension
Nursing Process: Analysis; *Test Plan:* PHYS

7 Answer: 1 *Rationale:* Poor nutritional intake, vomiting, diarrhea, and overuse of antacids are related to alcoholism and alcohol abuse. These can lead to hypophosphatemia. During oliguria the kidneys are unable to excrete phosphorus (option 2). Clients with prolonged (not short-term) gastric suction are more likely to experience hypophosphatemia (option 3). Prolonged or continuous use of aluminum containing antacids (not occasional use) leads to hypophosphatemia (option 4).
Cognitive Level: Analysis
Nursing Process: Assessment; *Test Plan:* PHYS

8 Answer: 3 *Rationale:* Calcium and phosphorus have an inverse relationship in the body. For this reason, when phosphorus levels are high, then calcium levels are low. The other responses do not address this relationship.
Cognitive Level: Application
Nursing Process: Assessment; *Test Plan:* PHYS

9 Answer: 2 *Rationale:* In clients with hyperphosphatemia from use of cytotoxic drugs, allopurinol (Zyloprim) may be ordered to decrease uric acid production, which prevents the formation of uric acid calculi in the kidney and uric acid nephropathy. Aluminum hydroxide (Amphogel) is an antacid that would be useful in binding phosphates (option 1); acetazolamide is a diuretic (option 3); and hydralazine (option 4) is an antihypertensive.
Cognitive Level: Analysis
Nursing Process: Analysis; *Test Plan:* PHYS

10 Answer: 1 *Rationale:* Food additives do tend to be high in phosphates. For this reason, clients should be taught to read food labels carefully. Vitamin D will enhance phosphorus absorption, not vitamin A (op-

tion 2). Aluminum-containing antacids decrease phosphorus absorption by binding to it (option 3). Soy-based foods are low in phosphorus (option 4).
Cognitive Level: Application
Nursing Process: Implementation; *Test Plan:* HPM

Posttest

1 Answer: 2 *Rationale:* Newborn levels of phosphorus are nearly twice those of an adult. Normal adult serum phosphate levels in the adult range from 2.5 to 4.5 mg/dL and newborn levels range from about 4.0 to 7.0 mg/dL (option 3). Phosphate levels vary throughout the day (option 1). Phosphorus is the second most abundant mineral in the body (option 4).
Cognitive Level: Comprehension
Nursing Process: Analysis; *Test Plan:* PHYS

2 Answer: 2 *Rationale:* Phosphorus and calcium have an inverse relationship in the blood (option 2). Phosphorus levels vary throughout the day (option 1). Phosphorus is the primary anion of intracellular fluid (option 3). Children have a greater rate of skeletal growth than adults and consequently have a higher level of serum phosphorus (option 4).
Cognitive Level: Comprehension
Nursing Process: Implementation; *Test Plan:* HPM

3 Answer: 4 *Rationale:* The kidneys are responsible for 90% of phosphate excretion. Phosphate is not excreted through the respiratory system or the intestines (options 1 and 3) but rather through the kidneys. When the serum phosphate level is high, the kidneys will excrete, not retain (option 2), excess phosphate in the urine.
Cognitive Level: Comprehension
Nursing Process: Analysis; *Test Plan:* HPM

4 Answer: 1 *Rationale:* Severe vomiting and diarrhea deplete the body's stores of many electrolytes including phosphorus. Prolonged use of aluminum and magnesium-containing antacids that bind to phosphorus (option 2) is a condition leading to hypophosphatemia. Balanced TPN solutions contain adequate levels of phosphorus (option 3). Vitamin D deficiencies lead to decreased intestinal absorption of phosphorus (option 4).
Cognitive Level: Analysis
Nursing Process: Assessment; *Test Plan:* PHYS

5 Answer: 2 *Rationale:* Hypophosphatemia results in decreased ATP production, decreasing enzyme levels of 2,3-DPG, which in turn keeps oxygen bound to hemoglobin and less available to the tissues. Clients with hypophosphatemia will experience hypoactive

bowel sounds (option 1), muscle weakness (option 3), and paresthesias and anemia due to RBC fragility from low ATP levels (option 4).
Cognitive Level: Analysis
Nursing Process: Assessment; *Test Plan:* PHYS

6 **Answer: 3** *Rationale:* Hypophosphatemia leads to a decline in 2,3-DPG levels, reducing the release of oxygen to the tissues. Clients are more likely to have complaints of apprehension than euphoria (option 1). Decreased gastric motility leads to anorexia in the hypophosphatemic client (options 2 and 4).
Cognitive Level: Application
Nursing Process: Assessment; *Test Plan:* PHYS

7 **Answer: 4** *Rationale:* The normal range for serum phosphorus levels is 2.5 to 4.5 mEq/L. Any level that falls below this range indicates hypophosphatemia, while any level that lies above this range indicates hyperphosphatemia.
Cognitive Level: Application
Nursing Process: Analysis; *Test Plan:* PHYS

8 **Answer: 2** *Rationale:* Chronic renal failure impairs the ability to excrete phosphorus normally, since the kidneys are the major organs for excretion of phosphorus. The other options are incorrect.
Cognitive Level: Analysis
Nursing Process: Analysis; *Test Plan:* PHYS

9 **Answer: 3** *Rationale:* Red meat is high in phosphorus content, along with dairy products, eggs, poultry, organ meats, legumes, and whole grains. For this reason, it should be limited in the diet when hyperphosphatemia is present. The other foods listed have less phosphorus content.
Cognitive Level: Analysis
Nursing Process: Evaluation; *Test Plan:* HPM

10 **Answer: 1** *Rationale:* Enemas can be high in phosphorus, thus making the client at risk for hyperphosphatemia if they are frequently used. The other products listed do not necessarily have large amounts of phosphorus in them.
Cognitive Level: Analysis
Nursing Process: Analysis; *Test Plan:* HPM

References

Corbett, J. (2000). *Laboratory tests and diagnostic procedures with nursing diagnoses* (4th ed.). Upper Saddle River, NJ: Prentice-Hall, Inc., pp. 135–136.

Ignatavicius, D., Workman, M., & Mischler, M. (1999). *Medical-surgical nursing: A nursing process approach* (3rd ed.). Philadelphia: W. B. Saunders, pp. 243–264.

Kozier, B., Erb, G., Berman, A., & Burke, K. (2000). *Fundamentals of nursing: Concepts, process, and practice* (6th ed). Upper Saddle River, NJ: Prentice-Hall, Inc., pp. 1302–1339.

LeMone, P. & Burke, K. (2000). *Medical surgical nursing: Critical thinking in client care* (2nd ed). Upper Saddle River, NJ: Prentice-Hall, Inc., pp. 99–162.

Wallach, J. (2000). *Interpretation of diagnostic tests* (7th ed.). Philadelphia: Lippincott, Williams & Wilkins, pp. 48, 72–73, 489–500.

Whitney, E.N., Cataldo, C.B., & Rolfes, S.R. (1998). *Understanding normal and clinical nutrition* (5th ed.). New York: West Wadsworth, pp. 423–424.

CHAPTER 8

Acid-Base Balance and Imbalances

Lynn Rhyne, MN, RN

CHAPTER OUTLINE

OBJECTIVES

▮ Review basics of acid-base physiology.

▮ Identify potential acid-base disturbances.

▮ Identify priority nursing diagnoses for acid-base disturbances.

▮ Discuss the therapeutic management of acid-base disturbances.

▮ Discuss nursing management of a client who is experiencing an acid-base disturbance.

[Media Link]

Use the CD-ROM enclosed with this text, or log onto the address given to access the free, interactive Companion Website created for this series. The CD-ROM and Companion Website accompanying this book offer additional practice opportunities and information—NCLEX Review, Case Studies, Glossary, In Depth with NCLEX, and more.

www.prenhall.com/hogan

REVIEW AT A GLANCE

acid *a substance that releases a hydrogen (H⁺) ion when dissolved in water*

base *a substance that will bind to a hydrogen (H⁺) ion when dissolved in water*

buffer *prevents major changes in the extracellular fluid (ECF) by releasing or accepting hydrogen (H⁺) ions*

compensation *the body process of using its regulatory mechanisms to return the pH to its normal level*

HCO₃⁻ *bicarbonate, an alkalotic substance; a direct reflection of the renal system's ability to compensate for pH changes*

metabolic acidosis *a gain of hydrogen (H⁺) ions or a loss of HCO₃⁻; pH decreases and HCO₃⁻ decreases*

metabolic alkalosis *a loss of hydrogen (H⁺) ion or a gain in HCO₃⁻; pH increases and HCO₃⁻ increases*

mixed acid-base disorder *occurs when two or more independent acid-base disorders occur at the same time*

PaCO₂ *the measurement of the CO₂ pressure that is being exerted on the plasma and is directly related to the amount of CO₂ being produced*

PaO₂ *measures the amount of pressure exerted by oxygen on the plasma*

pH *the negative logarithm of H⁺ ion concentration in mEq per liter*

respiratory acidosis *a condition that occurs in response to hypoventilation; carbon dioxide is retained and the pH is decreased*

respiratory alkalosis *a decreased level of CO₂; sometimes call a H₂CO₃ deficit; pH is elevated and PaCO₂ is decreased*

SaO₂ *the amount of oxygen attached to a hemoglobin molecule*

Pretest

1   A new RN orientee asks the nurse preceptor about acid-base imbalances. Which of the following responses by the preceptor best describes respiratory acidosis?

(1) "Respiratory acidosis occurs when a client is hyperventilating."
(2) "Respiratory acidosis occurs when the kidneys retain sodium bicarbonate, leading to acidosis."
(3) "This condition occurs when a client has inadequate ventilation, retains CO_2, and the pH drops."
(4) "This condition is a direct result of a rapid respiratory rate, which blows off too much carbon dioxide, making the pH of the blood drop."

2   A nurse is teaching a group of clients with chronic obstructive pulmonary disease (COPD) about the importance of the acid-base balance in relation to respiratory disease. Which of the following explanations reflects the nurse's understanding of acid-base balance and respiratory disease?

(1) "The pH is an indication of how well your body is adjusting to the acidosis that sometimes occurs with COPD."
(2) "Your lungs are the main organs that act as a buffer to bring your body back into correct acid-base balance when acidosis occurs with your disease."
(3) "Your kidneys are the first organ to act when you have an acid-base imbalance, so infections in the urinary system can affect your acid-base balance."
(4) "The body has many different structures that act to bring your acid-base balance back into alignment when you develop acidosis."

3   Which of the following arterial blood gases (ABGs) would the nurse expect to see when a client has apnea and develops acidosis?

(1) pH 7.42, $PaCO_2$ 48 mmHg, HCO_3^- 25 mEq/L
(2) pH 7.29, $PaCO_2$ 62 mmHg, HCO_3^- 23 mEq/L
(3) pH 7.36, $PaCO_2$ 42 mmHg, HCO_3^- 26 mEq/L
(4) pH 7.49, $PaCO_2$ 30 mmHg, HCO_3^- 35 mEq/L

4 Which of the following statements by a student nurse reflects correct understanding about the body's attempt to restore homeostasis during periods of acidosis?

(1) "The kidneys start to work within seconds after an imbalance occurs and are very effective in restoring the body to a correct acid-base balance."
(2) "The kidneys may not start to function immediately but are very effective as a buffer system to restore the acid-base balance."
(3) "The kidneys are not as effective as the lungs in restoring the acid-base balance because the bicarbonate ion is not a good buffer."
(4) "The kidneys are very slow to respond to any acid-base imbalance but are very effective in ridding the body of carbonic acid."

5 Which of the following ABG results would the nurse expect to see when a client is admitted with diarrhea that has lasted for four days?

(1) pH 7.50, $PaCO_2$ 60 mmHg, HCO_3^- 28 mEq/L
(2) pH 7.30, $PaCO_2$ 40 mmHg, HCO_3^- 18 mEq/L
(3) pH 7.40, $PaCO_2$ 38 mmHg, HCO_3^- 28 mEq/L
(4) pH 7.50, $PaCO_2$ 38 mmHg, HCO_3^- 32 mEq/L

6 The nurse has been caring for a client who has become extremely anxious and agitated. Which of the following assessment findings would the nurse expect to find in this client because of anxiety and agitation?

(1) Rapid, deep respiratory pattern
(2) Rapid, shallow respiratory pattern
(3) Rapid, irregular heart rate
(4) Slow, irregular heart rate

7 Which of the following laboratory values would the nurse expect to see in an anxious client?

(1) pH 7.45
(2) pH 7.38
(3) pH 7.50
(4) pH 7.20

8 The nurse anticipates which of the following responses in a client who develops metabolic acidosis?

(1) Heart rate will increase.
(2) Urinary output will increase.
(3) Respiratory rate will increase.
(4) Temperature will increase.

9 The nurse assesses a client with uncontrolled Type 1 diabetes mellitus for which of the following acid-base imbalances?

(1) Metabolic alkalosis
(2) Respiratory alkalosis
(3) Respiratory acidosis
(4) Metabolic acidosis

10 The client with COPD asks the nurse why a continuous pulse oximeter is ordered. Which of the following responses by the nurse is correct?

(1) "The pulse oximeter measures your CO_2 level so ABGs only need to be drawn once a day."
(2) "The pulse oximeter measures the oxygen saturation in your blood at any given time."
(3) "The pulse oximeter is being used so we don't ever have to draw ABGs on you while you are in the hospital."
(4) "The machine is used to adequately assess your ventilatory effort while you are in bed."

See pages 189–190 for Answers and Rationales.

I. Overview of Acid-Base Physiology

A. Nature of acids and bases

1. An **acid** is a substance that releases a H^+ ion when dissolved in water

2. A **base** is a substance that will bind to a H^+ ion when dissolved in water

3. Weak acids do not completely separate in water; they only release some of the H^+ ions

4. A weak base accepts the H^+ ion less easily but it is extremely valuable in preventing major alterations in the pH of the extracellular fluid (ECF)

B. Chemical buffer systems in the body

1. A **buffer** prevents major changes in the ECF by releasing or accepting hydrogen (H^+) ions

2. The major chemical buffers are found in the blood and include the carbonic acid-bicarbonate buffer system, the phosphate buffer system, and the protein buffer system

3. Chemical buffers are present in both intracellular fluid (ICF) and ECF

4. Buffers are found in all tissues of the body, including bone

5. Chemical buffers act within seconds to neutralize acids and bases and keep the pH within the narrow normal range of 7.35 to 7.45

6. Bicarbonate buffer system

   a. This system consists of a water solution that contains a weak acid, carbonic acid (H_2CO_3), and a bicarbonate salt, usually sodium bicarbonate ($NaHCO_3$)

   b. Normally the body maintains the pH by keeping the ratio of bicarbonate (**HCO_3^-**) to H_2CO_3 at a proportion of 20:1

      1) This ratio is changed if the pH goes up or down depending on the alteration

      2) Once compensation occurs, the ratio becomes stable again

   c. The bicarbonate/carbonic acid buffer system is linked to both the respiratory and renal systems

      1) H_2CO_3 is the respiratory compensatory component because it can dissociate into carbon dioxide (CO_2) and water, with CO_2 being exhaled by the lungs

      2) HCO_3^- is the primary renal compensatory component because it can be excreted by the kidneys

      3) This function is illustrated by the following equation:

      $$CO_2 + H_2O \leftrightarrow H_2CO_3 \leftrightarrow HCO_3^- + H^+$$

7. The phosphate buffer system buffers both ICF and ECF to maintain a normal pH

8. The protein buffer system acts in a similar manner to the bicarbonate-carbonic acid buffer system because it releases or accepts H^+ readily and can exist as either an acid or a base; it is a major intracellular buffer

9. The hemoglobin-oxyhemoglobin buffer system helps to maintain pH within normal range in both arterial and venous blood, which have different amounts of CO_2

C. Physiologic buffers in the body

1. Pulmonary regulation

   a. The lungs control the respiratory carbonic acid buffer system

   b. The lungs compensate for acid-base disturbances that are primarily metabolic in nature (lactic acidosis that occurs with exercise, for example)

   c. Under control of the medulla oblongata, the lungs increase or decrease the respiratory rate and depth in response to the amount of CO_2 in the ECF

   d. The respiratory system is extremely sensitive to changes in the pH and begins compensatory efforts within seconds to minutes

      1) These mechanisms can become quickly exhausted

      2) This system is not as efficient as renal compensatory efforts

   e. The elderly have a reduced amount of gas exchange during breathing and less alveolar membrane so CO_2 retention and increased H^+ ions are a problem

2. Renal regulation

   a. The kidneys control the metabolic buffer $NaHCO_3^-$ by excreting an acidic urine or an alkaline urine

   b. This system works within several hours to days, but is powerfully effective in that it can eliminate either acids or bases as needed

   c. The kidneys control the HCO_3^- in ECF by either reabsorbing or excreting the H^+ ion

      1) They can reabsorb HCO_3^- as needed

      2) They can secrete free H^+ ions into the renal tubules from the peritubular capillaries

      3) They can combine ammonia (NaH_3) with hydrochloric acid (HCl) to form ammonium (NH_4Cl), which is excreted by the kidneys; approximately 50% of excess H^+ can be excreted by this mechanism

   d. The kidneys can actually excrete the weak acids into the urine

   e. The body depends on the kidneys to excrete acids from cellular metabolism; thus the urine in normally acidic (average pH 6)

   f. Renal function decreases with age so elderly clients do not excrete H^+ ions or synthesize HCO_3^- as efficiently and therefore their acid-base imbalances are more difficult to correct especially if other conditions, such as pneumonia, fever, or infection occur

3. **Compensation** for an acid-base imbalance occurs when the body uses regulatory mechanisms to return the pH to its normal level by transforming acids and bases within the body; the pH is normal but there are abnormal amounts of CO_2 and/or HCO_3^-

   a. A primary metabolic disturbance will cause a respiratory compensation

   b. A primary respiratory disturbance will cause an acute metabolic response due to buffering system and a more chronic compensation due to renal function

   c. Complete compensation means that the buffers have achieved homeostasis and the pH is fully corrected

   d. Partial compensation means that the buffers are in the process of working to restore homeostasis

   e. Decompensation refers to a worsening state of acid-base imbalance

4. Correction of the acid-base imbalance occurs when the lungs and/or the kidneys eliminate the offending substance(s) from the body; the CO_2 and HCO_3^- levels are returned to normal, not just the pH

D. **Measurement of acid-base status:** assessed by using arterial blood gases (ABGs) (see Table 8-1)

   1. **pH:** the negative logarithm of H^+ ion concentration in mEq per liter

      a. The actual concentration of the H^+ ions is very small (< 0.0001 mEq/liter); therefore, it has a negative logarithm

      b. Because the pH is calculated as a negative value, there is an inverse relationship between the pH and the H^+ ion concentration; therefore, as the H^+ ion concentration increases, pH decreases

      c. The normal value for the pH in arterial blood is 7.35 to 7.45; in venous blood the pH is 7.32 to 7.42

      d. A pH less than 7.35 is termed acidotic

      e. Conversely, a pH greater than 7.45 is called alkalotic

Table 8-1 Arterial Blood Gas Interpretation	Blood Gas Values	Acidosis	Normal	Alkalosis
	pH	< 7.35	7.35–7.45	> 7.45
	$PaCO_2$ Abnormal with a normal HCO_3^- indicates a respiratory basis	> 45 mm Hg respiratory	35–45 mmHg	< 35 mmHg respiratory
	HCO_3^- Abnormal with a normal PaO_2 indicates a metabolic basis	< 22 mEq/L metabolic	22–26 mEq/L	> 26 mEq/L metabolic

2. **PaCO$_2$** (partial pressure of carbon dioxide): the measurement of the CO$_2$ pressure that is being exerted on the plasma and is directly related to the amount of CO$_2$ being produced

   a. The PaCO$_2$ is regulated by the lungs and indicates the amount of H$_2$CO$_3$ that is available to act as a buffer

   b. The PaCO$_2$ is the value that indicates whether the condition is a respiratory disturbance

   NCLEX!

   c. The normal value of PaCO$_2$ is 35–45 mm Hg

   d. Values less than 35 mm Hg are indicative of alkalosis

   e. Acidosis occurs when the value rises above 45 mm Hg

3. **PaO$_2$** (partial pressure of oxygen): measures the amount of pressure exerted by oxygen on the plasma

   NCLEX!

   a. The range of normal values for PaO$_2$ is 80–100 mm Hg for adults under 60 years of age

   b. For every year above 60, there is an expected decrease in PaO$_2$ of 1 mmHg

   c. If the PaO$_2$ drops dramatically, then the oxygen saturation also decreases greatly

4. **SaO$_2$:** refers to the percent of hemoglobin saturated with oxygen

   a. Since most oxygen is carried on hemoglobin, the total oxygen concentration is measured using the hemoglobin saturation (SaO$_2$)

   b. There is a relationship between the PaO$_2$ and SaO$_2$ that influences binding affinity and dissociation of oxygen and hemoglobin (see Figure 8-1)

   c. Acidosis causes a shift to the right on the oxyhemoglobin dissociation curve that results in a decreased affinity; oxygen is more easily released to the tissues

Figure 8-1

Oxygen-hemoglobin dissociation curve. The lower the PaO$_2$ level, the more readily hemoglobin will on-load or off-load oxygen.

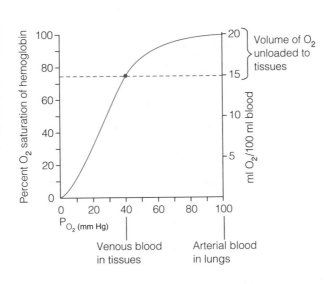

d. Alkalosis causes a shift to the left on the oxyhemoglobin dissociation curve that results in an increased affinity; oxygen is held more tightly and is less available to tissues

e. There are other factors that affect oxygen affinity, such as body temperature and transfusion of banked blood

5. Electrolyte interactions

NCLEX!

a. HCO_3^- is a direct reflection of the renal system's ability to compensate for pH changes

1) A decreased HCO_3^- level is indicative of acidosis

2) Alkalosis occurs when the HCO_3^- level rises above normal

b. The base excess (BE) is an indication of the amount of HCO_3^- available in the ECF

1) Either a negative or positive amount of HCO_3^- is available for use

2) Normal base excess ranges from a −3.0 to a +3.0 in adults

3) Values above + 3.0 indicate metabolic alkalosis

4) Metabolic acidosis exists when the value is below −3.0

c. Serum anion gap (AG) represents an attempt to calculate concentrations of anions (HCO_3, chloride [Cl], proteins, phosphates, and sulfates) and cations (sodium [Na^+], potassium [K^+], magnesium [Mg^{++}], calcium [Ca^{++}])

1) Normal range is 10–12 mEq/L

2) Calculated value is $Na^+ - [CL^- + HCO_3^-]$

3) Increased AG of > 12 mEq/L indicates metabolic acidosis (anion gap acidosis)

4) Normal AG can exist with a metabolic acidosis (non-anion gap acidosis) when there is a decrease in HCO_3^- balanced by an increase in Cl^-

5) Serum K^+ levels are also evaluated in connection with normal AG levels

6) Decreased AG can be seen in clients with low albumin levels or in conditions where there is an increase in unmeasured cations (multiple myeloma, lithium toxicity, or nephrotic syndrome)

d. Chloride levels are used to evaluate clients who are at risk for metabolic alkalosis

1) Urinary levels < 10 mEq/L are associated with chloride-responsive metabolic alkalosis

2) Chloride-responsive metabolic alkalosis is the more commonly occurring type and is usually seen with ECF volume depletion and renal and GI losses; bicarbonate retention occurs

3) Urinary levels >10 mEq/L are associated with chloride-resistant metabolic alkalosis

4) Chloride-resistant metabolic alkalosis is less common and is seen in clients with adrenal problems, hypertension, and Mg^{++} or K^+ depletion

E. Identification of simple acid-base disturbances (refer again to Table 8-1)

1. Interpret the pH

    a. Is the pH less than 7.35? This indicates acidosis

    b. Is the pH greater than 7.45? This indicates alkalosis

2. Identify primary cause—respiratory or metabolic

    a. Examine the $PaCO_2$ and the HCO_3^- values

    b. If the $PaCO_2$ is abnormal, then the problem is respiratory

    c. If the HCO_3^- is abnormal, a metabolic problem exists

3. Determine presence of compensation

    a. Determine if the $PaCO_2$ and HCO_3^- are decreased or increased as the body attempts to maintain the ratio of HCO_3^- to H_2CO_3 at 20:1

    b. Partial compensation exists when the pH remains abnormal but the parameter not associated with the pH changes (example: the pH indicates an acidotic state but the HCO_3^- is increased, indicating that the body is utilizing the buffer system to bring the pH back into line)

    c. Full or complete compensation occurs when the buffer system is working effectively and brings the pH back to a value of 7.35 to 7.45 (example: respiratory acidosis exists as indicated by an elevated $PaCO_2$; however, the pH is normal and the HCO_3^- is increased)

II. Respiratory Acidosis

A. *Respiratory acidosis*: a condition in which carbon dioxide is retained and the pH is decreased (see Table 8-2)

B. It occurs in response to hypoventilation, which occurs with respiratory depression, inadequate chest expansion, airway obstruction, or interference with alveolar-capillary exchange

C. Clinical presentation

1. Cardiovascular

    a. Hypotension

    b. Delayed cardiac conduction that can lead to heart block, peaked T waves, prolonged PR intervals, and widened QRS complexes

    c. Peripheral vasodilation with thready, weak pulse

    d. Tachycardia

    e. Warm, flushed skin related to the peripheral vasodilation as well as to impaired gas exchange

2. Respiratory

    a. Dyspnea

    b. May have hypoventilation with hypoxia

3. Central nervous system (CNS)

    a. Headache

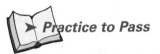

Practice to Pass

How would the nurse determine if a client was in uncompensated respiratory acidosis?

NCLEX!

NCLEX!

NCLEX!

Table 8-2	Clinical Picture	Acidosis	Alkalosis
Respiratory Alterations in Acid-Base Balance	pH	< 7.35	> 7.45
	$PaCO_2$	> 45	< 35
	HCO_3^-	Elevated with compensation	Decreased with compensation
	Signs and symptoms		
	Cardiovascular	Hypotension, heart block, peaked T waves, prolonged PR interval, weak and thready pulse, tachycardia, warm and flushed skin	Increased myocardial irritability, increased heart rate, increased sensitivity to digitalis preparations
	Respiratory	Rapid and shallow respiratory pattern	Dyspnea, chest tightness
	CNS	Headache, seizures, altered mental status, papilledema, decreased LOC, drowsiness, coma	Dizziness, anxiety, panic, tetany, convulsions, blurred vision
	Causes	Chronic obstructive pulmonary disease, sedative or barbiturate overdose, chest wall abnormalities, pneumonia, atelectasis, respiratory muscle weakness, underventilation	Hyperventilation caused by hypoxia, fear, fever, pain, exercise, anxiety, pulmonary embolus Mechanical overventilation Stimulated respiratory centers caused by septicemia, encephalitis, brain injury, salicylate poisoning
	Compensation	Kidneys eliminate H^+ ions and retain HCO_3^-	Kidneys conserve H^+ ions and excrete HCO_3^-

b. Seizures

c. Altered mental status

d. Papilledema

e. Muscle twitching

f. Decreased level of consciousness

g. Drowsiness that can progress to a coma

D. Diagnostic findings

1. pH decreased below 7.35

2. $PaCO_2$ elevated above 45 mm Hg

3. Hyperkalemia

E. Compensation

1. Increased rate and depth of respirations to blow off CO_2

2. Kidneys eliminate H^+ ions and retain HCO_3^- (urine pH less than 6)

3. HCO_3^- levels rise when the body is compensating for the acidosis

F. Priority nursing diagnoses

1. Ineffective breathing pattern related to hypoventilation

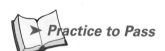

▶ Practice to Pass

Why is the nurse concerned about hyperkalemia in the client who has respiratory acidosis?

2. Impaired gas exchange related to alveolar hypoventilation

3. Sensory-perceptual alterations related to acid-base alterations

4. Anxiety related to breathlessness

5. Risk for injury related to decreased level of consciousness

6. Risk for decreased cardiac output related to dysrhythmias

G. Therapeutic management

1. Treatment is directed toward correcting the underlying cause and improving ventilation

2. It is important to implement pulmonary hygiene measures to clear the respiratory tract of mucus and purulent drainage

3. Provide adequate fluid intake to liquefy secretions

4. If indicated, administer supplemental oxygen cautiously to a client with chronic respiratory acidosis

   a. It is important to note that clients with chronic acidosis have compensated and are adjusted to living with higher PCO_2 levels

   b. Remember CO_2 levels are the mechanisms that stimulate the respiratory drive

   c. Oxygen administration at higher levels can lead to a decreased ventilatory drive and can cause further hypoxia

   d. Low flow oxygen is the expected treatment

   e. Collaborate with physician and respiratory therapist in the management of clients with chronic respiratory disease

5. Mechanical ventilation may be required to improve respiratory status and to decrease the CO_2 gradually to prevent alkalosis and seizures from occurring

H. Planning and implementation

1. Assess respiratory rate and depth

2. Monitor the client for complications and response to therapy

3. Take apical pulse and assess for tachycardia and irregularities

4. Assess level of consciousness

5. Monitor ECG for dysrhythmias

6. Draw serum electrolytes, especially potassium and ABGs

7. Administer oxygen as indicated and ordered

8. Administer medications as ordered

9. Provide good oral hygiene frequently

10. Keep side rails up, the bed at the lowest level, and the call bell within reach of the client

11. Maintain a calm, quiet environment

12. Assess color of skin, nail beds, and mucous membranes

13. If client is confused, orient frequently to person, place, and time

14. Position to facilitate maximum lung expansion

15. Provide adequate fluid intake

I. Medication therapy

1. The type of drug and route of administration depend on client's baseline condition and whether the disease is either acute or chronic with an acute exacerbation

2. Medications that could be used include:

    a. Bronchodilators to decrease bronchospasm

    b. Antibiotics to treat infections in the respiratory tract

    c. Respiratory agents to decrease viscosity of pulmonary secretions, such as acetylcystine (Mucomyst)

    d. Anticoagulants and thrombolytics to prevent or treat pulmonary emboli

3. Medications are usually administered IV in acute situations and then changed to PO as the client's condition stabilizes

4. Respiratory therapy often administers medications as part of the treatment plan; they are often called on a PRN basis to assist the client during acute episodes

J. Client education

1. Teach preventive measures to clients at risk

2. Teach deep breathing techniques

3. Teach signs and symptoms of infection to report to the healthcare provider

4. Report signs of infections, shortness of breath, fatigue, and increased pulse rate to healthcare provider

K. Evaluation

1. ABGs return to as near normal as possible for client

2. Anxiety level diminishes, leading to improved work of breathing with less effort

3. Client is oriented to person, place, and time

4. Client remains free of injury

5. No cardiac dysrhythmias occur

6. Level of consciousness improves

7. Respiratory pattern becomes deeper and rate decreases

III. Respiratory Alkalosis

A. *Respiratory alkalosis:* a condition in which pH is elevated and $PaCO_2$ is decreased

B. Occurs with hyperventilation and leads to a decreased level of CO_2; sometimes called an H_2CO_3 deficit

C. Other causes can include:

1. Respiratory center stimulation from fever, salicylate intoxication, and trauma to the CNS

2. Infection

3. Excessive mechanical ventilation

4. Refer back to Table 8-2

D. Clinical presentation

1. Cardiovascular

   a. Increased myocardial irritability; palpitations

   b. Increased heart rate

   c. Increased sensitivity to digitalis

2. Respiratory

   a. Rapid, shallow breathing

   b. Chest tightness and palpitations

3. CNS

   a. Dizziness

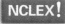

   b. Lightheadedness

   c. Anxiety, panic

   d. Tetany

   e. Convulsions

   f. Difficulty concentrating

   g. Blurred vision

   h. Numbness and tingling in extremities

   i. Hyperactive reflexes

E. Diagnostic findings

1. High pH (> 7.45)

2. Low $PaCO_2$ (< 35 mm Hg)

3. Hypokalemia

4. Hypocalcemia (as pH increases, calcium binding occurs in the serum and the calcium levels decrease)

F. Compensation

1. Kidneys conserve H^+ and excrete HCO_3^- (urine pH greater than 6)

2. Low HCO_3^- indicates the body is attempting to compensate

G. Priority nursing diagnoses

1. Sensory/perceptual alterations related to neurological deficits

2. Altered thought processes related to altered cerebral functioning

3. Ineffective breathing pattern related to hyperventilation

4. Risk for injury related to weakness or seizures

5. Risk for injury related to tetany

H. Therapeutic management

1. Treat the underlying cause

2. Have client rebreathe CO_2 by using a rebreather mask or a paper bag

3. Give oxygen therapy if the client is hypoxic

4. Medicate as needed with antianxiety drugs

I. Planning and implementation

1. Provide support and reassurance

2. Monitor vital signs and ABGs

3. Assist client to breathe more slowly

4. If needed, provide client with rebreather mask or paper bag to breathe into

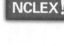

5. Protect from injury

6. Administer antianxiety medications as ordered

7. Monitor response to therapy

J. Medication therapy

1. Sedatives may be used to control hyperventilation due to anxiety

2. Antianxiety agents may also be ordered to control anxiety

K. Client education

1. Teach client relaxation techniques

2. Encourage client to attend stress management classes

3. Teach parents to keep aspirin and other salicylates out of reach of children and to keep syrup of ipecac available

L. Evaluation

1. Respiratory rate decreases

2. Numbness and tingling in extremities dissipates

3. ABGs return to normal

4. Anxiety diminishes

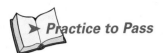

Practice to Pass

Why would a client with uncontrolled Type 1 diabetes develop metabolic acidosis and how can this be prevented?

NCLEX!

NCLEX!

NCLEX!

5. Client remains free from injury

IV. Metabolic Acidosis

A. *Metabolic acidosis:* an imbalance in which pH decreases and HCO_3 decreases

B. Occurs when acids other than carbonic acid accumulate in the ECF or when there is a loss of HCO_3^-

C. This condition rarely occurs spontaneously but rather is accompanied by other problems, such as GI conditions (starvation, malnutrition, and chronic diarrhea), renal (kidney failure), DKA, hyperthyroidism, trauma, shock, increased exercise, severe infection, and fever

D. Clinical presentation

  1. Cardiovascular

    a. Hypotension

    b. Dysrhythmias

    c. Peripheral vasodilation

    d. Cold, clammy skin

  2. Respiratory

    a. Deep, rapid pattern

    b. Kussmaul's respirations

  3. CNS

    a. Drowsiness

    b. Coma

    c. Headache

    d. Confusion

    e. Lethargy

    f. Weakness

  4. Gastrointestinal

    a. Nausea and vomiting

    b. Diarrhea

    c. Abdominal pain

E. Diagnostic findings

  1. pH less than 7.35

  2. HCO_3^- less than 22 mEq/L

  3. Hyperkalemia frequently seen

  4. ECG may show changes related to potassium levels

  5. Anion gap calculation increases

  6. Base excess decreases

F. Compensation

1. Lungs eliminate CO_2; kidneys conserve HCO_3^-

2. Urine pH less than 6

3. $PaCO_2$ decreases when compensation is occurring

G. Priority nursing diagnoses

1. Decreased cardiac output secondary to dysrhythmias and/or fluid volume deficits

2. Risk for sensory/perceptual alterations related to changes in neurological functioning secondary to acidosis

3. Risk for injury related to confusion, weakness, and drowsiness

4. Risk for fluid volume deficit related to excessive loss from the kidneys or gastrointestinal system

H. Therapeutic management

1. Treatment is aimed at correcting the underlying problem

2. Provide hydration to restore water, nutrients, and electrolytes

3. Administration of alkalotic IV solution (sodium bicarbonate or sodium lactate) may be indicated to correct acidosis

4. Mechanical ventilation is used only if other treatment modalities are ineffective

I. Planning and implementation

1. Monitor ABGs

2. Monitor intake and output

3. Measure daily weights

4. Assess vital signs, especially respiration for rate and depth

5. Assess level of consciousness

6. Assess gastrointestinal function

7. Monitor ECG for conduction problems

8. Monitor serum electrolytes

9. Protect from injury

10. Administer medications and IV fluids as ordered

J. Medication therapy: based on underlying cause

1. If cause is secondary to diabetic ketoacidosis, implement hydration with normal saline, regular insulin, and potassium

2. If diarrhea is the cause, treat with hydration and antidiarrheal agents

3. Administer $NaHCO_3$ cautiously and only when HCO_3^- levels are very low (below 16–18 mEq/L)

    a. Can cause metabolic alkalosis and hypokalemia

          b. The medication must be titrated closely so as to avoid further acid-base imbalances

  K. Client education

      1. Teach clients to seek healthcare if they have prolonged diarrhea

      2. Teach diabetic clients the importance of preventing occurrences of DKA and how to manage DKA should it occur

  L. Evaluation

      1. Client remains free from injury

      2. No dysrhythmias occur

      3. ABGs return to normal

      4. Fluid volume deficits are corrected

      5. Level of consciousness returns to normal

      6. Gastrointestinal upset is corrected

V. Metabolic Alkalosis

  A. *Metabolic alkalosis:* a condition in which there is an increased pH and increased HCO_3^-

  B. Occurs when there is a loss of H^+ ion (such as in vomiting or nasogastric suctioning) or an increase in the HCO_3^- level (such as with ingestion of bicarbonate-based antacids)

  C. See Table 8-3

  D. Clinical presentation

      1. Cardiovascular

          a. Tachycardia

          b. Dysrhythmias

          c. Hypertension

          d. Atrial tachycardia

          e. Premature ventricular contractions

      2. Respiratory

          a. Hypoventilation

          b. Respiratory failure

      3. CNS

          a. Dizziness

          b. Irritability

          c. Nervousness

          d. Confusion

          e. Tremors

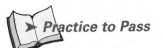

Practice to Pass

How would the nurse prevent the client from losing H^+ ions when nasogastric suctioning is being used?

NCLEX!

NCLEX!

NCLEX!

Table 8-3	Clinical Picture	Acidosis	Alkalosis
Metabolic Alterations in Acid-Base Balance	pH PaCO₂ HCO₃⁻	< 7.35 < 35 with compensation < 22	> 7.45 > 45 with compensation > 26
	Signs and symptoms Cardiovascular	Hypotension, dysrhythmias, peripheral vasodilation, cold, clammy skin	Tachycardia, dysrhythmias secondary to hypokalemia, hypotension, premature ventricular contractions, atrial tachycardia
	Respiratory	Deep, rapid respiratory pattern (Kussmaul's respirations)	Hyperventilation, respiratory failure
	CNS	Drowsiness, coma, headache, confusion, lethargy, weakness, nausea and vomiting, diarrhea, abdominal pain	Dizziness, irritability, nervousness, confusion, tremors, muscle cramps, tetany, hyperreflexia, paresthesias in fingers and toes, seizures
	Causes	Diabetic ketoacidosis, lactic acidosis, starvation, severe diarrhea, renal tubule acidosis, renal failure, GI fistulas, shock	Severe vomiting, excessive NG suctioning, diuretic therapy, hypokalemia, licorice, excessive NaHCO₃ use, excessive mineralcorticoids
	Compensation	Lungs eliminate CO₂; kidneys conserve HCO₃⁻	Lungs retain CO₂; kidneys excrete HCO₃⁻

    f. Muscle cramps

    g. Hyperreflexia

    h. Tetany

    i. Paresthesias in fingers and toes

    j. Seizures

  4. Gastrointestinal

    a. Anorexia

    b. Nausea and vomiting

    c. Paralytic ileus if hypokalemia occurs

E. Diagnostic findings

  1. pH greater than 7.45

  2. HCO₃⁻ above 26 mEq/L

  3. Hypokalemia

  4. Hypocalcemia (as pH increases, calcium binding occurs and serum calcium levels decrease)

  5. Hyponatremia and hypochloremia

  6. Urine chloride levels reveal whether client is chloride responsive (< 10 mEq/L) or chloride resistant > 10 mEq/L)

  7. Base excess increases

F. Compensation

1. Lungs retain CO_2; kidneys conserve H^+ and excrete HCO_3^-

2. $PaCO_2$ increases with compensation

3. Urine pH greater than 6

G. Priority nursing diagnoses

1. Fluid volume deficit related to excess gastrointestinal fluid loss

2. Decreased cardiac output related to fluid volume deficit and altered cardiac conduction secondary to hypokalemia and alkalosis

3. Knowledge deficit related to appropriate use of potassium-wasting diuretics and antacids

4. Risk for impaired gas exchange related to hypoventilation

5. Risk for injury related to hypotension secondary to fluid volume deficit

H. Therapeutic management

1. Treatment aimed at correcting underlying problem

2. Provide sufficient chloride to enhance renal absorption of sodium and excretion of HCO_3^-

3. Restore normal fluid balance

I. Planning and implementation

1. Assess level of consciousness

2. Assess vital signs, especially respiratory rate and depth

3. Administer medication and IV fluids as ordered

4. Monitor intake and output

5. Monitor response to therapy

6. Protect from injury

7. Monitor ECG for conduction abnormalities

8. Monitor ABGs

9. Monitor serum electrolytes

J. Medication therapy

1. Normal saline-based IV fluid replacement

2. Potassium supplementation if hypokalemic

3. Histamine-2 receptor antagonists such as cimetidine (Tagamet) or ranitidine (Zantac) to reduce production of H^+ ions and loss of H^+ ions from gastrointestinal drainage

4. If client is chloride responsive, then administer acetazolamide (Diamox) to increase renal bicarbonate excretion

5. If client is chloride resistant, then correct K^+ and Mg^{++} deficits with appropriate supplementation

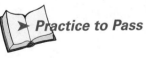

Practice to Pass

Why does the client with metabolic alkalosis have cardiac conduction problems that must be monitored?

NCLEX!

NCLEX!

NCLEX!

K. Client education

1. Teach clients to take antacids correctly

2. Teach signs and symptoms to report to healthcare provider for those at risk, especially the elderly

3. Teach signs and symptoms of hypokalemia to report to healthcare provider

L. Evaluation

1. Client remains free from injury

2. ABGs return to normal

3. Hypertension is corrected

4. Electrolytes restored to normal

5. Cardiac conduction abnormalities do not occur

6. Client states ways to prevent problem from reoccurring

VI. Mixed Acid-Base Disturbances

A. Identification and treatment of primary disorder

1. A **mixed acid-base disorder** occurs when two or more independent acid-base disorders occur at the same time

2. The pH is dependent on the type and severity of each simple disorder

3. Respiratory acidosis and alkalosis cannot occur concurrently; it is impossible to have hyperventilation and hypoventilation at the same time

4. Treatment is aimed at correcting the underlying cause of each disorder

5. When identifying acid-base imbalances, mathematical formulas can be used to assess degree of expected compensation

    a. The use of these equations is usually done on an intermediate level of acid-base balance

    b. However, it is important for the nurse to know that there are calculations that will identify the degree of compensatory changes

6. Anion gap and urine pH values will also assist in determining which imbalance is occurring

B. Chronic and superimposed acid-base disturbances

1. Mixed metabolic acidosis and respiratory acidosis

    a. Clients with acute pulmonary edema

    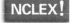

    b. Clients with cardiac arrest as a result of build-up of lactic acidosis and CO_2 retention due to inadequate ventilation

    c. pH values decrease and are more pronounced because of decreasing bicarbonate level coupled with increasing carbon dioxide level

2. Mixed metabolic alkalosis and respiratory acidosis

    a. Seen in clients with chronic obstructive pulmonary disease (COPD) secondary to treatment with potassium-wasting diuretics, severe vomiting, or development of diarrhea

    b. Seen in clients with COPD who have a quick improvement in ventilation

    c. pH values tend to become balanced because of an increase in both HCO_3 and PCO_2 values

  3. Mixed metabolic acidosis with respiratory alkalosis

    a. Seen in clients with a rapid correction of metabolic acidosis

    b. Seen in clients with salicylate intoxication

    c. Seen in clients with gram-negative septicemia

    d. pH values tend to become balanced because of decreases in both HCO_3 and pCO_2

  4. Mixed metabolic alkalosis and respiratory alkalosis

    a. Seen in clients postoperatively with severe hemorrhage

    b. Seen in clients who have massive transfusions

    c. Seen in clients with excessive NG drainage

    d. pH values increase and are more pronounced because of an increase in bicarbonate coupled with a decrease in carbon dioxide levels

  5. Mixed metabolic acidosis and metabolic alkalosis

    a. Seen in clients with gastroenteritis, vomiting, and diarrhea

    b. If imbalance is present in the same proportion, there is usually no change in values (pH, HCO_3, and pCO_2) even though there is volume depletion

  6. Chronic and acute respiratory acidosis

    a. Clients with chronic respiratory conditions with an acute condition superimposed can lead to increased pCO_2 levels, causing further pulmonary dysfunction and leading to serious consequences that can compromise both treatment and expected response to treatment

    b. Clients who have both a chronic and a superimposed acute respiratory acid-base imbalance should be closely monitored by a pulmonologist

    c. Respiratory therapy should be part of the collaborative healthcare team during the management of this client

C. Diagnostic and laboratory findings

  1. Increased pCO_2 with decreased pH

    a. Respiratory acidosis

    b. Respiratory acidosis with incompletely compensating metabolic alkalosis

    c. Respiratory acidosis with coexisting metabolic acidosis

  2. Increased pCO_2 with increased pH

    a. Metabolic alkalosis with incomplete compensating respiratory acidosis

        b. Metabolic alkalosis with coexisting respiratory acidosis

    3. Decreased pCO_2 with decreased pH

        a. Metabolic acidosis with incomplete respiratory alkalosis

        b. Metabolic acidosis with coexisting respiratory alkalosis

    4. Decreased pCO_2 with increased pH

        a. Respiratory alkalosis

        b. Respiratory alkalosis with incomplete compensating metabolic acidosis

        c. Respiratory alkalosis with coexisting metabolic alkalosis

    5. Normal pH values

        a. Increased pCO_2 leads to respiratory acidosis with compensated metabolic alkalosis

        b. Decreased pCO_2 leads to respiratory alkalosis with compensated metabolic acidosis

    6. Changes in anion gap levels and bicarbonate levels

    7. Abnormal serum electrolyte levels can reflect changes in acid-base balance

    8. ECG results may show electrolyte disturbances

    9. CXR may show underlying cardiac or pulmonary disease

   10. Hemoglobin and hematocrit levels can indicate oxygen-carrying potential

D. Priority nursing diagnoses

    1. Decreased cardiac output related to dysrhythmias secondary to fluid volume or potassium alterations

    2. Sensory/perceptual alterations related to acid-base imbalance

    3. Risk for injury related to neurological changes secondary to acid-base imbalances

E. Therapeutic management

    1. Treatment focuses on correcting the underlying causes of the disorder

    2. The mixed disorders must be treated before acid-base balance can be restored

    3. A collaborative team approach (including a pulmonologist, respiratory therapist, nurses, and dietitian) is needed to assist client in restoring acid-base balance, increasing activity tolerance, and improving physiological function

F. Planning and implementation

    1. Monitor vital signs

    2. Monitor ABGs, pulmonary function tests, pulse oximetry, and CXR

    3. Protect from injury

    4. Monitor level of consciousness

    5. Monitor ECG, H&H, and serum electrolytes

    6. Ensure adequate fluid intake

    7. Implement therapeutic measures as ordered

NCLEX!

NCLEX!

NCLEX!

NCLEX!

G. Medication therapy

  1. Therapy is aimed at resolving the underlying causes of disorders

  2. Administer oxygen per physician order and respiratory therapy guidelines

  3. The presence of chronic disease will influence selection of medications

H. Client education

  1. Clients with chronic respiratory conditions should report exacerbations to the healthcare provider

  2. Clients who experience fluid losses through emesis or diarrhea are at increased risk for acid-base imbalance and should notify the healthcare provider if the condition is not self-limiting

  3. Clients who are diabetic are at risk for acid-base imbalance due to alterations in glucose levels and should closely monitor serum glucose levels and use appropriate interventions to maintain normal levels

  4. Clients who have renal problems are prone to develop acid-base imbalance due to alterations in electrolyte levels; closely monitor renal status to identify potential disturbances and allow for intervention

I. Evaluation

  1. Client remains free from injury

  2. Mixed disorder is treated quickly and effectively

  3. ABGs return to normal

  4. ECG conduction problems do not occur

  5. Fluid volume is maintained

  6. Electrolytes return to normal

  7. Level of consciousness improves

  8. Client reports ways to prevent problem from reoccurring

Case Study

A 69-year-old client with chronic obstructive pulmonary disease (COPD) is admitted with an acute respiratory infection. You are the nurse assigned to the care of this client.

❶ What would this client's ABGs look like?

❷ What will you do to help improve the client's respiratory status?

❸ Why is a client with COPD given oxygen at a low flow rate?

❹ Why is this client's $PaCO_2$ different than a client who does not have COPD?

❺ What teaching does this client require in order to prevent development of metabolic alkalosis?

For suggested responses, see page 233.

Posttest

1 A client with COPD is admitted to the hospital with an exacerbation of the disease. ABG results are pH 7.30, PaCO₂ 51, and HCO₃⁻ 25. How would the nurse interpret these?

    (1) Respiratory acidosis, uncompensated
    (2) Respiratory alkalosis partially compensated
    (3) Respiratory acidosis, compensated
    (4) Metabolic acidosis, compensated

2 A client admitted to the Emergency Department following a motor vehicle accident with chest injuries complains that it hurts to breathe. The client's respiratory rate is 12 and very shallow. The nurse would anticipate which of the following results on ABGs?

    (1) pH 7.42, PaCO₂ 41 mmHg, HCO₃⁻ 23 mEq/L, SaO₂ 96%
    (2) pH 7.31, PaCO₂ 49 mmHg, HCO₃⁻ 24 mEq/L, SaO₂ 87%
    (3) pH 7.49, PaCO₂ 34 mmHg, HCO₃⁻ 30 mEq/L, SaO₂ 89%
    (4) pH 7.38, PaCO₂ 38 mmHg, HCO₃⁻ 22 mEq/L, SaO₂ 90%

3 What action can the nurse take initially when a client becomes anxious and starts to hyperventilate?

    (1) Tell the client to stop breathing so fast because he may pass out.
    (2) Give the client a sedative to decrease anxiety and stop hyperventilation.
    (3) Give the client a paper bag to breathe into.
    (4) Notify the physician.

4 The nurse would closely monitor a client with diabetic ketoacidosis (DKA) for which of following acid-base imbalances?

    (1) Metabolic acidosis
    (2) Metabolic alkalosis
    (3) Respiratory acidosis
    (4) Respiratory alkalosis

5 A 36-year-old female is admitted with vomiting and dehydration due to the flu for three days. ABGs are pH 7.46, PaCO₂ 50, HCO₃⁻ 33, SaO₂ 95%. What do these value indicate to the nurse?

    (1) Metabolic acidosis, uncompensated
    (2) Respiratory acidosis, compensated
    (3) Metabolic alkalosis, partially compensated
    (4) Metabolic alkalosis, uncompensated

6 A client is admitted to the Emergency Department in a full cardiac arrest. ABGs indicate a respiratory acidosis. How does the nurse respond to correct this condition?

    (1) Administer NaHCO₃ to correct the acidosis.
    (2) Administer epinephrine to get a heart rate so the acidosis can be corrected.
    (3) Ventilate client to "blow off" excess CO₂.
    (4) Start cardiac compressions.

7 Which of the following responses by the nurse is correct when trying to explain to a client why vomiting caused the development of a metabolic alkalosis?

    (1) "Vomiting causes you to lose a large amount of the base in your system and this in turn leads to alkalosis."
    (2) "When vomiting occurs, a large amount of HCO₃⁻ can be lost and this leads to metabolic alkalosis."
    (3) "Vomiting causes a loss of HCl from the stomach and a metabolic acidosis results from the loss of the acids in the GI fluids."
    (4) "Vomiting can cause a loss of gastric acids from the stomach and metabolic alkalosis develops from this loss."

8 A 68-year-old client is admitted with pneumonia. ABG results are pH 7.46, PaCO₂ 30, HCO₃⁻ 19, and SaO₂ 72. The nurse interprets this as:

    (1) Respiratory acidosis, uncompensated.
    (2) Respiratory alkalosis, partially compensated.
    (3) Respiratory alkalosis, uncompensated.
    (4) Metabolic alkalosis, partially compensated.

9 A 71-year-old client develops hypertension, tachy-cardia, and increased respirations two days after surgery. ABG results are pH 7.29, PaCO₂ 52, HCO₃⁻ 24, SaO₂ 95%. These indicate:

(1) Respiratory acidosis, uncompensated.
(2) Respiratory acidosis, partially compensated.
(3) Metabolic acidosis, uncompensated.
(4) Metabolic acidosis, partially compensated.

10 A 57-year-old client is admitted with a diagnosis of an acute myocardial infarction. ABG results are pH 7.36, PaCO₂ 29, HCO₃⁻ 20 and SaO₂ 100%. The nurse interprets that this client is:

(1) Well oxygenated with uncompensated respiratory alkalosis.
(2) Hypoxemic with compensated respiratory acidosis.
(3) Well oxygenated with compensated metabolic acidosis.
(4) Hypoxemic with compensated metabolic acidosis.

See pages 190–191 for Answers and Rationales.

Answers and Rationales

Pretest

1 **Answer: 3** *Rationale:* Respiratory acidosis is the direct result of hypoventilation due to certain conditions. This hypoventilation results in rising carbon dioxide levels and carbonic acid production. Respiratory alkalosis is associated with hyperventilation, making options 1 and 4 incorrect. Option 2 is incorrect as retained levels of sodium bicarbonate lead to alkalotic states.
Cognitive Level: Application
Nursing Process: Analysis; *Test Plan:* PHYS

2 **Answer: 1** *Rationale:* Clients with COPD are prone to develop acidosis as CO₂ levels are retained in the body. There is less surface area for gas exchange because the alveolar walls break down. In addition, the goblet cells overproduce mucus, making air movement out of the lung difficult. Consequently, CO₂ builds up. Clients who have chronic COPD learn to compensate for higher levels of CO₂ by increasing hydrogen (H⁺) ion excretion and retaining bicarbonate (HCO₃⁻). As COPD progresses, acidosis develops and the pH will drop. Option 2 is incorrect because the lungs are affected by the disease process and may not be able to correct the acid-base disturbance. Option 3 is incorrect because the renal response is not the primary mechanism by which acid-base imbalances are resolved. Option 4 is not correct—it is too vague and does not address the acid-base relationship of this disease process.
Cognitive Level: Application
Nursing Process: Analysis; *Test Plan:* HPM

3 **Answer: 2** *Rationale:* Apnea and hypoventilation result in rising carbon dioxide levels, which lead to acidosis. The ABG would likely reflect respiratory acidosis without compensation. Option 1 is incorrect because it reflects a normal pH, a slight increase in PaCO₂, and a normal HCO₃⁻ level. Option 3 is incorrect because it reflects normal values in all three parameters. Option 4 reflects an alkalotic state because the pH and HCO₃⁻ are elevated and the PaCO₂ is decreased.
Cognitive Level: Analysis
Nursing Process: Assessment; *Test Plan:* PHYS

4 **Answer: 2** *Rationale:* The kidneys respond more slowly to acid-base imbalances but are more effective than the lungs in restoring acid-base balance to the extracellular fluid. The primary response to acidosis is with lung compensation. Option 1 is incorrect because the kidneys do not respond immediately to correct acid-base imbalances. Option 3 is incorrect because the kidneys utilize several mechanisms to restore acid-base balance involving phosphate buffer salts, reabsorption of bicarbonate, and excretion of ammonia. The bicarbonate buffer system is a very strong buffer system in the body and also helps to regulate the respiratory response to acid-base balance. Option 4 is incorrect because the kidneys help to restore acid-base balance by reabsorbing bicarbonate by ionizing carbonic acid. Ion exchange occurs between Na⁺ and H⁺, which leads to bicarbonate formation, which is then absorbed into the blood.
Cognitive Level: Application
Nursing Process: Analysis; *Test Plan:* PHYS

5 Answer: 2 *Rationale:* Diarrhea leads to loss of bicarbonate from the intestinal tract. This can cause metabolic acidosis. With metabolic acidosis, the pH is low and the HCO_3^- is also decreased. Option 1 is incorrect because the pH is alkalotic, the $PaCO_2$ is elevated, and the HCO_3 is slightly elevated. These values reflect metabolic alkalosis. Option 3 is incorrect because the pH and $PaCO_2$ are within normal limits and the HCO_3^- is slightly elevated. These values do not reflect a cause for concern at this point in time. Option 4 is incorrect because the pH is alkalotic, the $PaCO_2$ is normal, and the HCO_3^- is slightly elevated. These results reflect metabolic alkalosis.
Cognitive Level: Analysis
Nursing Process: Assessment; *Test Plan:* PHYS

6 Answer: 2 *Rationale:* Clients who are extremely anxious tend to hyperventilate and have a rapid, shallow respiratory pattern. Cardiac rhythm and regularity are independent of respiratory function, and the rate may vary depending on the client's medical condition and/or treatment. A rapid deep respiratory pattern is associated with further respiratory compromise.
Cognitive Level: Application
Nursing Process: Assessment; *Test Plan:* PHYS

7 Answer: 3 *Rationale:* Anxious clients hyperventilate, which leads to alkalosis because of a depletion of carbon dioxide. Options 1 and 2 reflect normal pH values. Option 4 reflects acidemia and is associated with clients who hypoventilate.
Cognitive Level: Application
Nursing Process: Assessment; *Test Plan:* PHYS

8 Answer: 3 *Rationale:* A client with metabolic acidosis will have an increase in respiratory rate and depth in an attempt to compensate for the acidosis. Increases in heart rate, temperature, and urinary output are all metabolic responses that are not directly associated with maintaining acid-base balance. Initial compensation with metabolic acidosis will be via the lungs.
Cognitive Level: Application
Nursing Process: Assessment; *Test Plan:* PHYS

9 Answer: 4 *Rationale:* Due to a lack of insulin, diabetic clients are more likely to use fats as an energy source. During the metabolism of fats, free fatty acids are released, leading to accumulation of fatty acid fragments and the development of diabetic ketoacidosis. Diabetic clients are likely to develop metabolic acidosis characterized by decreased pH and HCO_3^- levels.
Cognitive Level: Application
Nursing Process: Assessment; *Test Plan:* PHYS

10 Answer: 2 *Rationale:* The pulse oximeter measures the amount of oxygen in the blood and is a good indication of oxygenation status. It is not meant to replace needed ABG monitoring, but rather it is used in conjunction with appropriate respiratory assessment to provide important information on a continuous basis. Pulse oximetry does not determine or reflect ventilatory effort regardless of client positioning.
Cognitive Level: Application
Nursing Process: Implementation; *Test Plan:* PHYS

Posttest

1 Answer: 1 *Rationale:* A pH of 7.30 indicates acidosis. A $PaCO_2$ of 51 indicates a respiratory acidosis is occurring. Since the $PaCO_2$ is elevated with a normal HCO_3^-, an uncompensated respiratory acidosis is occurring. Options 2 and 4 are incorrect because the pH value does not indicate that alkalosis could be present. Option 3 is incorrect because the bicarbonate level is normal, indicating that compensation has not taken place. With compensation, you would expect an increase in the bicarbonate level.
Cognitive Level: Analysis
Nursing Process: Analysis; *Test Plan:* PHYS

2 Answer: 2 *Rationale:* A client with a chest injury is likely to hypoventilate (have a shallow respiratory pattern) as a result of pain due to associated trauma. It is unknown at this time whether there are any internal injuries that could affect the client's oxygen saturation. This type of respiratory pattern is associated with respiratory acidosis. Options 1 and 4 reflect normal lab values. Option 3 reflects respiratory and metabolic alkalosis (increased pH and HCO_3^-, decreased pCO_2).
Cognitive Level: Analysis
Nursing Process: Analysis; *Test Plan:* PHYS

3 Answer: 3 *Rationale:* One of the first things a nurse should do when a client is hyperventilating is to give the client a paper bag to breathe into. This prevents the CO_2 level from decreasing and rebreathing the gas in the bag will also help to decrease the respiratory rate. Hyperventilation is associated with respiratory alkalosis. Although sedatives may be indicated to decrease anxiety and decrease hyperventilation, the use of a paper bag may stop the breathing pattern response by redirecting the client's focus. Telling the client that he or she may pass out may make the client change the breathing pattern, but it could also make it worse by increasing anxiety. Notifying the physician may be indicated to further assist in client treatment

but the initial response should be to interrupt the present breathing pattern of the client.
Cognitive Level: Application
Nursing Process: Implementation; *Test Plan:* PHYS

4   **Answer: 1** *Rationale:* DKA is associated with an increase in acid production. Diabetic clients with DKA are unable to metabolize glucose and the liver responds with an increase in fatty acid metabolism. These fatty acids are oxidized leading to ketone body formation and increased acidity. Option 2 is incorrect because metabolic alkalosis might occur as a response to overtreatment of the primary disturbance. Options 3 and 4 are not associated with DKA.
Cognitive Level: Application
Nursing Process: Assessment; *Test Plan:* HPM

5   **Answer: 3** *Rationale:* The pH indicates alkalosis and the HCO_3^- is elevated, indicating a metabolic basis. The $PaCO_2$ is slightly elevated, indicating that compensation is occurring. Options 1 and 2 are incorrect because the client's pH reflects alkalosis. Option 4 is incorrect because compensation is occurring due to the increased CO_2 level.
Cognitive Level: Analysis
Nursing Process: Analysis; *Test Plan:* PHYS

6   **Answer: 3** *Rationale:* During a cardiac arrest, the client develops profound respiratory acidosis and needs to be ventilated, first with bag-valve-mask device and then by mechanical means once intubation is accomplished. Other interventions will be instituted during the course of the code, but the nurse should always respond to any emergency situation with the ABCs (airway, breathing, and circulation).
Cognitive Level: Application
Nursing Process: Implementation; *Test Plan:* PHYS

7   **Answer: 4** *Rationale:* When vomiting occurs, HCl (a strong acid) is lost from the body. Excessive loss of GI fluids is the most common cause of metabolic alkalosis. Options 1, 2, and 3 are incorrect because

vomiting is associated with acid loss. Vomiting causes further acid depletion and leads to bicarbonate excess.
Cognitive Level: Application
Nursing Process: Analysis; *Test Plan:* PHYS

8   **Answer: 2** *Rationale:* The slightly elevated pH (alkalosis), the low $PaCO_2$ (respiratory origin) and the low HCO_3^- indicate compensation is starting but is not yet fully complete, since the pH is still abnormal. In addition, SaO_2 level is decreased significantly, which is not consistent with aging alone. Option 1 is incorrect because the pH is alkalotic. Option 3 is incorrect because in an uncompensated respiratory alkalosis, the bicarbonate level would be normal. Option 4 is incorrect because the bicarbonate level is not elevated.
Cognitive Level: Analysis
Nursing Process: Analysis; *Test Plan:* PHYS

9   **Answer: 1** *Rationale:* The pH is low (acidosis) and $PaCO_2$ high (respiratory origin). The HCO_3^- is normal, indicating that compensation has not occurred. The client is experiencing hyperventilation but blood gases reveal a respiratory acidosis, probably because of prior hypoventilation. Option 2 is incorrect because the bicarbonate level has not increased in an attempt to restore balance. Options 3 and 4 are incorrect because the bicarbonate levels are within normal limits and yet the $PaCO_2$ level is still elevated.
Cognitive Level: Analysis
Nursing Process: Analysis; *Test Plan:* PHYS

10   **Answer: 3** *Rationale:* The pH is normal (but is nearer to the acidotic end), while the $PaCO_2$ is low (compensation has occurred), and the HCO_3^- is low (indicating metabolic origin). The oxygen saturation of 100% indicates the blood is well oxygenated, making options 2 and 4 incorrect because the client is not hypoxemic. Since the pH is within normal limits, it is more likely that there are mixed acid-base disorders occurring that are compensating each other. Since the $PaCO_2$ and HCO_3^- are low, metabolic acidosis is occurring with a respiratory alkalosis.
Cognitive Level: Analysis
Nursing Process: Analysis; *Test Plan:* PHYS

References

Ball, J. & Bindler, R. (1999). *Pediatric nursing: Caring for children* (2nd ed.). Stamford, CT: Appleton & Lange, pp. 324–337.

Horne, M. M. & Bond, E. F. (2000). Fluid, electrolyte, and acid-base imbalances. In S. M. Lewis, M. M. Heitkemper, & S. R. Dirksen (Eds.), *Medical-surgical nursing: Assessment and management of clinical problems* (5th ed.). St. Louis: Mosby, pp. 342–346.

Horne, C. & Derrico, D. (1999). Mastering ABGs: The art of arterial blood gas measurement. *Nursing 99*(8), 26–32.

Kozier, B., Erb, G., Berman, A., & Burke, K. (2000). *Fundamentals of nursing: Concepts, process, and practice* (6th ed.). Upper Saddle River, NJ: Prentice-Hall, Inc., pp. 1315–1321.

LeMone, P. & Burke, K. (2000). *Medical-surgical nursing: Critical thinking in client care* (2nd ed.). Upper Saddle River, NJ: Prentice-Hall, Inc., pp. 149–161.

Pagana, K. D. & Pagana, T. J. (2001). *Mosby's diagnostic and laboratory test reference* (5th ed.). St. Louis: Mosby, pp. 111–119.

Patton, K. T. & Thibodeau, G. A. (2000). *Mosby's handbook of anatomy and physiology.* St. Louis: Mosby, pp. 532–544.

Smeltzer, S. C. & Bare, B. G. (2000). *Brunner & Suddarth's medical-surgical nursing* (9th ed.). Philadelphia: Lippincott, pp. 229–232.

Williams, B. R. & Baer, C. L. (1998). *Essentials of clinical pharmacology in nursing* (3rd ed.). Springhouse, PA: Springhouse, pp. 624–628.

Wong, F. (1999). A new approach to ABG interpretation. *Nursing 99*(8), 34–36.

Workman, M. (1999). Interventions for clients with electrolyte imbalances. In D. Ignatavicius, M. Workman, & M. Mishler (Eds.), *Medical-surgical nursing across the health care continuum* (3rd ed.). Philadelphia: W. B. Saunders, pp. 283–303.

CHAPTER 9

Replacement Therapies for Fluid and Electrolyte Imbalances

Bernadette VanDeusen, MSN, RN

CHAPTER OUTLINE

Fluid Therapies

Diagnostic and Laboratory Findings

Selection of Fluid and Electrolyte Therapies

OBJECTIVES

- Review concepts of hydration therapy.
- Review assessment data and diagnostic testing used to evaluate fluid balance.
- Identify specific solutions used for the treatment of fluid imbalance.
- Identify priority nursing diagnoses for clients receiving fluid and electrolyte replacement therapy.
- Discuss the therapeutic management of a client receiving fluid replacement therapy.
- Discuss the nursing management of a client receiving fluid replacement therapy.

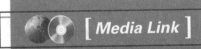

[Media Link]

Use the CD-ROM enclosed with this text, or log onto the address given to access the free, interactive Companion Website created for this series. The CD-ROM and Companion Website accompanying this book offer additional practice opportunities and information—NCLEX Review, Case Studies, Glossary, In Depth with NCLEX, and more.

www.prenhall.com/hogan

REVIEW AT A GLANCE

ABO blood typing *blood typing system that identifies naturally occurring antigens and antibodies located on the membrane of the RBCs and helps to identify correct recipient and donor for administration of blood products*

anaphylaxis *a severe, potentially life-threatening allergic reaction accompanied by itching, urticaria, bronchospasm, laryngeal edema, hypotension, and vascular collapse*

autologous transfusion *represents the donation of blood by an individual for use during perioperative or postoperative period or for use as a salvage method during the perioperative phase*

colloid *a high molecular weight substance that pulls fluids out of the intracellular and interstitial space and expands the intravascular volume*

crystalloid *a solution containing small molecules that is able to pass through a semipermeable membrane; may be hypotonic, isotonic, or hypertonic*

cytomegalovirus (CMV) negative blood *blood that does not carry CMV, a herpes virus that, after infecting an individual, remains in the leukocytes; if transfused into an immunocompromised recipient, can cause severe illness*

fresh frozen plasma (FFP) *a blood product removed from whole blood that contains all the coagulation factors and liquid plasma portion*

granulocytes *consist of basophils, eosinophils, and neutrophils (with platelets or platelet-poor) that are used to treat acquired neutropenia or severe infections that do not respond to conventional antibiotic therapy; infusion of these is currently not approved by the FDA but is undergoing clinical investigation and therefore may occur in the clinical setting*

hemolytic transfusion reaction *the most serious and potentially life-threatening reaction usually stemming from administration of ABO or Rh-incompatible blood and resulting in chills, low back pain, hemoglobinuria, renal failure, and shock*

homologous transfusion *the donation of blood for other clients or for their own use (designated homologous transfusion); can also be called allogenic*

human leukocyte antigen (HLA) allo-immunization *the process by which an individual exposed to HLA antigens via nonleukocyte-depleted blood develops antibodies to those antigens that limit the effectiveness of future platelet transfusions*

irradiated blood *blood that is exposed to radiation to kill cells that might initiate transfusion graft vs. host disease (TGVHD) in the immunocompromised individual*

leukocyte depleted blood *packed red blood cells and platelets that have been filtered to remove leukocytes to decrease the incidence of transfusion-related febrile reactions, CMV transmission, and HLA alloimmunization*

leukopheresis *the process by which leukocytes are extracted from withdrawn blood, which is then retransfused into the donor*

packed red blood cells (PRBCs) *a blood product that provides same number of RBCs as whole blood but with most of the plasma removed, leading to a solution with an increased hematocrit*

transfusion graft vs. host disease (TGVHD) *condition in which donor lymphocytes attack the immunocompromised individual, resulting in an erythematous (sunburn) rash, liver dysfunction, and pancytopenia*

type and cross-match *process by which the recipient's blood is typed to determine ABO blood group and Rh factor and the recipient's serum is mixed with donor RBCs to check for the presence of antibodies to the donor's minor antigens*

type and screen *process whereby blood antigens and antibodies are determined but no blood product is physically held for the client*

Pretest

1 A trauma victim admitted to the Emergency Department is hemorrhaging, in shock, and has lost a significant percentage of blood volume. There is no time to perform a cross-match. Which of the following actions should be implemented immediately?

(1) Transfuse type AB, Rh-positive blood.
(2) Transfuse albumin to expand the remaining plasma volume.
(3) Transfuse type O, Rh-negative blood.
(4) Transfuse platelets to restore adequate clotting ability.

2 A client with gastrointestinal bleeding suddenly develops diaphoresis and a rapid and thready pulse, and the nurse is finding it difficult to hear a blood pressure. Which of the following intravenous fluids does the nurse anticipate the physician will order STAT?

(1) Dextrose in water (D_5W)
(2) Normal saline (0.9% NaCl)
(3) ½ normal saline (0.45% NaCl)
(4) Dextrose 5% in 0.45% sodium chloride

3 A client with pretransfusion hemoglobin and hematocrit values of 9 grams and 27%, respectively, received two units of packed red blood cells on the evening shift. Which of the following post-transfusion laboratory results would the nurse anticipate seeing the following morning?

(1) 13 g, 30%
(2) 15 g, 39%
(3) 11 g, 33%
(4) 12 g, 36%

4 Which of the following interventions should the nurse include in a plan of care for a client who has had too much warfarin (Coumadin)?

(1) Monitor for bleeding, check prothrombin time (PT) or International Normalized Ratio (INR), and prepare to administer fresh frozen plasma.
(2) Monitor for bleeding, check partial thromboplastin time (PTT) or activated PTT (aPTT), and prepare to administer cryoprecipitate.
(3) Monitor for bleeding, check PT/INR, and prepare to administer albumin.
(4) Monitor for bleeding, check aPTT/PTT, and prepare to administer platelets.

5 Which of the following intravenous solutions would the nurse refrain from administering to a client who is at risk for increased intracranial pressure?

(1) 0.9% Sodium chloride (NS)
(2) Lactated Ringer's (LR)
(3) Dextrose 2.5% in water
(4) Dextrose 5% in normal saline

6 Which of the following changes in laboratory values would the nurse anticipate after administering isotonic intravenous fluids to a client with a hypertonic plasma?

(1) Increased serum osmolality, increased blood urea nitrogen (BUN), and decreased hematocrit (HCT)
(2) Decreased serum osmolality, decreased BUN, and decreased HCT
(3) Increased serum osmolality, increased BUN, and increased HCT
(4) Decreased serum osmolality, decreased BUN, and increased HCT

7 A client with a history of congestive heart failure (CHF) has been carefully rehydrated with normal (0.9%) saline for isotonic dehydration related to overzealous diuresis. Which of the following statements by the client indicates that the nurse's discharge teaching has been effective?

(1) "I will increase my salt intake and double up on my fluid intake."
(2) "I will take my diuretic pill every fourth day."
(3) "I will weigh myself daily and notify the doctor if I develop a fever or diarrhea."
(4) "I will drink only one glass of water a day so I can eventually stop taking my pill."

8 A female client with type B, Rh-negative blood has been exposed to Rh-positive blood in the past. The nurse will evaluate that instruction regarding blood compatibility has been effective when the client makes which of the following statements?

(1) "I'm aware that I can safely receive type B positive and type O positive blood."
(2) "I'm aware that I can safely receive type B negative and type O negative blood."
(3) "I'm aware that I can safely receive type AB negative and type O negative blood."
(4) "I'm aware that I can safely receive type A positive and type O positive blood."

9 A client in need of a blood transfusion is concerned about the possibility of disease transmission. Which of the following statements by the nurse is accurate and may help to alleviate some anxiety for the client?

(1) "All blood products are absolutely safe after testing and there is no need to worry."
(2) "If you do not want the transfusion, do not sign the consent. Perhaps the physician can give you some iron pills."
(3) "More sophisticated screening tests have made the blood supply safer and the risk of infection, while it exists, is very low."
(4) "Have a family member or friend donate blood for you because this will guarantee its safety."

10 Which of the following blood products does the nurse anticipate the physician will order for a client diagnosed with hemophilia?

(1) Whole blood
(2) Packed red blood cells (PRBCs)
(3) Fresh frozen plasma (FFP)
(4) Albumin

See pages 220–221 for Answers and Rationales.

I. Fluid Therapies

A. Crystalloids: solutions that contain small molecules and are able to pass through semipermeable membranes (flowing readily from the vascular to interstitial space and cells)

1. Isotonic solutions

   a. Have approximately the same concentration (osmolality) as that of the extracellular fluid (ECF), thereby remaining within the ECF space

   b. Are given to expand the ECF volume

   c. Have no net effect on cellular dynamics because of their osmolarity

   d. Examples: normal saline (NS or 0.9 NaCl), Lactated Ringer's (LR), and dextrose 5% in water (D_5W); note that D_5W is considered hypotonic after metabolism of dextrose occurs

2. Hypotonic solutions

   a. Osmolality is lower than that of serum plasma

   b. Are given to reverse dehydration

   c. With regard to cellular dynamics, cause cells to swell and possibly burst

   d. Fluid shifting occurs with administration as fluids shift out of the blood vessels and into the interstitial space, causing ECF volume depletion

   e. Due to fluid shifting effects, hypotonic fluids should be administered cautiously

   f. Examples: ½ NS (0.45% NaCl), dextrose 2.5% in water ($D_{2.5}W$)

3. Hypertonic solutions

   a. Osmolality is higher than that of serum plasma

   b. Are given to increase the ECF volume and decrease cellular swelling

NCLEX!

NCLEX!

    c. With regard to cellular dynamics, cause cells to shrink and contribute to ECF volume overload

    d. Should be administered cautiously due to fluid shifting and potential for vein irritation due to high osmolar concentration

    e. Examples: 5% dextrose in 0.9% NaCl (D_5NS), 10% dextrose in water ($D_{10}W$), and 3% NaCl

B. Colloids: solutions that contain high molecular weight proteins or starch, do not cross the capillary semipermeable membrane, and remain in the intravascular space (pulling fluid out of the intracellular and interstitial space) for several days, assuming that the client has an intact capillary membrane; although colloids contain no clotting factors, they can affect the coagulation process—this fact must be considered in reference to certain treatment therapies

    1. Albumin

      a. Major plasma protein available in two forms: 5% (isotonic—equivalent to 12.5 g or 250 mL) and 25% (hypertonic—equivalent to 25 g or 50 mL)

      b. Normal human serum albumin is derived from donor plasma and is heat treated for viral inactivation (free from hepatitis; no known risk for acquired immunodeficiency syndrome [AIDS])

      c. Changes in albumin concentration affect cellular dynamics

        1) Increased albumin concentration results in fluid moving back into the capillaries from the interstitial space

        2) Decreased albumin concentration results in fluid leaking through the capillary walls into the interstitial space (edema)

        3) Clients suffering from underlying medical/nutritional problems (malnutrition, cirrhosis, or nephritic syndrome) can have chronically low albumin levels

      d. Comparison with crystalloid solutions

        1) Remain in the vascular space longer than crystalloids

        2) More expensive than crystalloids

        3) May cause febrile reactions

        4) Because they remain in the intravascular space for a longer period of time, they are more likely to cause circulatory overload than crystalloid solutions

      e. Indications and contraindications

        1) Primary clinical use is as volume expander when treating hypovolemic shock from trauma or surgery

        2) Given as a volume expander in a client who needs whole blood while the cross-match is being done

        3) Used to support blood pressure during a hypotensive episode, create diuresis in fluid volume excess, and facilitate remobilization of fluid from third-space fluid shifts

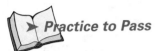

Practice to Pass

The physician has ordered 0.9% NaCl IV at 250 mL per hour for your newly admitted client in diabetic ketoacidosis. How will you evaluate the effectiveness of this IV therapy for this client?

NCLEX!

NCLEX!

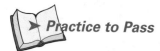

Practice to Pass

The physician has just ordered 25% albumin STAT for a 75-year-old female client in hypovolemic shock. Detail your priority assessments, interventions, and expected outcomes for the client.

NCLEX!

NCLEX!

4) Also used to treat burns, trauma, acute liver failure, hypoproteinemia, overzealous diuresis in clients with cirrhosis or nephrotic syndrome and to prevent and treat cerebral edema

5) Are contraindicated in severe anemia and avoided in clients who are dehydrated

6) Are given cautiously to clients with cardiac and pulmonary problems or in clinical situations where there is increased capillary leakage (sepsis, trauma, or burns)

f. Administration and nursing actions

1) Use glass bottle with administration set and filter that requires vented tubing

2) Should be used within a 4-hour time frame, as there are no preservatives

3) Requires dedicated line for infusion

4) Dose and rate of infusion are based on client's blood volume and underlying condition; infuse as rapidly as tolerated in clients with hypovolemic shock to replace vascular volume; in a client with normal blood volume, infuse 5% albumin at 2–4 mL/minute and 25% albumin at 1 mL/minute

5) Assess for urticaria, fever, and manifestations of fluid volume overload; monitor vital signs and breath sounds of all clients regardless of underlying condition and rate of administration

2. Dextran

a. A glucose solution with colloidal activity similar to albumin that expands the plasma volume by pulling fluid from the interstitial to intravascular space, thereby promoting dehydration of tissues

b. No risk of transfusion-related illnesses (not extracted from human plasma)

c. Increased likelihood of hypersensitivity reactions during the first minutes of administration due to presence of polysaccharide-reacting antibody

d. Available in two strengths

1) Dextran 40—low molecular weight dextran (refer to Box 9-1 for specific drug information)

2) Dextran 70—high molecular weight dextran (refer to Box 9-2 for specific drug information)

e. Alterations of diagnostic tests

1) Can affect **type and cross-match** (process by which compatibility between donor and recipient blood is determined) due to presence of Rouleaux formation

2) Can result in false increases in blood glucose, total protein, total bilirubin, and urine specific gravity

3) Can increase liver enzymes, such as AST and ALT levels

4) Can alter coagulation indices and increase bleeding times

NCLEX!

Box 9-1

Specific Information Related to Dextran 40

- Acts as a hypertonic colloidal solution that rapidly expands the plasma volume.
- Stays in the vascular space for up to 12 hours, depending on renal clearance (half-life of 2 to 6 hours).
- Appropriate for all types of shock states and acts as an adjunct to restore volume.
- Parenteral infusion is given via dedicated line because it has a high incompatibility profile.
- Will alter clotting factors because it has antiplatelet activity (decreases the adhesiveness of RBCs and improves peripheral blood flow).
- Can lead to false elevations in some laboratory tests and interfere with blood typing.
- Used prophylactically during surgical procedures that present a high risk for clotting to prevent DVT and PE and can be used for pump priming in extracorporeal circulation.
- Contraindicated in clients who have defined hypersensitivities, renal failure, cardiac failure, severe anemia, pregnancy, and clients receiving anticoagulant therapy.
- Clients with chronic liver disease, severely dehydration, or at risk for developing renal or cardiac failure require cautious use and monitoring if therapy is indicated by the physician.

f. Administration and nursing actions

1) Draw blood for type and cross-match (especially) and other labs as needed prior to beginning the dextran infusion if possible; at minimum, notify laboratory personnel that the client is receiving dextran

2) Obtain baseline hematocrit prior to dextran infusion and maintain HCT > 30% during course of therapy or notify physician of decreased volume

NCLEX!

3) Assess for signs and symptoms of **anaphylaxis** (tightness in chest, wheezing, bronchospasm, and urticaria)

4) Dextran 1 (Promit) is usually given IV prior to infusion of dextran to prevent formation of immune complexes by site binding on the antibody

5) Maintain hydration of client with supplemental IV fluids

6) Observe for signs and symptoms of bleeding

Box 9-2

Specific Information Related to Dextran 70

- Has higher molecular weight that is broken down more slowly in the body.
- Interferes with coagulation because it can prolong bleeding time, increase platelet adhesiveness, and increase blood viscosity.
- Can lead to false elevations in some laboratory tests and interfere with blood typing.
- Shows volume expansion within minutes with a duration of 12 hours (half-life of 12 hours).
- Give parenteral infusion via a dedicated line because it has a high incompatibility profile.
- Use in emergency situations to treat impending or existing hypovolemic or hemorrhagic shock as a result of burns, trauma, or surgery.
- Contraindicated for clients who have severe coagulopathy, known sensitivity to dextran, and severe cardiac or renal failure.

7) Monitor pertinent labs including HCT, serum chemistries, and serum protein levels on a frequent basis

3. Hetastarch (Hespan, Hextend)

a. Synthetic colloid made from cornstarch and available in a 6% solution (approximates albumin and dextran in terms of colloidal activity) that is diluted in 500 mL of NS (Hespan) and 6% solution that is diluted in 500 and 1,000 mL of an electrolyte-lactated solution (Hextend)

b. Expands the plasma and is used in shock precipitated by hemorrhage, trauma, burns, and sepsis; will stay in the vascular space up to 36 hours but the plasma volume expansion starts decreasing at about 24 hours; causes osmotic diuresis

c. Hespan is also used in the process of **leukopheresis** (the process by which leukocytes are extracted from withdrawn blood) when **granulocytes** are being harvested from a donor in order to be transfused into a neutropenic client

d. Alterations of diagnostic tests

1) Will not interfere with blood typing or cross-matching but can dilute clotting factors; PT, PTT, and clotting times may be transiently prolonged

2) Serum amylase will increase after Hespan administration (up to 4 times normal levels)

3) Can increase serum bilirubin levels but total bilirubin levels usually remain normal

e. Excretion is both renal and hepatic; do not administer to clients in renal failure with oliguria or anuria; use caution in clients with liver disease

f. Use caution in clients with CHF or bleeding disorders; contraindicated in severe bleeding disorders

g. Administration and nursing actions

1) Use opened containers immediately; contains no preservatives

NCLEX!

2) Monitor every client receiving Hespan for signs of hypervolemia (increased blood pressure, dyspnea, and bounding pulse)

3) Monitor for transient changes in PT and PTT; check serum amylase level prior to beginning the infusion

NCLEX!

4) Assess for adequate tissue perfusion; expect an increased urine output as Hespan causes osmotic diuresis; the increased urine output is not an indicator of adequate blood volume

NCLEX!

5) Be alert to signs and symptoms of anaphylaxis and intervene accordingly (stop infusion; provide oxygen; hydrate with NS; administer epinephrine, steroids; antihistamines as ordered; be prepared to intubate and maintain circulatory support)

6) Clients who are diabetic or who have acid-base imbalances due to increased lactate levels should not be given this medication because it can worsen the alkalosis (Hextend) or contribute to lactic acidosis

4. Plasma protein fraction (PPF)

   a. Major component is albumin with immunoglobulins and sodium; used to expand the intravascular volume

   b. Indicated for emergency treatment of hypovolemic shock, burns, and low protein states; functions as a blood-product volume expander

   c. Monitoring parameters include vital signs (hemodynamic—central venous pressure [CVP] if possible) and urine output during the first hour at a frequency of every 5 to 15 minutes

   d. Monitor clients closely for potential fluid volume overload, pulmonary edema, or heart failure

   e. Monitor serum protein, electrolytes, and hemoglobin and hematocrit during course of therapy

   f. Contraindicated in clients with CHF, history of bypass surgery, allergic reactions to albumin, and severe anemia

C. **Blood and blood products**

   1. **Packed red blood cells (PRBCs)**

      a. Prepared from whole blood with each unit approximately 250 mL (some plasma, leukocytes, and platelets from the whole blood are still present)

      b. Platelets and leukocytes are not viable but can cause problems for the recipient in that they contain human leukocyte antigens (HLAs); recipient can form antibodies against these antigens (HLA alloimmunization); this can create problems with future transfusions especially when receiving platelets

      c. Typically, PRBCs are **leukocyte depleted** (blood is filtered to remove leukocytes) to minimize the possibility that HLA alloimmunization will occur

      d. Contain the same red blood cell concentration as whole blood from which they are derived; advantage is client receives the same increase in oxygen-carrying capacity without being exposed to risk of fluid volume overload as with whole blood

      e. Increase colloidal oncotic pressure; pull fluids from extravascular to intravascular space and increase plasma volume

      f. Identification methods used for transfusion therapy

         1) Recipient's blood must be typed to determine **ABO blood typing** and Rh factor to ensure that the client receives compatible blood

         2) Recipient must not have antibodies to donor's major antigens on the RBCs (refer to Table 9-1)

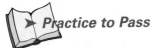

Practice to Pass

A client receiving Hespan for hypovolemia related to hemorrhage becomes very pale and diaphoretic, complains of chest tightness, and begins wheezing. Physical examination reveals hives covering the client's chest. What are your immediate nursing actions?

Table 9-1	Client Blood Type (recipient)	Donor Blood That Can Be Safely Administered	Rationale
ABO Compatibility System and Safe Transfusion	Type A	Type A Type O	Client has no anti-A antibodies. *Universal donor.* Donor has no antigens for recipient to react to.
	Type B	Type B Type O	Client has no anti-B antibodies. *Universal donor.* Donor has no antigens for recipient to react to.
	Type AB	Type A, B, or AB Type O	*Universal recipient.* Client has no anti-A or anti-B antibodies. *Universal donor.* Donor has no antigens for recipient to react to.
	Type O	Type O	*Universal donor.* Donor has no antigens for recipient to react to.

Note: Rh status must also be determined as part of the blood typing procedure. Rh-positive clients can receive Rh-positive and Rh-negative blood. Rh-negative clients can only receive Rh-negative blood.

3) Cross-matching: to detect the presence of recipient antibodies to the donor's minor antigens

    a) Recipient's serum is mixed with donor's RBCs; if antibodies to donor's antigens present, agglutination will occur (no match)

    b) If no antibodies to the donor's RBCs present, no agglutination (desired)

    c) Takes approximately 20 minutes to perform; type and cross-match is good for 48 hours only; must be repeated if time expires and the client needs blood; blood is physically held for a specific client

4) A **type and screen** can be used to identify blood type, surface antigens, and Rh factor but blood is not physically held; this process can be used in non-emergency situations in which it is helpful to know specific blood typing information but one does expect that blood will have to be administered

NCLEX!

5) In an emergency situation, type O negative blood (universal donor) can be administered to a client, foregoing the type and cross-matching procedure

6) May transmit viruses; additional tests for donated blood: hepatitis A, B, C, HIV, syphilis, ALT level (increased may be suspicious for hepatitis)

g. Specific treatments related to blood processing

1) **Irradiated blood:** blood is treated with radiation that kills donor cells that may attack the immunocompromised client (bone marrow transplant recipients, clients with Hodgkins disease, leukemia, intrauterine neonatal transfusion, or in clients who are being aggressively treated with chemotherapy)

    a) Goal is to prevent the transmission of **transfusion graft vs. host disease (TGVHD)**—donor lymphocytes attack recipient, cause liver dysfunction and bone marrow suppression, and can be fatal

    b) Leukocyte-depleted (Leukopor) blood will not prevent TGVH disease

2) **Cytomegalovirus (CMV) negative blood:** for immunocompromised clients including AIDS clients; CMV remains in a latent state in donor's leukocytes if previously infected with the virus; transfer of the leukocytes to immunocompromised recipients could cause severe illness; leukodepletion may eliminate CMV

h. One unit of PRBCs should raise hemoglobin 1 gram and hematocrit by 3% (assuming there is no ongoing blood loss if bleeding was either a cause or a contributing factor)

i. Are expensive as compared to other colloids and crystalloids (collecting, testing, and screening blood and all the special processing contribute heavily to the expense)

j. Indications

1) To improve oxygen-carrying capacity in clients with symptomatic anemia

2) To restore blood loss as a result of hemorrhage (gastrointestinal or trauma related) or surgical blood loss

k. Transfusion options

1) **Autologous transfusion** (to self) may be planned prior to surgical procedure (preoperative donation) or blood may also be collected and reinfused during or after surgery (perioperative, intraoperative, or postoperative blood salvage)

2) **Homologous transfusion** (or allogenic) represents blood collected from clients for use for other clients (volunteer), or for themselves (designated)

3) The blood collected for homologous transfusion undergoes testing for antibodies, pathologic organisms (HIV, CMV, hepatitis variants, HTLV, and syphilis)

4) Minimum standards are set by the American Association of Blood Banks (AABB) regarding criteria for donor requirements citing age, baseline hemoglobin and hematocrit, vital signs, weight, no evidence of transmittable disease or drug use, and frequency of blood donation

l. Administration (refer to Box 9-3)

1) Pretransfusion: verify the order and follow hospital policy and procedure with regard to all transfusion therapy; ensure that client has received informed consent and has signed the consent form

2) Start an IV if one not already in place; use an 18- to 20-gauge angiocath, which is preferred

3) Note that if the client is elderly with small fragile veins, you may use a 22- to 24-gauge angiocath without an infusion pump (force created by the pump through a small gauge catheter may cause cells to lyse); blood

Box 9-3	• Obtain informed consent for transfusion therapy.
Principles of Transfusion Therapy	• Have IV access ready prior to retrieving blood from the blood bank using appropriate tubing with NS as the priming solution.
	• Follow hospital policy and procedure regarding blood typing, acquisition of unit from blood bank, and verification of orders with two registered nurses.
	• Identify client at the bedside confirming client name and identification (ID) number, blood bank identification band (if used), unit number, blood type, and expiration date.
	• Remain at client's bedside during the first 15 minutes of transfusion therapy and monitor vital signs per protocol.
	• Obtain followup blood work to determine response to transfusion therapy.

will infuse more slowly but RBCs will remain intact; blood bank may be able to split the unit into two bags (one bag can infuse while the other remains properly refrigerated in the blood bank); check hospital policy for managing the elderly client with fragile veins

NCLEX!

4) Administer blood with normal saline only so as to prevent cell lysis; obtain 500 cc of NS and Y tubing and prime Y tubing that contains blood filter; additional filters may be required, such as Pall filter, depending on blood product used and/or general health condition of client; may connect to client and run at KVO (to keep vein open) rate if blood will arrive soon

5) Once blood bank indicates that the blood is ready, premedicate the client if ordered; common premedications are diphenhydramine (Benadryl), acetaminophen (Tylenol), and occasionally a corticosteroid or H_2 receptor blocker; premedication may be indicated to minimize allergic potential and symptom management; furosemide (Lasix) can be given either as premedication or in between units in order to minimize risks of potential fluid volume overload from administration

6) Obtain blood from blood bank following hospital procedure and record baseline vital signs

NCLEX!

7) Two RNs must verify identification of pertinent blood unit information (type, Rh factor, unit number, expiration date, matching with client's blood identification bracelet and original physician order)

NCLEX!

8) Prior to hanging any blood product, inspect for discoloration and/or bubbling that could indicate bacterial contamination; if there is any suspicion, then return blood unit to blood bank

9) In preparation for blood administration, don gloves and hang blood, keeping the spike and blood bag opening sterile, prime filter and tubing with blood; make sure that filter is completely filled with blood; may use pump for administration of blood if hospital policy permits

NCLEX!

10) Remain with the client for the first 15 minutes of therapy and monitor vital signs as per policy (refer to Box 9-4)

Box 9-4

Timing Issues Relevant to Transfusion Therapy

- Transfusion should be started within 30 minutes of the time that the unit is checked out of the blood bank.
- Remain with the client during the first 15 minutes of the transfusion and monitor accordingly for signs and symptoms of possible transfusion reaction.
- Stop blood if any signs or symptoms of a transfusion reaction occur and notify the physician.
- Run each unit over 2 hours unless otherwise ordered by the physician.
- Blood cannot hang more than 4 hours at room temperature because this can lead to cellular breakdown of the blood product.

11) If client will receive another unit of blood, check to see if physician has ordered a diuretic in between units if client is at risk for fluid volume overload

12) Lab work (hemoglobin and hematocrit) should be ordered two hours post-transfusion in order to assess client's response to therapy

NCLEX!

m. Clients who undergo multiple transfusions are at risk for developing additional electrolyte problems; these may include hyperkalemia or increased ammonia levels (because of cellular release from stored blood products) and hypocalcemia (because of chelation of calcium with citrate anticoagulant used as a blood preservative)

NCLEX!

n. Clients may still experience a transfusion reaction, regardless of all the precautions that are used to prevent such an occurrence (refer to Box 9-5)

2. Platelets

a. Require ABO typing only but Rh matching preferred; if no ABO compatible platelets are available, mismatched platelets may be given, which can lead to potential allergic reactions; HLA-matched platelets are recommended to decrease the likelihood of allergic reactions

b. Can be random donor (pooled platelets from 6 to 10 donors) or single donor

c. Are stored at room temperature for up to five days with frequent gentle agitation of bag to keep platelets viable; half-life of platelets is three to four days; platelet transfusion may be repeated every one to three days

Box 9-5

Transfusion Reaction Principles

- Stop blood immediately if you suspect client is exhibiting a significant reaction.
- Monitor client's vital signs, keep IV access with NS (switch tubing), and insert indwelling urinary catheter if needed.
- Give old tubing and remaining blood product to lab for investigation.
- Notify physician and lab for followup blood draws and report client's condition.
- Keep client warm and provide supplemental oxygen at low flow rates.
- Medicate as ordered following hospital policy and procedure and emerging physician orders.

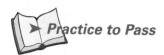

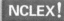

d. If platelet count $< 20,000/\text{mm}^3$ and client is experiencing major bleeding, platelets may be needed; 1 platelet concentrate (1 unit) should increase recipient platelet count by approximately 5,000 to $10,000/\text{mm}^3$; usual dose is 6 to 10 units of concentrate

e. Clients receiving platelets over a long period of time develop antibodies to the HLA antigens found on the surface of the circulating platelets (causing antigen-antibody reaction, febrile reaction, and platelet destruction); over time the client's platelet count is less responsive to platelet transfusions because alloimmunization is occurring; in response to the platelet administration, the count would show little or no rise after transfusion; actions to decrease likelihood of reaction include the following:

   1) Use single-donor platelet transfusions from the onset of therapy

   2) Use WBC filters to minimize infusion of WBCs as this will help to decrease antibody production

   3) Try to find HLA-matched donor platelets for the recipient

   4) Premedicate with diphenhydramine (Benadryl), acetaminophen (Tylenol), or hydrocortisone (Cortef) to decrease possibility of a reaction

   5) Fever, infection, and active bleeding can modify the effectiveness of the transfusion

f. Indications and contraindications

   1) Thrombocytopenia resulting from decreased platelet production (aplastic anemia, leukemia), increased platelet loss (bleeding), increased platelet destruction (hypersplenism in cirrhosis, transfusion reaction), and increased use or consumption as in disseminated intravascular coagulopathy (DIC)

   2) Clients undergoing needed surgery with a platelet count less than $100,0000/\text{mm}^3$ or experiencing platelet dysfunction and/or coexisting coagulation disorders

   3) Not indicated for idiopathic thrombocytopenic purpura (ITP) unless client is actively bleeding because administered platelets will also be destroyed

   4) Avoid administering platelets when client is febrile

g. Administration and nursing actions

   1) Premedicate as ordered, especially if client has a history of platelet transfusion reaction

   2) Obtain IV access with 20- to 22-gauge angiocath, Y tubing, and NS to prime tubing

   3) Begin platelet transfusion slowly and observe for signs of a reaction; adjust rate to 1–2 mL/minute and infuse each unit over 5 to 10 minutes as tolerated (platelets tend to clump, which is why they should be infused quickly)

4) A poor 15-minute platelet count indicates HLA antibodies are present, indicating need to use HLA matched platelets; if there is a good 15-minute count but poor 24-hour count, this suggests consumption (fever, sepsis) but client does not need HLA-matched platelets

5) Administer single donor platelets if at all possible for all clients; if client will receive multiple transfusions, use single donor platelets and use a leukodepletion filter (some platelets may be prepared as leukodepleted; check the bag label); if client will receive aggressive chemotherapy or a transplant, check for anti-HLA antibodies first so that blood product administration can be carefully planned

3. Whole blood

   a. One unit of donated whole blood can be broken down into one unit of packed cells, one unit of platelets, and one unit of fresh frozen plasma to replace whichever component(s) the client may need

   b. Not routinely used; indicated for treatment of acute massive hemorrhage and loss of > 25–30% of blood volume; may also be used with cardiac surgeries, trauma situations, or major burns

   c. Must be ABO and Rh compatible

   d. Increases colloidal oncotic pressure and plasma volume, increases red cell mass, and improves tissue oxygenation; however, it can result in fluid volume overload

   e. Should not be administered to clients with chronic anemia who only need RBCs and should have a normal blood volume

   f. Stored whole blood is high in potassium

   g. Administration and nursing actions

   1) One unit equals approximately 500 mL; use an 18- to 20-gauge angiocath and Y tubing; use only NS as primer; infuse over 2 to 4 hours

   2) Observe for signs and symptoms of a transfusion reaction, such as **hemolytic transfusion reaction** (refer to Table 9-2), fluid volume overload, hypothermia, electrolyte disturbances, citrate toxicity (citrate is a preservative used in blood), and infection

   3) Expect a 1-gram increase in hemoglobin and a 3–4 percent rise in hematocrit for each unit of whole blood infused, assuming no further bleeding

4. Fresh frozen plasma (FFP)

   a. Derived from one unit of donated whole blood whereby plasma is separated from the RBCs and then frozen; contains clotting factors and fibrinogen, but no platelets; volume of each unit is approximately 225 mL

   b. Must know the client's ABO group to ensure client's RBCs are compatible with antibodies that may be present in the plasma; group AB FFP may be administered if client's blood type is unknown; Rh matching (although not required) is preferred

   c. Increases colloidal oncotic pressure and moves fluid into the vascular space

Table 9-2	Transfusion Reactions			

Type	Etiology	Clinical Presentation	Nursing Actions	Prevention
Hemolytic	ABO or Rh incompatibility. Most severe and potentially life threatening but accounts for a very small percentage. Severe antigen-antibody reaction due to clumping of cells.	Chills, low back pain, headache, chest pain, tachycardia, dyspnea, hypotension, nausea, vomiting, restlessness, anxiety, shock, flank pain, and oliguria. Symptoms occur during first 30 minutes of infusion or in response to 100–200 cc of incompatible blood.	*Stop transfusion immediately.* Keep IV line open with NS and new tubing. Follow ABCs. Notify appropriate personnel (blood bank, physician, and lab). Follow hospital protocol. Medicate per protocol.	Follow established protocol. Verify orders. Monitor client during therapy.
Blood contamination (bacterial)	Organisms that survive the cold such as *pseudomonas* or *staphylococcus*.	Sudden chills, fever, dry flushed skin, headache, abdominal pain, lumbar pain, nausea, vomiting, diarrhea, hypotension, and/or signs of renal failure.	*Stop transfusion immediately.* Keep IV line open with NS and new tubing. Follow ABCs. Notify appropriate personnel (blood bank, physician, and lab). Follow hospital protocol. Medicate per protocol.	Change administration set and filter per protocol (per unit). Infuse unit over prescribed time period. Do not run blood unit > 4 hours. Maintain sterile technique.
Febrile (nonhemolytic)	Most common transfusion reaction. Sensitizations to HLA antibodies or plasma occur.	Mild reaction—chills and fever. Severe reaction—high fever, chills, headache, tightness in chest, palpitations, tachycardia, facial flushing, or flank pain. Symptoms can occur within 30 minutes but may start as late as 1–2 hours post-transfusion.	Physician may note parameters to run blood even if the client presents with slight temperature elevation. Validate order prior to hanging to be aware of parameters. With a severe reaction, *stop the transfusion* and proceed with hospital protocol for a hemolytic reaction.	Keep client warm. For clients with prior history of this reaction, premedicate with acetaminophen (Tylenol), or diphenhydramine (Benadryl), administer leukocyte-poor blood products, HLA-compatible products, or washed RBCs.
Allergic	Sensitivity reaction, antigen-antibody reaction to plasma proteins. IgE molecules on mast cells react to form histamine release.	Mild reaction involves uriticaria and hives. Severe reaction involves chills, fever, facial and airway swelling, SOB, wheezing, loss of consciousness, shock, or possible cardiac arrest.	Mild reactions—follow hospital policy and procedure, slow down transfusion, notify the physician, medicate as ordered. Severe reaction—*stop transfusion.* Follow hospital policy and protocol. Medicate as ordered. With critical situations, client may need to be intubated and managed by in-house physician.	Premedication for clients who have history of allergic reactions or multiple transfusions. Washed RBCs, leukocyte-depleted products, and additional filters may be needed on a routine basis for transfusion therapy.

Note: It is critical to follow agency policy and procedure for ALL transfusion therapies. Many reactions can be prevented or minimized if correct administration techniques are instituted and prompt assessment and monitoring of the client is done. Remain at the client's bedside during the first 15 minutes of any transfusion therapy. Have all necessary equipment readily available should the client experience a reaction (additional tubing and oxygen setup).

d. May cause fluid volume overload, hypersensitivity reaction, or hemolytic reactions

e. Indications

    1) Replaces plasma volume in hemorrhage and/or hypovolemic shock

    2) Replaces clotting factors for the client with a known (specific clotting factor may not be available) or unknown deficiency

    3) Indicated for the following clinical conditions: liver disease with significantly impaired clotting factor synthesis, DIC with active bleeding, prolonged PT/INR with active bleeding or when immediate surgery is needed, and dilutional coagulopathy (substantial volume overload)

f. Administration and nursing actions

    1) Use as soon as possible after it is thawed or within 6 hours (takes about 30 minutes to thaw)

    2) Use a 20- to 22-gauge angiocath, NS not required (no RBCs present)

    3) Administer as rapidly as possible, suggested rate is 4 to 10 mL/minute; most units are completed in 1 to 2 hours

    4) Observe for signs and symptoms of allergic or febrile reaction and fluid volume overload; there is also a risk for hepatitis transmission

    5) Clients receiving large amounts of FFP may become hypocalcemic due to citric acid binding with calcium in the plasma; observe for signs and symptoms of hypocalcemia; may need calcium gluconate intravenously

5. Cryoprecipitate

a. Derived from one unit of FFP and contains Factor VIII (antihemophilia factor), Factor XIII (Von Willebrand factor), and fibrinogen

b. ABO compatibility testing is not required; however, may cause ABO incompatibility; donor plasma and recipient RBCs should be ABO compatible (because some donor plasma is present and plasma contains the antibodies); if client's (recipient) blood group is unknown, type AB cryoprecipitate is preferred; Rh matching is not required (Rh factor is on the RBC and RBCs are not being transfused)

c. Used to treat hemophilia A, Von Willebrand disease, hypofibrinogenemia, DIC (will quickly raise fibrinogen level), and massive transfusion with hemodilution

d. Possibility of hepatitis or HIV transmission exists

e. Administration and nursing actions

    1) Use within 6 hours once thawed; usual dose is 6 to 10 units

    2) Use 20- to 22-gauge angiocath and standard blood filter

    3) Administer as rapidly as tolerated (10 mL/min)

6. Granulocytes

a. Harvested by leukopheresis from a single donor; must be transfused within 24 hours after obtaining from donor

---

NCLEX!

NCLEX!

NCLEX!

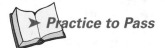

Practice to Pass

A client with disseminated intravascular coagulopathy (DIC) is receiving platelets, fresh frozen plasma, and packed red blood cells. What laboratory results will you review in evaluating the effectiveness of the transfusions? How does the disease process complicate the clinical picture?

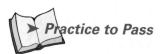

b. Each unit consists of granulocytes, lymphocytes, platelets, and RBCs in plasma

c. Donor must be ABO and Rh compatible (RBCs present in unit); it is preferable to be HLA compatible as well

d. Granulocytes are not FDA approved at the current time and are being used in clinical research trials to support febrile neutropenic clients who are not responding to other methods (antibiotic therapy or neupogen injections) to improve white blood cell (WBC) count

e. Infusion can cause fever, allergic reaction, severe chills, mild hypertension, disorientation, and hallucinations; premedicate with diphenhydramine (Benadryl), steroids, and antipyretics

f. Use an 18- to 20-gauge angiocath and Y tubing with standard inline filter; no microaggregate filter is used because it would trap the WBCs; administer slowly, generally 50 mL/hour within 4 hours

g. Treat chills with antipyretics or blankets; treat hypertension if needed; only discontinue transfusion if client has severe respiratory distress

h. Generally given for at least 4 to 5 days, one unit/day or until infection resolves

II. Diagnostic and Laboratory Findings

A. Serum or plasma osmolality

1. Hydration status affects serum/plasma osmolality and specific parenteral therapies can affect osmolality due to nature of solution (tonicity of fluid) and crystalloid or colloid status

2. Increases are seen in dehydration, hyperglycemia, and in conditions where BUN is also increased; decreases are seen in clinical states resulting in overhydration

3. Allows nurse to assess client's baseline hydration status and evaluate response to replacement therapy

B. Serum chemistries

1. Blood urea nitrogen (BUN) and creatinine levels are indicators of renal function; BUN is also affected by hydration status

   a. Increased levels seen in dehydration (BUN only), renal disease, and gastrointestinal bleeding, due to retention of urea; decreased levels are seen in clinical states that result in overhydration

   b. Creatinine is a more accurate indicator of renal dysfunction than BUN because it is a constant metabolic end product and reflects glomerular filtration rate

   c. Creatinine is generally unaffected by fluid intake; however, marked fluid volume deficit can decrease glomerular filtration and slightly increase the creatinine level

   d. Adequate renal function needs to be determined before fluid and electrolyte replacement begins (except in the case of a fluid challenge to check the kidneys' responsiveness); abnormal renal function can put the client at risk for fluid volume overload and electrolyte disturbances

2. Electrolytes

   a. Sodium (Na^+) and chloride (Cl^-) concentration should be considered in replacement therapies because they are part of the content of many crystalloid fluids; specific parenteral solutions (hypotonic or hypertonic) can result in fluid shifting and impact serum and urinary levels

   b. Potassium (K^+) is usually considered in replacement therapies as an additive being used to restore normal serum levels; it is important to know the client's baseline, trend pertinent laboratory values, and administer replacement according to protocol

   c. Critical laboratory values exist for both hypokalemic and hyperkalemic states with resultant effects on the cardiac system

   d. Acid-base imbalances can arise from alterations in potassium and chloride levels and the client should be properly monitored using serial arterial blood gases (ABGs)

   e. Calcium levels can be affected by replacement therapies, such as multiple blood unit administration (citrate anticoagulant resulting in hypocalcemic state), that require calcium administration; calcium levels should be correlated with serum albumin levels because binding occurs that could affect the results

   f. Specific therapies such as diuretic administration, prolonged infusion of hypotonic fluids, dehydration states (malnutrition), overhydration, and underlying disease states can further impact serum electrolyte levels and response to replacement therapies

4. Serum glucose

   a. Regulation of serum glucose levels is necessary in order to maintain normal cognitive function and prevent adverse health conditions that result in coma

   b. Since many IV solutions contain dextrose, the client must be evaluated and monitored closely for possible effects on blood glucose; in addition, other medications (such as dextran, diuretics, and steroids) and parenteral therapies (such as TPN) can lead to increases in blood glucose

5. Serum albumin

   a. Major protein in plasma that regulates colloidal oncotic pressure and maintains intravascular integrity

   b. Hydration status affects albumin level with dehydration leading to increased albumin levels; decreased albumin from volume excess leads to fluid shifting and third spacing of fluids

   c. It is important to know the albumin level when evaluating serum calcium level, since calcium exists in the body in both ionized and nonionized forms and the ionized form is bound to protein; a low albumin level can therefore be accompanied by hypocalcemia

C. Blood counts and clotting studies

1. RBC count

   a. Normal range: male 4.7–6.1 million/mm^3, female 4.2–5.4 million/mm^3

b. Hydration states can affect RBC count; dehydration falsely elevates the RBC count and overhydration decreases the RBC count

c. CBC with differential and a peripheral smear will provide pertinent information relative to RBC indices and morphology

2. Hematocrit

a. Packed cell volume with normal range for males 42 to 52%; females 37 to 47%, which is usually three times the hemoglobin value

b. Hydration status can affect serum values due to hemoconcentration (seen in dehydration causing falsely high values) and hemodilution (seen in overhydration causing decreased values)

c. Serial hematrocrit levels are drawn for a client with ongoing bleeding

d. In a healthy client, transfusion is generally not needed if hemoglobin is > 8 g/dL and hematocrit is above 24% (variation depends on age and any underlying clinical condition)

e. Each unit of PRBCs will increase hematocrit by 3%; a unit of whole blood will increase hematocrit by 3 to 4%

3. Hemoglobin

a. Normal range for males is 14 to 18 g/dL and for females is 12 to 16 g/dL

b. Serial hemoglobin levels are drawn in client with ongoing blood loss

c. Hydration can affect serum values (dehydration causes false high and overhydration decreases concentration, causing a lower value)

d. Each unit of PRBCs or whole blood will increase hemoglobin by 1 gram

4. Platelets

a. Normal range is 150,000 to 400,000/mm^3

b. Increased levels are seen with iron deficiency anemia (IDA) and decreased levels are seen with hemorrhage or coagulation disorders

NCLEX!

c. Each unit of platelets administered should increase the platelet count by approximately 5,000 to 10,000/mm^3 unless alloimmunization has occurred

d. Dextran has antiplatelet activity

5. Prothrombin time (PT)

a. Used to evaluate the competence of the extrinsic coagulation pathway and final common coagulation pathway

b. If the clotting factors making up the pathway are inadequate, the PT is prolonged

c. Normal range is 11.0 to 12.5 seconds

NCLEX!

d. Vitamin K is necessary to make prothrombin; drug interaction is seen with sodium warfarin (Coumadin) anticoagulant therapy because it interferes with the production of vitamin K-dependent clotting factors, thus prolonging PT and increasing risk for bleeding; assess client for signs and symptoms of bleeding; INR may be monitored instead of PT to determine effectiveness of warfarin therapy

        e. Inadequate clotting may require the transfusion of FFP, cryoprecipitate, or administration of vitamin K depending on cause and urgency of the situation

        f. Hespan can transiently prolong the PT

   6. Partial thromboplastin time (PTT)

        a. Used to evaluate the intrinsic clotting system and final common pathway

        b. Normal range for PTT is 60 to 70 seconds, and for activated PTT (aPTT) is 30 to 40 seconds

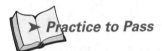

        c. Used to monitor heparin therapy; therapeutic range for heparin is 1.5 to 2.5 times the control in seconds; PTT >100 seconds or aPTT >70 seconds greatly increases risk of bleeding

        d. PTT may be abnormally prolonged due to hemophilia A or B, DIC, liver disease, or biliary obstruction

        e. Assess for signs and symptoms of bleeding

        f. FFP or cryoprecipitate may be indicated to restore missing clotting factors and vitamin K in the case of biliary obstruction

        g. Hespan can transiently prolong PTT

   7. Antibody and immunoglobulin testing

        a. Direct antiglobulin test (direct Coomb's) pertains to detection of immunoglobulins on the RBC surfaces and can be used to investigate hemolytic transfusion reactions, aid in the differential diagnosis of hemolytic anemia, and test for hemolytic disease of the newborn

        b. Antibody screening (indirect Coomb's) pertains to determination of Rh-positive antibodies in maternal blood and assists with identification of ABO incompatibility in the newborn

        c. HLA antigens are identified on surface of circulating platelets, WBCs, and most tissue cells; this can be used to match blood products to minimize reactions (such as **HLA alloimmunization**) and identify disease processes

D. Daily weights and body surface area (BSA)

   1. Clients receiving IV fluids should be weighed daily (before breakfast and after voiding; use same scale; have client wear similar clothing each time—i.e., hospital gown)

   2. One kg (2.2 lbs) of body weight is approximately equal to one liter of IV fluid; abrupt changes in weight are an important clue to changes in fluid status

   3. Despite a weight gain, a client may have a significant fluid volume deficit if there is third spacing of fluid; thorough client system assessment is critical; a weight loss is generally expected during diuretic therapy and a weight gain is expected when a client is being rehydrated for a fluid volume deficit

   4. Calculation of BSA provides a more accurate determination of fluid needs for a client with critical needs; a nomogram is used to assist in calculating BSA from height and weight data

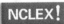

Practice to Pass

An elderly client with a history of CVA was admitted with fluid volume deficit related to inadequate intake and fever. What instructions will you include in discharge teaching for the client and the home health aide assigned to the client's care?

III. Selection of Fluid and Electrolyte Therapies

A. Replacement therapies

1. Oral

   a. May be indicated if fluid loss is not excessive, client is not vomiting, client has intact gag and swallowing reflexes and adequate GI absorption, client has intact thirst mechanism, and is able to drink

   b. Physician may write an order to "push fluids" for clients with actual or potential fluid volume deficits (fever, mild diarrhea)

   NCLEX!

   c. In choosing oral fluid replacement, it is important to consider client preferences, offer fluids frequently, and assist clients with impaired swallowing by proper positioning (upright with head and neck flexed forward slightly) and providing thickened liquids or semisolid foods such as jello, pudding, or milk shakes

   NCLEX!

   d. It is critical to keep an accurate record of intake and output, trend results, and notify the physician accordingly if imbalances occur

2. Parenteral

   a. Indicated when client is unable to take PO fluids due to clinical presentation, when client is NPO and requires maintenance to replace insensible losses, to provide nutrients and electrolytes when GI tract is not functional, or to replace abnormal losses (GI suction, vomiting, diarrhea, fever, hemorrhage)

   NCLEX!

   b. Infusion rate affected by maintenance and/or replacement need and underlying condition of client (administer cautiously in clients with congestive heart failure and renal failure)

   c. Refer to Table 9-3 for information about the use of crystalloid fluid therapy

   d. The physician bases the use of specific blood component therapy on individualized assessment of the client's underlying health status, current medical status, and the client's own personal decision (i.e., religious beliefs) to allow transfusion therapy

B. Monitoring parameters

1. Daily weights

2. Intake and output (I & O)

   a. Maintain fluid restriction or orders to increase fluids

   NCLEX!

   b. Properly label and time all IV solutions; run and maintain at ordered rate

   c. Measure the client's entire intake and output from all sources

      1) Intake—by mouth, all IV fluids (includes IV meds), tube feedings

      2) Output—urine (urinal, bedpan, foley, graduated container, incontinence—approximate amount), nasogastric drainage, wounds, diarrhea, and emesis

   NCLEX!

   d. Accurately record findings and review 24-hour totals for several days to determine trends in fluid balance

Table 9-3	Hypotonic Fluids	Isotonic Fluids	Hypertonic Fluids
Crystalloid Fluid Replacement Therapy	Indicated for cellular dehydration, hyperosmolar states (due to severe hyperglycemia), and to treat hypernatremia. Hypotonic fluids provide free water that assists with renal excretion of wastes.	Indicated for hypovolemia (ECF volume deficit), and postoperative fluid management. Isotonic fluids dilute the vascular compartment and lower hemoglobin and hematocrit concentrations.	Indicated for electrolyte replacement, hyponatremia, and to correct fluid shifting because this leads to cellular dehydration.
	Do not give to clients with increased ICP (can increase cerebral edema), abnormal fluid shifts (third spacing), hypotension (can lower BP further), or during code situations (can worsen neurological outcome).	Do not give lactated solutions to clients with liver disease; monitor client for signs and symptoms of FVE. Cautious use in clients with CHF or RF because they are already prone to developing FVE.	Do not give to clients who are already at risk for cellular dehydration (hyperosmolar serum). Cautious use in clients with cardiac or renal failure.

    e. Use trended I & Os in conjunction with daily weights, labs, and knowledge of underlying pathophysiology to determine if client is responding appropriately to IV therapy

    f. Monitor for extremes such as fluid intake greatly exceeding output or output greatly exceeding intake (remember, however, this could be part of the resolution of the problem, i.e., client receiving diuretics for fluid volume excess may have output that greatly exceeds intake with eventual balancing of intake and output; correspondingly, a client in hypovolemic shock may have intake greatly exceeding output in order to build up vascular volume)

    g. Correlate intake and output trend with changes in client's weight; generally, weight gain occurs when intake exceeds output and weight loss occurs when output exceeds intake

    h. Notify the physician of any significant imbalance

    i. In general, high urine output indicates intravascular fluid volume excess; low urine output with high specific gravity indicates intravascular fluid volume deficit; low urine output with low specific gravity indicates renal disease

  2. Trending of pertinent labs

    a. Review pertinent laboratory and diagnostic test results related to specific replacement therapies

    b. Look for improvement of underlying condition as evidenced by lab results and other assessment findings

    c. In general, if a client is being appropriately treated for an isotonic fluid volume deficit, the following should be seen:

      1) An increase in urinary output

      2) A decrease in urine specific gravity

      3) An increase in body weight

NCLEX!

4) An increase in blood pressure (if client was hypotensive)

5) A decreased pulse rate

6) Improved skin turgor and moist mucous membranes

7) Decreased BUN, serum osmolality, and hematocrit

NCLEX!

  d. If client is being appropriately treated for a fluid volume excess, the following should be seen:

1) Improvement in breath sounds

2) Increase in urine output (in response to diuretics), hematocrit, BUN, and serum osmolality

3) Decreased weight

4) Decrease in blood pressure if client's BP was elevated

5) Decrease in or resolution of edema

C. Priority nursing diagnoses

1. Fluid volume deficit (FVD)

2. Fluid volume excess (FVE)

3. Risk for impaired gas exchange

4. Risk for decreased cardiac output

5. Risk for altered tissue perfusion: cerebral, renal

D. Therapeutic management

1. Carefully evaluate client's individualized fluid and electrolyte needs

2. Give appropriate IV fluid(s) as maintenance and/or replacement therapy

3. Monitor client responses to therapy on a daily basis or more often in unstable clients with review of pertinent labs, daily weights, intake and output, and comprehensive client physical assessments

4. Prevent complications (fluid volume excess, dehydration)

E. Planning and implementation

1. Assist client to maintain and/or restore adequate plasma, cellular, or intracellular volume

    a. Encourage oral fluid intake if client able to ingest liquids

    b. Include ample fluids that client enjoys at the bedside

NCLEX!

    c. Infuse appropriate IV solution at ordered rate

NCLEX!

    d. Assess client each shift or at least daily for signs and symptoms of adequate hydration (moist mucous membranes, elastic skin turgor, no complaints of thirst, vital signs within normal limits, adequate urine output, level of consciousness within normal limits)

    e. Monitor vital signs frequently

NCLEX!

    f. Carefully record intake and output from all sources and weigh client daily

      g. Review pertinent laboratory results on a daily basis; closely follow any trends and interpret their significance

      h. Administer fluid challenge if needed to help determine renal status for clients with underlying clinical conditions, such as heart failure or respiratory failure, who may be at risk for developing FVE due to inability to handle fluids

  2. Support client in achieving adequate oxygen-carrying capacity and coagulation status as needed

      a. Administer compatible blood and blood products, carefully applying knowledge of transfusion principles and following agency procedure

NCLEX!

      b. Assess the client for signs of improved oxygenation: respirations with greater ease, increased tissue perfusion, improved capillary refill, increased activity tolerance, improved oxygen saturation, and possibly increased alertness

      c. Assess the client for signs of improved coagulation status: decreased bleeding, decreased petechiae, ecchymosis, no gingival oozing, guiac-negative stool

  3. Prevent potential complications of IV therapy in client

      a. Maintain a sterile IV system when priming tubings and administering IV fluids

NCLEX!

      b. Observe the IV insertion site regularly for signs of infection or phlebitis

NCLEX!

      c. Be alert to signs and symptoms of fluid volume overload (pulmonary congestion, shortness of breath, elevated vital signs, edema, and weight gain)

      d. Infuse hypertonic solutions (selected crystalloids and colloids) slowly

NCLEX!

      e. Be alert to signs and symptoms of fluid volume deficit (dry mucous membranes, thirst, weight loss, increased heart rate, decreased blood pressure, poor perfusion, orthostatic hypotension)

      f. Do not infuse hypotonic solutions (D_5W, ½NS) in clients at risk for increased intracranial pressure or third-space fluid shifts

NCLEX!

      g. Premedicate clients as ordered prior to transfusions of blood or blood products; carefully assess for signs or symptoms of transfusion reaction and intervene accordingly

F. Client education

  1. Explain need for increased oral intake if appropriate

  2. Teach client how to follow sodium and fluid restriction if appropriate

  3. Teach client to weigh self daily

  4. Review signs and symptoms of dehydration with client

  5. Instruct client to change positions slowly if any signs of dizziness or lightheadedness occur

  6. Review signs and symptoms of overhydration with client

7. Instruct client to report to the nurse any pain, swelling, leaking, redness, or hardness (induration) at IV site

8. Explain rationale for blood/blood product transfusion and procedure to client

9. Verify that client has received informed consent prior to transfusing blood

10. Teach client to inform the nurse immediately if he or she experiences signs or symptoms of transfusion reaction (chills, fever, nausea, abdominal cramps)

G. Evaluation

1. Client exhibits adequate hydration status demonstrated by warm dry skin, moist mucous membranes, no complaints of excessive thirst, capillary refill < 3 seconds, regular strong peripheral pulses, stable weight, vital signs and urine output within normal limits, no edema and clear lung sounds

2. Client exhibits adequate oxygenation and coagulation status as demonstrated by: no bleeding; vital signs within normal limits; adequate perfusion with improved capillary refill; hemoglobin, hematocrit, platelets, PT, and PTT within normal limits for client; and improved activity tolerance

3. Client experiences no significant adverse effects from transfusion of blood or blood products

---

Case Study

S.W., a 35-year-old female client with severe anemia, tachycardia, and shortness of breath, is admitted to your unit. The physician has ordered 2 units of packed red blood cells (PRBCs).

❶ What assessments will you make before transfusing the blood?

❷ What are priority nursing diagnoses for S.W.?

❸ What will you teach S.W. about the transfusion prior to beginning it?

❹ What steps will you follow to administer the transfusion safely?

❺ How will you evaluate the effectiveness of the transfusion for S.W?

For suggested responses, see page 233.

Posttest

1   A client with dry skin and mucous membranes is weak, has orthostatic blood pressure changes, and has decreased urine output. The client's serum osmolality, however, is normal. Which of the following IV fluids would the nurse anticipate being prescribed for this client?

(1) 5% Dextrose in water
(2) ½ Normal saline
(3) 10% Dextrose in water
(4) Normal saline

2 A client receiving a transfusion of packed RBCs suddenly sounds hoarse, begins wheezing, is diaphoretic and short of breath, and reports palpitations. Blood pressure is 76/52. What is the priority nursing action?

(1) Stop the transfusion.
(2) Infuse the normal saline rapidly to maintain intravascular volume.
(3) Administer epinephrine and steroids.
(4) Maintain the client's airway and notify the physician.

3 Which of the following would the nurse anticipate after infusion of 25% albumin to a client in hypovolemic shock?

(1) Increase in heart rate
(2) Decrease in blood pressure
(3) Decrease in peripheral perfusion
(4) Increase in blood pressure

4 Which of the following actions should the nurse take when a client is receiving a granulocyte transfusion?

(1) Administer the granulocytes rapidly.
(2) Premedicate with an antihistamine, a steroid, and a antipyretic.
(3) Attach a microaggregate filter to the IV tubing.
(4) Check lymphocyte count following the transfusion.

5 Which of the following laboratory tests should the nurse monitor closely in an elderly client with congestive heart failure (CHF) who is receiving IV albumin?

(1) Platelet count
(2) Hematocrit
(3) Serum bilirubin
(4) Prothrombin time

6 The nurse is conducting a class for oncology clients who frequently receive blood products. The nurse is correct in teaching that if a client becomes alloimmunized, the most effective way to increase the platelet count would be to:

(1) Transfuse single-donor platelet units.
(2) Transfuse HLA-matched donor platelets.
(3) Use a WBC filter to minimize infusion of WBCs.
(4) Premedicate the client with diphenhydramine (Benadryl) and acetaminophen (Tylenol).

7 A physician has ordered Dextran for a client while waiting for the results of the type and cross-match. The nurse is aware that the advantage of using Dextran to expand the plasma volume is that it:

(1) Contains no risk of transfusion-related illnesses.
(2) Has a decreased risk for anaphylaxis as compared to hetastarch or albumin.
(3) Promotes hydration of tissues.
(4) Has no effect on clotting factors.

8 Which of the following interventions should the nurse include in developing a plan of care for a client receiving Hespan?

(1) Draw specimen for type and cross-match prior to beginning Hespan infusion.
(2) Monitor client for signs of hypovolemia.
(3) Expect decreased urine output as body begins conserving plasma volume.
(4) Monitor for transient changes in PT, PTT, and clotting times.

9 A client will receive 2 units of packed red blood cells (PRBCs). The nurse places highest priority on teaching the client which of the following?

(1) The rationale for the transfusion
(2) Overview of the procedure so the client will know what to expect
(3) Signs and symptoms to report to the nurse if they should occur
(4) Frequency with which vital signs will be taken so as not to alarm the client

10 A client with severe anemia is to receive 4 units of packed red blood cells (PRBCs) with premedication therapy and wants to know what effect premedication will have on the likelihood that he will experience a transfusion reaction. The best response by the nurse to the client's concern would be:

(1) "Hives and airway swelling may occur due to an allergic reaction but will be minimized by medications your doctor has ordered for you."

(2) "You have no need to worry because your doctor has ordered medications to prevent a reaction."

(3) "Chilling and fever caused by previous exposure to blood or blood products may occur but these are minimized by medications your doctor has ordered for you."

(4) "Shortness of breath and kidney problems could occur caused by incompatible blood but these would be minimized by medications your doctor has ordered for you."

See pages 221–222 for Answers and Rationales.

Answers and Rationales

Pretest

1 Answer: 3 *Rationale:* A client who is hemorrhaging and in shock requires immediate restoration of oxygen-carrying capacity. With no time available for cross-match, universal donor blood (type O, Rh-negative) is administered. Option 1 is incorrect because type AB, Rh-positive blood can only be given to type AB, Rh-positive recipients. Option 2 is incorrect because albumin has no oxygen-carrying capacity, which is essential in a trauma client. In addition, it would remain in the intravascular space and would not assist in restoring blood volume and maintaining adequate circulation. Option 4 is incorrect because platelets may be administered if needed, but they are not oxygen-carrying cells, which is the first priority.
Cognitive Level: Analysis
Nursing Process: Implementation; *Test Plan:* PHYS

2 Answer: 2 *Rationale:* Normal saline is an isotonic solution that will replace lost vascular volume and promote perfusion. All of the other options are incorrect because they are either hypotonic or act as hypotonic solutions in the bloodstream, providing free water that moves into the interstitial space and cells. Administration of these fluids can cause further fluid shifting, which will not help to replace lost volume or promote perfusion. In addition, when blood is available, it can be hung with the normal saline. Dextrose will cause lysis of red blood cells.
Cognitive Level: Analysis
Nursing Process: Analysis; *Test Plan:* PHYS

3 Answer: 3 *Rationale:* Each unit of PRBCs should raise the hemoglobin by 1 gram and hematocrit by 3%. Option 3 is the only option illustrating the ex- pected increase. The nurse should be aware of expected responses to therapy in order to validate that treatment has been effective.
Cognitive Level: Application
Nursing Process: Assessment; *Test Plan:* PHYS

4 Answer: 1 *Rationale:* Coumadin depresses the synthesis of vitamin K–dependent clotting factors in the liver, resulting in a prolonged PT/INR (extrinsic coagulation pathway). FFP contains the needed clotting factors and will reverse the PT/INR. The PT/INR needs to be adjusted to the therapeutic range for client's underlying condition. Option 2 is incorrect because the aPTT/PTT measures the intrinsic coagulation pathway. Options 3 and 4 are incorrect because neither albumin nor platelets will restore clotting factors.
Cognitive Level: Analysis
Nursing Process: Planning; *Test Plan:* SECE

5 Answer: 3 *Rationale:* A client at risk for increased intracranial pressure must guard against increasing cerebral edema. Dextrose 2.5% in water is a hypotonic solution that provides significant free water that moves into the cells, thereby increasing cerebral edema. The other options may be indicated depending on physician preference and/or overall client condition.
Cognitive Level: Analysis
Nursing Process: Planning; *Test Plan:* PHYS

6 Answer: 2 *Rationale:* The client's plasma is hypertonic (very concentrated) to begin with and thus serum osmolality, BUN, and hematocrit would be elevated from hemoconcentration. Once isotonic fluids are administered, the plasma concentration should decrease and all three laboratory test results should

show a corresponding decrease. Option 1 is incorrect because you would expect to see an improvement upon administration of isotonic fluids and BUN and serum osmolality remain increased. Option 3 is incorrect because these findings would be consistent in a client who has not been treated for hypertonic dehydration. Option 4 is incorrect because you would expect to see a decrease in hematocrit with the administration of isotonic fluid therapy.
Cognitive Level: Analysis
Nursing Process: Assessment; *Test Plan:* PHYS

7 **Answer: 3** *Rationale:* Abrupt changes in weight are an important clue to changes in fluid status. Unusual losses, i.e., fever or diarrhea, are significant; they need to be reported and may help the client prevent a fluid volume deficit (FVD) in the future, especially since the client is taking a diuretic. Option 1 is incorrect because increasing salt and fluids may put the client at significant risk for fluid volume excess (FVE) considering the history of CHF. Options 2 and 4 may put the client at risk for FVE or FVD, respectively.
Cognitive Level: Application
Nursing Process: Evaluation; *Test Plan:* HPM

8 **Answer: 2** *Rationale:* A client with type B blood can only receive type B (client/recipient has no anti-B antibodies) and type O (contains no antigens for recipient to react to). Since the client is Rh-negative and has been previously exposed to Rh-positive blood, the client may have antibodies to Rh-positive blood. Therefore only Rh-negative blood should be administered. Option 1 is incorrect because the client cannot receive type O positive blood due to the identified negative Rh factor. Options 3 and 4 are incorrect because they each contain at least one incompatible blood type component (type A antigens and type O positive blood).
Cognitive Level: Analysis
Nursing Process: Evaluation; *Test Plan:* HPM

9 **Answer: 3** *Rationale:* Option 3 is accurate and realistic and may help the client with decision making. Option 1 is not accurate and offers false reassurance to the client. Option 2 is incorrect because it involves giving "medical" advice, is nontherapeutic, and may increase client anxiety due to questioning of treatment plan. Option 4 is incorrect because it may delay treatment and there is no evidence that designated donor blood is safer.
Cognitive Level: Analysis
Nursing Process: Implementation; *Test Plan:* PSYC

10 **Answer: 3** *Rationale:* FFP is derived from one unit of whole blood and contains the clotting factors that the client needs plus fibrinogen. Option 1 is incorrect because even though whole blood contains some clotting factors, it is deficient in others and is indicated for significant acute blood loss (which is not the client's problem). Option 2 is incorrect because improved oxygen-carrying capacity (rendered by the infusion of packed red cells) is something the client does not need. Hemophilia is a clotting disorder that requires clotting factor replacement. Option 4 is incorrect because albumin contains no clotting factors.
Cognitive Level: Application
Nursing Process: Assessment; *Test Plan:* PHYS

Posttest

1 **Answer: 4** *Rationale:* The client is manifesting signs and symptoms of dehydration. Since the serum remains isotonic, this is isotonic dehydration or hypovolemia. Appropriate treatment is with an isotonic fluid to replace fluid volume. Options 1 and 2 are incorrect because they are hypotonic solutions and would cause fluid shifting leading to cellular edema (client's cells are normal size and free water is not needed for cells). Option 3 is incorrect because the solution is hypertonic and will cause further fluid shifting leading to cellular dehydration.
Cognitive Level: Analysis
Nursing Process: Analysis; *Test Plan:* PHYS

2 **Answer: 1** *Rationale:* The client is experiencing a severe allergic/anaphylactic reaction. The nurse should first stop the infusion of any more blood. Next, the nurse should maintain the client's airway, administer oxygen, and infuse NS through a clean IV tubing (one not contaminated with blood) to maintain the intravascular volume and prevent vascular collapse. Hospital protocol may include the administration of epinephrine and steroids. It is always critical to follow current standards of care and hospital protocols during transfusion therapy.
Cognitive Level: Analysis
Nursing Process: Implementation; *Test Plan:* SECE

3 **Answer: 4** *Rationale:* 25% albumin is a hypertonic colloid solution that will expand the plasma volume. This increase in plasma volume should increase blood pressure, which in turn will decrease the strain on the heart and thereby decrease heart rate. The increase in volume will not lower blood pressure or decrease peripheral perfusion; rather, it will have the opposite effect.
Cognitive Level: Application
Nursing Process: Assessment; *Test Plan:* PHYS

4 **Answer: 2** *Rationale:* A client receiving granulocytes is expected to experience fever and chills due to high potential for development of allergic reactions. Option 1 is incorrect because granulocytes should be administered slowly and client should be premedicated with medications indicated above. Option 3 is incorrect because a microaggregate filter would trap the granulocytes and nullify the transfusion. Option 4 is incorrect because, although lymphocytes are present in the transfusion, they are granulocytes and the neutrophil count is the appropriate laboratory value to trend.
Cognitive Level: Analysis
Nursing Process: Implementation; *Test Plan:* SECE

5 **Answer: 2** *Rationale:* A client with CHF has a compromised cardiac pump and therefore already has an increased risk for fluid volume excess or overload. Albumin is a hypertonic colloid solution that can cause circulatory overload. This represents a double risk, then, for a client with CHF. The hematocrit would decrease as the plasma volume increases (hemodilution). All of the other options are incorrect because the platelet count, PT, PTT, and serum bilirubin will be unaffected by albumin administration.
Cognitive Level: Analysis
Nursing Process: Assessment; *Test Plan:* PHYS

6 **Answer: 2** *Rationale:* Clients may develop HLA antibodies in response to previous transfusions of blood that are not leukodepleted. Since platelets carry class 1 HLA antigens, the HLA antibodies will quickly destroy them. Therefore, attempting to match the donor's platelet antigens with the recipient's and then transfusing these platelets should increase the platelet count. All of the other options are incorrect because they will not reverse alloimmunization.
Cognitive Level: Analysis
Nursing Process: Implementation; *Test Plan:* HPM

7 **Answer: 1** *Rationale:* Dextran is a glucose solution that is not extracted from human plasma and therefore presents no risk of transmission of viruses.

Option 2 is incorrect because Dextran has a higher risk for anaphylaxis than hetastarch and albumin. Options 3 and 4 are incorrect because Dextran promotes dehydration of tissues due to its hyperosmolar effect and does affect clotting factors.
Cognitive Level: Comprehension
Nursing Process: Assessment; *Test Plan:* PHYS

8 **Answer: 4** *Rationale:* Hespan can dilute clotting factors and therefore create transient changes in PT, PTT, and clotting times. Option 1 is incorrect, because Hespan will not interfere with blood typing and cross-matching. Option 2 is incorrect because Hespan expands the plasma volume and thus can cause hypervolemia. Option 3 is incorrect—urine output will be increased because Hespan causes osmotic diuresis.
Cognitive Level: Analysis
Nursing Process: Planning; *Test Plan:* PHYS

9 **Answer: 3** *Rationale:* The nurse's highest priority is client safety; therefore, it is imperative that the client know what to report to the nurse should a reaction occur, i.e., chilling, fever, itching, shortness of breath, back pain. All of the other options should be explained to the client to promote understanding and comfort but are not the highest priority.
Cognitive Level: Analysis
Nursing Process: Implementation; *Test Plan:* HPM

10 **Answer: 3** *Rationale:* Option 3 describes a mild nonhemolytic febrile reaction, which is the most common reaction, and one that may be minimized through premedication. Option 1 is incorrect because hives are a common occurrence but airway swelling is not, and will probably not be managed by premedication alone. Option 2 is incorrect because it gives false reassurance and is nontherapeutic. Option 4 is incorrect because it suggests a possible hemolytic reaction that is uncommon and will not be minimized by premedication.
Cognitive Level: Analysis
Nursing Process: Implementation; *Test Plan:* PSYC

References

Corbett, J. (2000). *Laboratory tests and diagnostic procedures with nursing diagnoses* (5th ed.). Upper Saddle River, NJ: Prentice-Hall, Inc., pp. 24–33, 48–53, 303–325.

Corrigan, A. M. & Pelletier, G. (2000). Transfusion therapy. In A. M. Corrigan, G. Pelletier, & M. Alexander (Eds.), *Intravenous Nurses Society core curriculum for intravenous nursing* (2nd ed.). Philadelphia: Lippincott, Williams & Wilkins, pp. 277–293.

De Loughery, T. (1999, March 15). Blood products and their indications, pp. 1–10. Retrieved October 27, 2000 from the World Wide Web: *http://www.ohsu.edu/somhemonc/handouts/deloughery/printtxn.html.*

Gahart, B. L. & Nazareno, A. R. (2000). *Intravenous medications* (17th ed.). St. Louis: Mosby, pp. 19–21, 213–215, 296–299, 493–495, 759.

Green-Nigro, C. (1999). Management of persons with problems of the immune system. In W. Phipps, J. Sands, & J. Marek (Eds.), *Medical-surgical nursing: Concepts and clinical practice* (6th ed.). St. Louis: Mosby, pp. 2175–2180.

Hadaway, L. (2001). Deliver safer peripheral I.V. therapy. *Nursing 2001: Education Directory*, 8.

Josephson, D. L. (1999). *Intravenous infusion therapy for nurses: Principles and practice.* Albany, NY: Delmar, pp. 107–127, 333–367.

Kozier, B., Erb, G., Berman, A., & Burke, K. (2000). *Fundamentals of nursing: Concepts, process and practice* (6th ed.). Upper Saddle River, NJ: Prentice-Hall, Inc., pp. 1327–1335, 1351–1362.

LeMone, P., & Burke, K. (2000). *Medical-surgical nursing: Critical thinking in client care* (2nd ed.). Upper Saddle River, NJ: Prentice-Hall, Inc., pp. 169–177, 385–389.

Lilley, L. & Aucker, R. (2001). *Pharmacology and the nursing process* (3rd ed.). St. Louis: Mosby, pp. 393–400.

Metheny, N. (2000). *Fluid and electrolyte balance: Nursing considerations* (4th ed.). Philadelphia: Lippincott, Williams, & Wilkins, pp. 26–34.

Pagana, K. & Pagana, T. (1998). *Mosby's manual of diagnostic and laboratory tests.* St. Louis: Mosby, pp. 118–120, 133–142, 178–179, 225–226, 251–256, 319–399, 443–444.

Phillips, L. D. & Kuhn, M. A. (1999). *Manual of IV medications* (2nd ed.). Philadelphia: Lippincott, Williams & Wilkins, pp. 302–306.

Reeves, C., Roux, G., & Lockhart, R. (1999). *Medical-surgical nursing.* New York: McGraw-Hill, pp. 193–200.

Smith, S., Duell, D., & Martin, B. (2000). *Clinical nursing skills: Basic to advanced skills* (5th ed.). Upper Saddle River, NJ: Prentice-Hall, Inc., pp. 863–865, 875–881.

Springhouse. (1998). *Nursing IV drug handbook* (6th ed.). Springhouse, PA: Author, pp. 74–82, 559–560, 593–597, 689–692, 695.

Weinstein, S. M. (2001). *Plumer's principles and practice of intravenous therapy* (7th ed.). Philadelphia: Lippincott, Williams & Wilkins, pp. 411–451.

Wilson, B., Shannon, M., & Stang, C. (2001). *Nursing drug guide 2001.* Upper Saddle River, NJ: Prentice-Hall, Inc., pp. 677–678, 1013–1015.

Appendix

➤ *Practice to Pass Suggested Answers*

Chapter 1

Page 7: *Solution*—Hypotonic fluids (D_5W, ¼NS, ½NS) are contraindicated because they provide free water that is pulled into cells. Cerebral cells absorb such water more rapidly than other cells, which would worsen cerebral edema in a client who has sustained a head injury and insult to the brain.

Page 12: *Solution*—3% saline is very hypertonic with a high concentration of sodium. It will increase serum sodium levels and draw water from the cells into the vascular space, causing hypervolemia, hypernatremia, and cellular dehydration. Only limited doses in very controlled amounts should be infused. The infusion should be controlled with an infusion pump and the client should be closely monitored for the development of circulatory overload, pulmonary edema, rising serum sodium levels, and cerebral cell dehydration. Frequent monitoring should include:

- Vital signs and pulse oximetry
- Neurological assessment
- Respiratory assessment
- Hourly urine output
- Serum electrolyte levels

Page 20: *Solution*—This client's clinical manifestations are indicative of hypovolemia and impending shock. Hemorrhage from trauma is causing an isotonic fluid loss that is primarily ECF. Isotonic intravenous fluids remain in the ECF and are used to expand vascular volume. The client needs large volumes of isotonic fluids (normal saline, Ringer's solution, or lactated Ringer's) infused rapidly to increase vascular volume and prevent shock. If hemorrhage is massive, blood infusions may be needed to restore volume.

Page 22: *Solution*—This elderly client should be monitored closely for signs of hypervolemia and circulatory overload due to reduced cardiac and renal reserves consistent with the aging process. Monitoring should include (1) I & O, (2) observing for signs of venous congestion (neck vein distention, delayed hand vein emptying), (3) peripheral edema, and (4) pulmonary congestion (tachypnea, dyspnea, moist lung crackles). Daily weights will reveal acute weight gain.

Page 23: *Solution*—Explain in simple terms that the child is losing water and minerals and needs both replaced. Suggest that she give the child small sips of a commercial oral rehydration solution (e.g., Pedialyte, Infalyte) frequently to replace the fluid and electrolytes lost through diarrhea and vomiting. Explain that this is a balanced solution that does not provide too much sugar or salt, which can make diarrhea worse. She should also be advised to continue a regular diet as soon as the child will eat food. This will help resolve the diarrhea and provide calories, protein, fluid, and electrolytes as well.

Page 26: *Solution*—The half-strength formula is a hypotonic solution that provides excess free water. If given on a regular basis, it could lead to hypotonic fluid volume excess and water intoxication as the fluid is pulled into cells. This should be explained in simple terms that the mother can understand. If finances are a problem, she should be referred to a community agency that can help her obtain assistance in getting formula for the baby.

Page 28: *Solution*—This is an elderly person with a history of heart disease who is receiving intravenous fluid therapy at a fairly rapid rate. Awakening at night with dyspnea and a cough signals possible fluid overload and impending pulmonary edema. The nurse should first slow the IV rate to 10–20 mL/hour to maintain IV access without infusing much fluid. The next actions should include focused assessment of respiratory status, providing emergency supplemental oxygen, and notifying the physician. This client may need intravenous diuretics and other rapid interventions to prevent acute pulmonary edema.

Page 30: *Solution*—The fluid should be controlled with an infusion pump to prevent accidental fluid overload in this infant. An infant's small body size and immature kidneys put him or her at higher risk for fluid volume overload if fluids are infused too rapidly. Monitoring should include (1) checking the intravenous infusion frequently, (2) I & O, (3) serial weights, and (4) vital signs in an effort to prevent accidental overinfusion of fluid and early detection of clinical signs of fluid overload.

Chapter 2

Page 40: *Solution*—Since serum sodium level is the primary determinant of plasma osmolality, it is easy to get a rough estimate of a client's plasma osmolality if the serum sodium level is known. Taking the known serum sodium level and doubling that figure gives a rough estimate of plasma osmolality. This can be helpful in the clinical setting to evaluate a client's osmolar state.

Page 41: *Solution*—The chief regulation of sodium occurs in the kidneys where it is reabsorbed along with chloride. The reabsorption of these two electrolytes plays an important role in water balance. Renal regulation of sodium is influenced as a response to different volume states.

Page 42: *Solution*—Water will shift from the ECF (area of lower volume of solutes) to the ICF (area of higher volume of solutes) in an attempt to restore equilibrium. This results in a decreased circulating plasma volume and an increase in cellular swelling.

Page 45: *Solution*—The pathophysiologic effects of hyponatremia are primarily seen in the central nervous system and result in neurological depression. Muscular weakness is seen as neuromuscular involvement occurs. Nausea and other GI complaints are seen as gastrointestinal involvement occurs. These effects are due to fluid shifting between the ECF and ICF as cellular swelling occurs.

Page 46: *Solution*—A client who is NPO and on NG suctioning is at risk for hyponatremia due to restricted oral replacement and the loss of gastric secretions. Clients who are on prolonged NPO status should have their hydration level maintained via parenteral routes. In addition, the loss of gastrointestinal secretions can lead to further electrolyte and fluid losses that will require adequate replacement therapies. Monitoring and recording intake and output is essential in the care of this client. Amount, color, and consistency of NG drainage should be monitored for potential electrolyte and fluid imbalances.

In addition, bowel sounds should be assessed on this client to see if there is resumption of normal peristalsis. Client should be in a safe position with the NG tube secure so as to prevent further complications related to potential aspiration. The suction equipment should be monitored for the correct setting and the canister changed as needed. Placement and verification of the NG tube

should be evaluated at least once a shift (if not more in case there is medication administration) to validate correct placement.

Page 53: *Solution*—The following measures should be instituted in taking care of a client with hypernatremia:

- Monitor neurological status, LOC, and observe for potential seizures.
- Keep the bed in the low position, side rails up, and the call bell in place.
- Assist with ambulation and mobility as needed.
- Make sure that environment is safe so as to prevent risk of falls and injury to client.

Chapter 3

Page 64: *Solution*—Potassium (K^+) in the intracellular fluid (ICF) is important for conduction of electrical impulses, which make the muscles in the body work. Too much or too little potassium can be detrimental to health by affecting neuromuscular excitability, acid-base balance, and cardiac contractility. Elevated or decreased levels can lead to the development of cardiac arrhythmias, which can be life threatening. It is very important to have a K^+ level in the normal therapeutic range so as to avoid compromise.

Page 67: *Solution*—Since potassium never leaves the body in relative hypokalemia, it is important to monitor the client closely to ensure that rebound hyperkalemia doesn't occur with treatment. Remember, a serum potassium level that is low does not indicate where the potassium loss has occurred. Clients who have relative hypokalemia may be at risk to develop hyperkalemia due to over-aggressive treatment. It is important to adequately assess clients who may be exhibiting hypokalemia as a result of water intoxication, alkalosis states, and increased insulin secretion.

Page 68: *Solution*—Clients who are hypokalemic may be weak and have muscle cramps. Clients should be assisted when ambulating in order to provide support and maintain balance. Have call bell in reach and side rails up when the client is in bed. Assist client to change position slowly to minimize the risk of orthostatic hypotension. Monitor client's level of consciousness and his or her respiratory, cardiac, and GI status. Administer medications as ordered to restore normal serum levels. Monitor client's labs accordingly to evaluate response to treatment.

Page 71: *Solution*—When KCl is administered intravenously, it should be diluted in enough solution to deliver no more than 10 mEq/mL. No more than 40 mEq should be added to a liter of solution when using a peripheral line. If a solution contains more than 20mEq/hr the client should be on continuous ECG monitoring with serum levels checked q 4–6 hours. Potassium should be infused using an infusion pump to ensure accurate rate of administration. Close monitoring of the IV site should be done because KCl is very irritating to veins. If the site is red or infiltrated, the IV must be discontinued to prevent damage to the vessel.

Page 73: *Solution*—Foods that are high in potassium include potatoes, bananas, watermelon, yogurt, and acorn squash. These are considered good sources because they contain the most K^+

per kilocalorie. Potassium is found in whole grains, meats, milk, fruits, vegetables, grains, and legumes and is present in most foods in the Western diet. It is important for the nurse to note that ingestion of large amounts of licorice can lead to hypokalemia and the client's dietary selections should be monitored for this. In addition, it is important to note if the client is using salt substitutes because they are usually high in K^+. It is also important to assess the client for use of dietary (nutritional) supplements for their potential effects on K^+ levels. Collaboration with a dietitian is essential in the management of these clients.

Page 75: *Solution*—Potassium is forced out of the cells and into the extracellular spaces during massive tissue destruction. Potassium enters the vascular space and hyperkalemia develops. Cellular trauma can lead to the release of large levels of K^+ and all clients should be monitored closely for potential problems as a result of hyperkalemia.

Chapter 4

Page 89: *Solution*—The parathyroid hormone, activated vitamin D, and calcitonin tightly control serum calcium levels. When there are alterations in any of these systems, disturbances in calcium levels can occur, leading to hypo- or hypercalcemia.

Page 93: *Solution*—Predisposing clinical conditions that can lead to calcium imbalances are related to inadequate intestinal absorption, deposition of ionized calcium into bone or soft tissue, or decreases in PTH and vitamin D levels. All of these factors can lead to decreased physiologic availability of calcium.

Page 96: *Solution*—Calcium plays an important role in determining the speed of ion fluxes through nerve and muscle membranes. The effects of too little calcium lead to an increase in nervous system irritability. This irritability is exhibited by tetany, as well as Chvostek's and Trousseau's signs, and may develop into seizures.

Page 100: *Solution*—The therapeutic response to calcium gluconate therapy can be evaluated by resolving signs of tetany and a return to serum calcium levels in the range of 8 to 9 mg/dL. Appropriate nursing interventions for a client receiving this type of therapy should include evaluating the IV site for signs of extravasation that can happen with calcium gluconate or calcium chloride, close titration of dose, and continuous ECG monitoring.

Page 102: *Solution*—Differences in the CNS as a result of hypocalcemia include clinical manifestations such as depression, anxiety, irritability, delusions, hallucinations, and convulsions. Hypercalcemia produces clinical manifestations such as lethargy, subtle personality changes, or acute changes such as psychosis, stupor, and possibly coma. Similarities in the CNS as a result of altered calcium levels (hypo- and hypercalcemia) result in clinical manifestations such as memory impairment and confusion.

Page 107: *Solution*—Foods to avoid are cheeses, milk, and other dairy products; canned salmon and sardines; rhubarb; spinach and other dark green leafy vegetables; and tofu. Calcium supplements and antacids such as Oscal and TUMS should be avoided.

During the nursing assessment, the client should be questioned as to food likes and dislikes and for any history of peptic ulcer disease or gastric distress because this increases the likelihood of increased use of calcium-containing antacids and calcium-rich foods.

Chapter 5

Page 116: *Solution*—Good sources of magnesium include green leafy vegetables, nuts, legumes, seafood, whole grains, bananas, oranges, cocoa, and chocolate.

Page 118: *Solution*—Because the two function together to help run the sodium-potassium pump, a change in one effects a change in the other.

Page 119: *Solution*—Maalox, Mylanta, Riopan, Gaviscon, Gelusil, and Di-Gel are common brand-name antacids that are high in magnesium.

Page 121: *Solution*—Cardiovascular symptoms include hypotension, flushing and sweating, arrhythmias, and possibly cardiac arrest.

Page 122: *Solution*—Calcium gluconate is an antagonist of magnesium and is given as an emergency treatment for severe hypermagnesemia.

Chapter 6

Page 134: *Solution*—In metabolic alkalosis, chloride is decreased because the kidneys retain bicarbonate and excrete chloride. Increased bicarbonate in the body leads to potassium and sodium depletion that affects extracellular volume depletion, resulting in accompanying chloride loss.

Page 136: *Solution*—Hypochloremia reflects a decrease in serum chloride, < 95 mEq/L. Chloride levels are usually not altered independently but rather are seen in conjunction with other electrolyte and acid-base imbalances. It is important to check serum sodium and potassium levels and assess client's acid-base status to help establish the etiology of the chloride deficit. In addition, it is important to ascertain clinical factors that would lead to chloride deficit such as disease states, GI loss, endocrine disturbance, and volume expansion in order to more clearly describe the hypochloremic state. Depending on the serum value, the following strategies can be used for correction: (1) increase intake of foods high in chloride or (2) administer sodium chloride intravenously, or potassium chloride if potassium level is also low.

Page 137: *Solution*—A Medrol dose pack is a steroid that causes sodium and chloride retention and fluid volume excess. Lasix (furosemide) is a loop diuretic that promotes sodium, chloride, potassium, and water excretion. The Medrol dose pack would be most likely to cause an increase in serum chloride levels.

Page 137: *Solution*—The nurse should assess the client for deep, rapid, vigorous respirations. A client who is hyperchloremic should present with metabolic acidosis with a normal anion gap.

In addition, to increase respiratory rate and depth, the client may also experience headache, drowsiness, and confusion. Depending on the state of acidosis, signs and symptoms will vary as the client attempts to return to normal acid-base balance by using compensatory mechanisms. The client can progress into shock states with accompanying dysrhythmias, so careful monitoring is critical to maintain client safety and establish favorable clinical outcomes.

Page 139: *Solution*—The client is likely experiencing hyperchloremia, since high fever, severe vomiting, and diarrhea would lead to a state of dehydration. Hyperchloremia is associated with dehydration states because fluid losses contribute to severe electrolyte deficiencies. The client is also likely to be suffering from both sodium and potassium losses. Remember, chloride imbalance states usually do not exist independently but rather occur together with sodium, potassium, and water imbalances.

Chapter 7

Page 148: *Solution*—Phosphorus is abundant in fish, poultry, eggs, red meat, and organ meats, such as brain, liver, and kidney. It is also found in dairy products such as milk. Legumes, whole grains, and nuts are other rich sources of phosphorus.

Page 151: *Solution*—The client may report circumoral and fingertip/extremity numbness and tingling. The client may also exhibit muscle weakness, parasthesias, tremors, spasms, and signs of tetany.

Page 154: *Solution*—When giving potassium phosphate, do not exceed a rate of infusion greater than 10 mEq/hr; give the dose slowly over 2 to 6 hours as ordered. Watch for complications of IV administration, including tetany from hypocalcemia, hypotension from too rapid an infusion rate, and formation of calcium and phosphorous deposits in the tissues.

Monitor infusion site for signs of infiltration, which may lead to tissue necrosis or sloughing.

Page 157: *Solution*—The client may exhibit any of the following manifestations:

- Metastatic calcification, including oliguria, corneal haziness, conjunctivitis, irregular heart rate
- EKG changes and conduction disturbance, tachycardia, deposits of calcium phosphate in the cardiac tissues
- Numbness and tingling around the mouth and in the fingertips, muscle spasms, tetany
- Decreased calcium
- Anorexia, nausea, vomiting
- Muscle weakness, hyperreflexia, and tetany

Page 158: *Solution*—Phosphate-binding medications contain either aluminum, magnesium, or calcium as the cation that binds to the phosphate anion. Products that bind phosphate will have one of these or may have aluminum and magnesium together, since they have opposing effects on the GI tract.

Chapter 8

Page 173: *Solution*—The nurse would examine the client's ABG results. With uncompensated respiratory acidosis, the pH is less than 7.35, $PaCO_2$ is greater than 45 mm Hg, and the HCO_3^- is normal (22–26 mEq/L). In a client with respiratory acidosis, compensation would involve the kidneys retaining bicarbonate and returning it to the ECF. Compensation would reflect an increase in the bicarbonate level.

Page 174: *Solution*—As acidosis occurs, H^+ ions move into the cell and potassium moves into the ECF, elevating the serum potassium level. Hyperkalemia can cause serious cardiac conduction defects and can be fatal. When someone is acidotic, the potassium level must be monitored closely. Transcellular shifting of potassium is affected by acid-base balance. With acidosis, H^+ is excreted and K^+ is retained leading to hyperkalemia. With alkalosis, K^+ is excreted and H^+ is retained leading to hypokalemia.

Page 179: *Solution*—Clients with Type 1 diabetes require insulin to control glucose levels. When there is insufficient insulin, fats are metabolized and free fatty acids accumulate, which can result in the development of diabetic ketoacidosis. Control of glucose levels with adequate insulin is the best prevention.

Page 181: *Solution*—Monitoring the amount of NG drainage and replacing the amount lost with an equal amount of an electrolyte solution can prevent excessive H^+ ion loss. It is important to account for intake and output and correlate with serum electrolyte levels. If fluids and electrolytes are being removed via suction, then the client may be at risk to develop further electrolyte imbalance, which could be complicated by acid-base disturbances.

Page 183: *Solution*—Conditions leading to the development of metabolic alkalosis result in depleted potassium levels, which can significantly affect cardiac function. Transcellular shifting of potassium is also affected by acid-base balance. Clients who are alkalotic have decreased potassium levels and are likely to become even more hypokalemic. Hypokalemia affects cardiac conduction leading to the development of dysrhythmias that can become life-threatening. These clients must be monitored closely so prompt management and intervention can be implemented.

Chapter 9

Page 197: *Solution*—The client has a very hyperosmolar serum and is experiencing osmotic diuresis and dehydration. 0.9% NaCl (normal saline) will begin to replace the fluid volume that is being lost as a result of the osmotic diuresis. Serum osmolality should begin to decrease (insulin is needed, of course). Although one might expect serum sodium to be high in this dehydrated client, a good amount of sodium is being lost in the urine as a result of the osmotic diuresis. Therefore, the serum sodium is low to begin with and should increase with 0.9% NaCl IV replacement. Blood pressure should increase, heart rate should decrease, and perfusion should improve.

Page 198: *Solution*—Priority assessments include obtaining baseline and frequent vital signs and determining adequacy of organ perfusion by assessing level of consciousness (LOC), urine output, and skin color. It is important to be alert to the fact that the client may develop possible dehydration or fluid overload due to the cellular dynamic effects of the hypertonic albumin. It is equally important to monitor the client for the possibility of a febrile reaction. Priority interventions include maintaining a patent airway and providing adequate ventilation and oxygenation. Albumin should be infused as rapidly as the client will tolerate, while paying close attention to lung sounds for possible pulmonary edema and for other indications of fluid volume excess. The client may be at greater risk for fluid volume excess (FVE) if there is a significant cardiac history. Even without a cardiac history, given the client's age, there may be some cardiac insufficiency due to the normal aging process. It is therefore important to place the client in a supine position with legs elevated in order to maximize organ perfusion. If the client cannot tolerate this position due to respiratory compromise, then position the client with the head elevated at 30 to 45 degrees. If the client is at risk for increased intracranial pressure (if head injury present), the head of the bed should be elevated to 30 degrees. Keep the client warm. If trauma occurred or may have occurred, observe for increased bleeding especially as the blood pressure rises. Monitor hemoglobin, hematocrit, electrolytes, and serum albumin. Expected outcomes for this client include an increased colloidal oncotic pressure with a corresponding increase in cardiac output, increased blood pressure, decreased heart rate, decreased respiratory rate, improved organ perfusion, increased urine output, increased serum albumin, and decreased hematocrit.

Page 201: *Solution*—Stop the infusion, because the client may be experiencing an anaphylactic reaction. Maintain the client's airway and provide high flow oxygen. Enlist assistance and have one colleague bring the crash cart and another notify the physician. Administer epinephrine per hospital protocol. Quickly change the IV line at the hub and infuse 0.9% normal saline (NS) to help maintain blood volume. The client should be attached to a cardiac monitor and pulse oximetry. Heart rate, respiratory rate, and oxygen saturation are monitored continuously and blood pressure readings should be taken frequently. Additional medications such as diphenhydramine (Benadryl), methylprednisolone sodium succinate (Solumedrol), and aminophylline (Theophylline) may be ordered by the physician. The client may need to be intubated. The physician may order additional IV fluids. A vasopressor, i.e., dopamine, may be ordered if the client is unable to maintain an adequate blood pressure. Once the client has stabilized, continue to observe the client for several hours. Once it has been determined that the client is allergic to the Hespan, the client should be advised to wear a Medic-Alert™ bracelet indicating the allergy.

Page 206: *Solution*—An appropriate response to the client's concern would be to tell the client, "The chemotherapy that you are receiving to treat the leukemia puts you at increased risk for infection. Specially treating the blood you will receive helps to ensure that it will not be a source of infection for you while you are at increased risk."

Page 209: *Solution*—Laboratory results to review in evaluating the effectiveness of transfusion therapy for a client with DIC include hemoglobin, hematocrit, RBC count, platelet count, partial thromboplastin time (PTT), prothrombin time (PT) or International Normalized Ratio (INR), and fibrinogen level. While transfusions of PRBCs, platelets, fresh frozen plasma (FFP), and possibly cryoprecipitate will help to replenish blood components, additional blood loss may occur through the presence of this coagulopathy. The presence of DIC complicates the clinical picture because unless the underlying mechanism is identified and treated, replacement therapies are aimed at supportive management and are not curative. Therefore lab values are bound to plunge again and again until the underlying cause is identified and treated.

Page 210: *Solution*—The nurse should first explain to the client what the transfusion is for, what to expect during the transfusion (chilling, fever, and allergic reaction), and answer any questions that the client might have. To safely administer granulocytes to this client, the nurse should begin by premedicating the client as ordered by the physician, generally with diphenhydramine (Benadryl), steroids, and an antipyretic. When hanging the unit, the nurse must verify that it is ABO and Rh compatible because it contains RBCs and is preferably HLA-compatible. The nurse is also aware that the granulocytes must be administered within 24 hours after being collected and are maximally effective when given as soon as possible after collection. The nurse must use a standard in-line filter (not a microaggregate filter, which will trap the WBCs) and administer the transfusion slowly, generally at a rate of 50 mL per hour for 4 hours. Monitor the client for expected side effects. Cover the client with a warm blanket to prevent chilling. Monitor the client for hypertension and treat it if needed. Only discontinue the transfusion if client develops severe respiratory distress. Be aware that granulocytes are generally administered for at least 4 to 5 days, one unit a day or until the infection resolves.

Page 213: *Solution*—If the client has any difficulty swallowing as a result of a prior stroke, it is important that the home health aide assists the client to an upright position with the head and neck flexed slightly forward. Liquids should be thick or semi-solid (gelatin, pudding, and milk shakes). The home health aide should offer the client fluid frequently and consider preferences when purchasing and preparing the fluids. It is also important that cold fluids are served cold and hot fluids are served hot. The client and home health aide must be aware if fluid restriction is necessary due to underlying CHF and/or renal insufficiency and maintain the limits of that restriction. The home health aide should keep a record of the client's intake and output and note the characteristics of urine output. It is important that daily weights be obtained. The aide should examine the client's skin and mucous membranes for signs of adequate hydration. The client should be instructed to report any excess thirst to the aide. All abnormal losses from fever, diaphoresis, or diarrhea, for example, should be reported to the physician. Last but not least, the client and aide should be instructed about good handwashing techniques and protecting themselves from infection.

➤ *Case Study Suggested Answers*

Chapter 1

1. Questions to ask the mother include:
   - How high has the fever been, how many times has the infant vomited, how many stools has the infant had today?
   - Has the infant been able to keep any food or fluids down?
   - When did the infant last urinate?
   - Is the infant acting "normal"? Are there any changes in behavior or activity?
   - Has there been any weight lost in the past two days?
   - Have you used any treatments or medicines at home? If so, which ones and how often? What effect did they have?

2. Serious fluid imbalance is indicated by:
   - Assessing infant's level of alertness, activity, interaction and response to others (lethargy, listlessness, and/or reduced activity/interaction are signs of serious dehydration).
   - Counting heart rate (tachycardia is an early sign of fluid volume deficit in infants).
   - Observing skin and mucous membranes (dry oral mucosa and tongue, furrowed tongue, no tears when crying are all signs of fluid volume loss).
   - Palpating fontanels (sunken fontanels are a sign of significant fluid volume loss).

3. Control the fluid rate with an infusion pump to prevent accidentally infusing a volume too large for the child's size. Explain all procedures to the parents and provide emotional support. Monitor the child for signs of improvement as well as fluid overload.

4. Give the child small, frequent sips of a commercial oral rehydration solution (e.g., Pedialyte, Infalyte) to replace both fluid and electrolyte losses without giving excess sugar or salt, which can make diarrhea worse. Resume regular foods as soon as the infant will eat them. Once the infant is eating and the diarrhea is getting better, add a variety of fluids the infant likes, avoiding those with high sugar or salt content.

5. The BRAT diet is a transition diet used to assist clients when they have gastrointestinal tract alterations (nausea, vomiting, or diarrhea). It is not meant for long-term use as it does not provide adequate amounts of required nutrients and calories. Once the infant is able to keep food and fluids down, it is important to progress the client's diet back to the original pattern.

Chapter 2

1. Client's past medical history (PMH) reveals hypertension diagnosed six weeks ago with prescription of hydrochlorothiazide and low-sodium diet. Current findings related to history of present illness (HPI) or chief complaint reveals dizziness, nausea, weakness, abdominal cramps, and headache. Onset of symptoms three days ago with worsening by today indicates that the client's condition is becoming more acute. These findings suggest that the client might be experiencing a sodium deficit. The use of a thiazide diuretic can lead to sodium deficit and the increase in neurological complaints of dizziness, weakness, and headache are consistent with hyponatremia.

2. Questions that should be asked prior to performing a physical examination should include:
   - Are you taking your diuretic as ordered? Clarify information relative to dosage, frequency, and compliance with treatment regimen.
   - Have you ever experienced these kinds of symptoms before?
   - Are there any contributory health problems that could affect your overall condition? Do you suffer from any acute or chronic disease process?
   - Are you taking any other medications, either prescription or OTC?
   - Have you been experiencing thirst?
   - Have you had excessive perspiration or sweating in the last few days?
   - You stated that you have been dizzy. Can you explain what that means to you? Are you having blurred vision? Are you having difficulty concentrating?
   - Can you tell me where you feel your headache and describe the type of discomfort that you experience (obtain pain characteristics)?
   - Have you taken any medication today to relieve any of your symptoms?
   - Obtain an accurate intake and output record from the client for the past 24 hours.

3. Clinical findings consistent with hyponatremia are tachycardia, hypotension, dry mucous membranes, muscular weakness, and flat neck veins. This data would be consistent with physical examination findings.

4. Based on the data obtained thus far and knowledge of fluid and electrolytes, the nurse expects a Na level < 135 mEq/L (which would indicate hyponatremia), a serum osmolality < 280 mOsm/kg (which would indicate decreased plasma osmolality), a serum chloride level < 97 mEq/L (which would indicate hypochloremia), and a specific gravity of < 1.008 (which would indicate a decreased ability to concentrate urine).

5. Discharge teaching that should be included in the plan of care for this client includes:
   - Teach the client the signs and symptoms of hyponatremia (such as abdominal cramps, nausea, muscle weakness) so that he will be able to identify potential problems and report to his healthcare provider.
   - Teach the client the importance of drinking liquids containing sodium during periods of heavy sweating and/or high environmental temperatures as the client's occupation requires him to be outdoors.
   - Teach the client to comply with regularly scheduled lab/diagnostic tests to monitor sodium and other electrolyte levels while taking diuretic therapy.

- Teach the client about low-sodium diet instructions and verify that client is meeting dietary goals. Referral to a dietician for followup if needed.
- Teach client the importance of safety upon ambulation as diuretic therapy and hyponatremia can lead to hypotension. Discuss slow change of positioning and monitor BP during therapy.
- Teach the client to keep all regularly scheduled healthcare appointments and report findings immediately to healthcare provider so that prompt recognition and treatment of symptoms can be started.

Chapter 3

1. The nurse should question this client closely about any medications that the client is taking (both prescription and over-the-counter). Particular attention should be given if the client is taking potassium supplements and/or digitalis preparations. The nurse should question this client about any acute or chronic disease process that could increase the risk for developing hypokalemia. In addition, any recent medical or surgical treatment should be explored with the client. The nurse should question this client regarding diet history. The nurse should also question the client regarding signs and symptoms of hypokalemia.

2. The client could manifest many other signs and symptoms, such as fatigue, muscle weakness, leg cramps, nausea, vomiting, paralytic ileus, paresthesias, polyuria, weak and irregular pulse, hyperglycemia, and ECG changes consistent with hypokalemia.

3. A serum chemistry panel should be drawn for this client since episodes of diarrhea are associated with potential fluid and electrolyte depletion. Magnesium levels and calcium levels should be looked at closely because hypokalemia often occurs in conjunction with losses of these two electrolytes. Arterial blood gases might be drawn to determine acid-base status, which could be influenced by loss of GI fluids leading to the development of metabolic alkalosis. ECG monitoring is indicated for this client because the client is complaining of cardiac effects. Depending on ECG baseline, additional labs might be ordered if further cardiac compromise was suspected (cardiac enzymes). If the client continues to have diarrhea, then a stool sample should be obtained for culture and sensitivity.

4. The client would be given either oral or parenteral potassium supplements depending on the baseline potassium level. If the level was low (below 3.0 mEq/L), then IV potassium would be the treatment of choice until the level reached 3.0 mEq/L; then oral supplements would be sufficient. Even at higher levels, some clients are unable to consume sufficient potassium to raise serum levels. These clients might have to remain on IV therapy with KCl in addition to oral supplements. If the diarrhea continues and the stool sample identifies a specific pathogen, then further medical treatment may be warranted by using either anti-biotic therapy to treat the organism; otherwise, antidiarrheal agents may be ordered to prevent excess fluid loss.

5. Teaching for this client should include information related to the nature of the complaint. As the client's clinical presentation denotes hypokalemia, the client should be given information relative to signs and symptoms of hypokalemia and to report to the healthcare provider if these should occur. Client teaching should further include specifics regarding whether the client's diet therapy and/or current medications contribute to potassium balance in the body. Since the client will most likely be started on K^+ supplementation, the client should be aware of potential interactions and adequate sources of potassium in the diet in order to maintain serum levels. Regarding the most effective teaching methods for the client, it is important to individualize so that the client can have both verbal and written information. Including significant family members may be warranted in order to reinforce information and help others participate in the client's healthcare upon discharge. Teaching should be an ongoing process started upon admission and continuing to discharge. In addition, follow-up reinforcement should be included so that the client continues with prescribed therapy.

Chapter 4

1. These signs and symptoms are caused by hypercalcemia from osteocytic activity of malignancy.

2. The chief cause appears to be osteoclastic bone resorption, mediated by PTH or other substances secreted by the tumor. The result is that more calcium is released from the bone into the ECF.

3. Isotonic saline diuresis will lead rapidly to increased renal excretion, depending upon renal function. Biphosphonate drugs (pamidronate, Aredia) are now first line therapy with saline diuresis because they inhibit osteoclasts from resorbing bone. Plicamycin (Mithramycin) is extraordinarily effective in clients with hypercalcemia that results from skeletal metastasis.

4. Priority nursing interventions include:
   - Monitor for signs of continuing hypercalcemia.
   - Monitor for signs of impending hypocalcemia from overcorrection secondary to treatment.
   - Monitor client carefully for signs of heart failure from saline diuresis.
   - Monitor for side effects of biphosphonate therapy.
   - Monitor for side effects of plicamycin.
   - Move the client with great care to avoid pain or fractures.
   - Pain management therapy should be an integral part of the treatment plan.

5. There will be an absence of the presenting clinical manifestations. Calcium and phosphorus levels will normalize. Serum creatinine will indicate effectively functioning kidneys and a urine output of 2 to 3 L/day. There are minimal side effects of medication therapy. There are no signs of

heart failure. Fluid volume is stable with signs of overhydration. The client will state a reduction in pain and the client is moved or ambulated without increased pain.

Chapter 5

1. The client has low weight for height. This leads to questions about starvation, dietary habits, anorexia, bulimia, and diabetes.

2. Data should also be gathered about alcohol use and over-the-counter medications, including diuretics, laxatives, enemas, and diet aids.

3. The client should have measurement of electrolytes, magnesium and calcium levels, and an electrocardiogram (ECG).

4. Depending on the findings, dietary evaluation, mental health counseling, and endocrinology evaluation could be indicated.

5. Instructions would include to avoid foods high in magnesium, antacids, laxatives, enemas, and magnesium supplements if there are high magnesium levels. Instructions would further include avoiding alcohol, diuretics, hyperglycemia, and treating unresolved vomiting or diarrhea if there were low magnesium levels.

Chapter 6

1. The following questions should be posed to the client upon admission:
   - How long have you been vomiting?
   - Can you estimate the amount, color, and frequency of emesis?
   - Have you been experiencing any nausea?
   - What methods have you used to help during the time you have been experiencing GI symptoms?
   - Have you noticed any muscle tremors, twitching, or breathing problems?
   - Have you had any other symptoms such as dizziness or excessive sweating?
   - Have you been running a fever?
   - Are you being treated for any medical condition at the present time?
   - Are you taking any medications, either prescription or OTC at the present time or recently?

   This is just a partial listing of questions that could be posed to the client to provide a more accurate assessment.

2. Reported vital signs reveal a BP within normal limits but at the lower end of the normal range. It would be pertinent to obtain a height and weight on the client and to correlate BP findings with client history and physical status. Assess the client for muscle tremors and twitching and maintain safety precautions so as to prevent fall injuries if the client is feeling dizzy. Assess client's skin turgor for evidence of dehydration and document findings.

3. Nursing diagnoses that could apply to this client include:
   - Alterations in acid-base balance related to GI losses
   - Alterations in fluid and electrolyte balance related to GI losses
   - Altered nutrition; less than body requirements related to altered intake pattern
   - Impaired skin integrity related to fluid losses
   - Risk for injury related to volume and electrolyte depletion

4. Interventions to implement would be to verify physician orders with the expectation that pertinent lab/diagnostic tests, such as a serum chemistries, would be ordered for the client to establish both a baseline and evaluate response to treatment. Since the client is dehydrated, and unable to keep down solid foods, parenteral administration of fluids would be required to rehydrate the client and correct fluid and electrolyte imbalances. The client would most likely be experiencing chloride, sodium, and potassium deficits in addition to volume deficits. If the client continues to experience vomiting and/nausea, then the use of anti-emetics may be indicated to prevent further fluid and electrolyte loss.

5. Discharge instructions would focus on maintaining hydration levels and electrolyte balance. Dietary instructions would include foods that are high in sodium, chloride, and potassium; these may be necessary to restore balance. The client should also receive instructions regarding the importance of early intervention in cases of severe GI symptoms so as to avoid hospitalization and to institute prompt treatment.

Chapter 7

1. Mr. G. will have hyperphosphatemia because the chronic renal failure will prevent his kidneys from eliminating excess phosphates.

2. As the kidneys fail, the nephrons (the functional units of the kidney) are not able to perform their intended functions adequately. Since the kidneys ordinarily eliminate excess phosphorus, this substance is retained in the bloodstream, leading to high phosphorus levels.

3. Many foods are naturally rich in phosphorus, making dietary management somewhat difficult. Mr. G. should avoid foods that are especially rich in phosphorus, such as fish, poultry, eggs, red meat, organ meats, dairy products, legumes, whole grains, and nuts.

4. Hemodialysis will compensate for the lack of functioning of the kidneys and help to eliminate excess phosphates from the bloodstream.

5. Mr. G. will be receiving a phosphate-binding agent as part of his medication therapy. The active ingredient in the medication that is ordered will be either aluminum, magnesium, or calcium. Currently, calcium-based products are popular for use in clients with renal failure because a client with this diagnosis often has concurrent hypocalcemia. Mr. G. should also be taught to read the labels of over-the-counter medications and products and avoid using those that are high in phosphorus or phosphate content.

Chapter 8

1. Due to the chronic nature of COPD and acute onset of URI, this client would most likely have ABG values consistent with respiratory acidosis. Compensation may or may not have occurred depending on the client's baseline status and nature of acute exacerbation. Due to retention of acids, the pH would be low and the $PaCO_2$ would be elevated.

2. The client with COPD should be taught ways to get rid of as much CO_2 as possible. The client should be taught purse-lipped breathing and to take bronchodilators as ordered by the physician to promote dilation of the bronchial tree. The client should also be taught the signs and symptoms of infection and to get the pneumonia and flu vaccines yearly since these two conditions could exacerbate the respiratory condition.

3. A client with COPD becomes insensitive to CO_2 elevations as a respiratory stimulus. Due to the chronic nature of this disease process, compensation has taken place and high levels of oxygen affect the respiratory center. When an oxygen concentration is too high, it will actually knock out the client's stimulus to breathe.

4. Because of chronic lung disease, this client's alveoli have been unable to get rid of excess CO_2. As a result, clients with COPD show chronically high CO_2 levels on ABG results. This is considered a normal/abnormal finding in clients with chronic COPD. A client who does not have COPD retains the normal response stimulus of CO_2 for ventilatory drive. Clients without airway disease are able to ventilate and perform gas exchange using normal mechanisms. They are able to maintain CO_2 balance by breathing patterns and are not subject to CO_2 retention.

5. Clients with COPD frequently develop cardiac problems along with their lung disease. Potassium-wasting diuretics are used to treat both conditions. When potassium is lost, hydrogen ions tend to move out of the cell into the blood creating an alkalotic state. The client should be taught the signs and symptoms of hypokalemia and metabolic alkalosis, and to report potential problems to the physician. Clients should eat foods high in potassium, if not already on a potassium supplement. Clients should also be taught to notify the physician immediately if severe diarrhea develops as this might cause the development of metabolic alkalosis.

Chapter 9

1. The nurse should check baseline vital signs, heart rhythm, and lung sounds as well as assess for other signs and symptoms of anemia. It is also important for the nurse to know the type of anemia the client has, its cause, and the client's current hematocrit and hemoglobin (as well as total RBC count and RBC indices if available). The client should be asked whether she's ever had transfusion of blood or a blood product before, when that was, and whether she had a reaction. Ensure that the client has given informed consent after speaking with the physician and that all transfusion-related questions have been answered.

2. The following are priority nursing diagnoses: Impaired gas exchange, Ineffective breathing pattern, Altered tissue perfusion, and Activity intolerance. While the blood is transfusing, the client may also be at Risk for injury. Knowledge deficit may also be appropriate as the client needs to understand the reason for the transfusion (to improve the oxygen carrying capacity of the blood), procedures that will be done during the transfusion process (identification of blood product, frequent vital signs, length of transfusion therapy, and signs and symptoms of transfusion reactions) and post-transfusion procedures (followup blood work and continued observation).

3. Prior to beginning the transfusion, it is important to determine that the client has informed consent and has signed the consent form. It is important to answer all questions regarding the administration of this blood product. If the client has additional questions or concerns that are beyond the scope of nursing practice, the physician should be notified. If there are no questions or if the client's questions have been answered to satisfaction, then the nurse should apprise the client of the steps that will be taken during the blood transfusion procedure. The client will be typed and crossed for two units of PRBCs by the lab. Once the type and cross-match has been completed, an IV site will be established for the transfusion. The blood unit will be brought to the floor and two RNs will verify the original order and (at the bedside) check the client's blood bank band with the unit in order to verify information concerning the blood unit (name, unit number, type and Rh, and expiration date). The client will be monitored throughout the course of therapy with frequent vital signs and observation. If any additional medication is ordered either as a premedication or in between units, the nurse will administer it per the physician's order. Following completion of the transfusion of the units, lab work will be drawn to see how the client responded to the therapy.

4. Following hospital policy and procedure will help to maintain safe transfusion therapy, but it alone may not prevent the occurrence of a transfusion reaction. In order to maintain transfusion safety, it is important to remain with the client during the first 15 minutes of any transfusion therapy to assess for potential transfusion reactions. If the client should develop any signs or symptoms of a transfusion reaction, stop or slow the transfusion depending on type of reaction and hospital policy, attend to the client, and notify the physician and the blood bank when appropriate. Using proper equipment, monitoring parameters, and assessing the client (not merely the equipment) will promote transfusion safety in the clinical setting.

5. In order to evaluate the effectiveness of transfusion therapy, the nurse should expect a decrease in heart rate, respiratory rate, improvement of clinical symptoms (decrease in shortness of breath and increased tissue perfusion) and increased activity tolerance. Diagnostic results post transfusion should reflect an increase of 2 grams in hemoglobin and a 6% increase in hematocrit.

Credits

Chapter 1

Fig. 1-1   Art, From *Medical Surgical Nursing: Critical Thinking in Client Care*, by Priscilla LeMone, Karen M. Burke, Edition 2, © 2000 by Prentice-Hall, Inc., Upper Saddle River, New Jersey; Page 101, Fig. 5-1; Artist: Nea Hanscomb.

Fig. 1-2   Art, From *Fundamentals of Nursing: Concepts, Process, and Practice*, by Barbara Kozier, Glenora Erb, Audrey Berman, and Karen Burke, Edition 6, © 2000 by Prentice-Hall, Inc., Upper Saddle River, New Jersey; Page 1304, Fig. 48-3; Artist: Nea Hanscomb.

Fig. 1-3   Art, From *Fundamentals of Nursing: Concepts, Process, and Practice*, by Barbara Kozier, Glenora Erb, Audrey Berman, and Karen Burke, Edition 6, © 2000 by Prentice-Hall, Inc., Upper Saddle River, New Jersey; Page 1305, Fig. 48-5; Artist: Nea Hanscomb.

Fig. 1-4   Art, From *Fundamentals of Nursing: Concepts, Process, and Practice*, by Barbara Kozier, Glenora Erb, Audrey Berman, and Karen Burke, Edition 6, © 2000 by Prentice-Hall, Inc., Upper Saddle River, New Jersey; Page 1305, Fig. 48-6; Artist: Nea Hanscomb.

Fig. 1-5   Art, From *Medical Surgical Nursing: Critical Thinking in Client Care*, by Priscilla LeMone, Karen M. Burke, Edition 2, © 2000 by Prentice-Hall, Inc., Upper Saddle River, New Jersey; Page 105, Fig. 5-6; Artist: Nea Hanscomb.

Fig. 1-6   Art, From *Medical Surgical Nursing: Critical Thinking in Client Care*, by Priscilla LeMone, Karen M. Burke, Edition 2, © 2000 by Prentice-Hall, Inc., Upper Saddle River, New Jersey; Page 105, Fig. 5-5; Artist: Nea Hanscomb.

Chapter 2

Fig. 2-1   Art, From *Fundamentals of Nursing: Concepts, Process, and Practice*, by Barbara Kozier, Glenora Erb, Audrey Berman, and Karen Burke, Edition 6, © 2000 by Prentice-Hall, Inc., Upper Saddle River, New Jersey; Page 1315, Fig. 48-11 A & B; Artist: Nea Hanscomb.

Chapter 3

Fig. 3-1   Art, From *Medical Surgical Nursing: Critical Thinking in Client Care*, by Priscilla LeMone, Karen M. Burke, Edition 2, © 2000 by Prentice-Hall, Inc., Upper Saddle River, New Jersey; Page 126, Fig. 5-10 A-C; Artist: The Left Coast Group.

Chapter 8

Fig. 8-1   Art, From *Medical Surgical Nursing: Critical Thinking in Client Care*, by Priscilla LeMone, Karen M. Burke, Edition 2, © 2000 by Prentice-Hall, Inc., Upper Saddle River, New Jersey; Page 1332, Fig. 32-8; Artist: Nea Hanscomb.

Index